This report contains the collective views of an international group of experts and does not necessarily represent the decisions or the stated policy of the United Nations Environment Programme, the International Labour Organisation, or the World Health Organization.

Environmental Health Criteria 194

ALUMINIUM

First draft prepared by Dr H. Habs, Dr B. Simon and Professor K.U. Thiedemann (Fraunhofer Institute, Hanover, Germany) and Mr P. Howe (Institute of Terrestrial Ecology, Monks Wood, United Kingdom)

Published under the joint sponsorship of the United Nations Environment Programme, the International Labour Organisation, and the World Health Organization, and produced within the framework of the Inter-Organization Programme for the Sound Management of Chemicals.

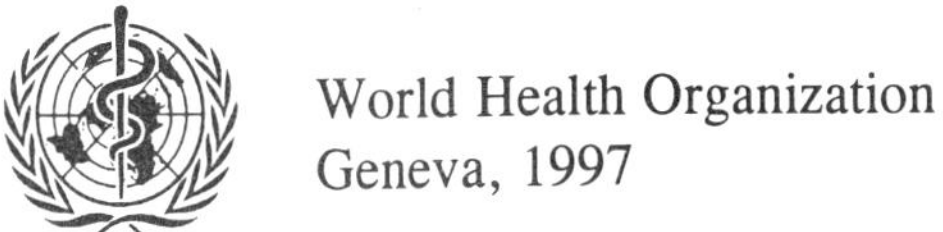

World Health Organization
Geneva, 1997

The **International Programme on Chemical Safety (IPCS)**, established in 1980, is a joint venture of the United Nations Environment Programme (UNEP), the International Labour Organisation (ILO), and the World Health Organization (WHO). The overall objectives of the IPCS are to establish the scientific basis for assessment of the risk to human health and the environment from exposure to chemicals, through international peer-review processes, as a prerequisite for the promotion of chemical safety, and to provide technical assistance in strengthening national capacities for the sound management of chemicals.

The **Inter-Organization Programme for the Sound Management of Chemicals (IOMC)** was established in 1995 by UNEP, ILO, the Food and Agriculture Organization of the United Nations, WHO, the United Nations Industrial Development Organization and the Organisation for Economic Co-operation and Development (Participating Organizations), following recommendations made by the 1992 UN Conference on Environment and Development to strengthen cooperation and increase coordination in the field of chemical safety. The purpose of the IOMC is to promote coordination of the policies and activities pursued by the Participating Organizations, jointly or separately, to achieve the sound management of chemicals in relation to human health and the environment.

WHO Library Cataloguing in Publication Data

Aluminium.

(Environmental health criteria ; 194)

1.Aluminium - toxicity   2.Aluminium - adverse effects
3.Environmental exposure   I.Series

ISBN 92 4 157194 2   (NLM Classification: QV 65)
ISSN 0250-863X

The World Health Organization welcomes requests for permission to reproduce or translate its publications, in part or in full. Applications and enquiries should be addressed to the Office of Publications, World Health Organization, Geneva, Switzerland, which will be glad to provide the latest information on any changes made to the text, plans for new editions, and reprints and translations already available.

PRINTED IN FINLAND
97/PLL/11539 – VAMMALA – 5000

CONTENTS

NOTE TO READERS OF THE CRITERIA MONOGRAPHS

Every effort has been made to present information in the criteria monographs as accurately as possible without unduly delaying their publication. In the interest of all users of the Environmental Health Criteria monographs, readers are requested to communicate any errors that may have occurred to the Director of the International Programme on Chemical Safety, World Health Organization, Geneva, Switzerland, in order that they may be included in corrigenda.

*　　*　　*

A detailed data profile and a legal file can be obtained from the International Register of Potentially Toxic Chemicals, Case postale 356, 1219 Châtelaine, Geneva, Switzerland (telephone no. + 41 22 - 9799111, fax no. + 41 22 - 7973460, E-mail irptc@unep.ch).

*　　*　　*

This publication was made possible by grant number 5 U01 ES02617-15 from the National Institute of Environmental Health Sciences, National Institutes of Health, USA, and by financial support from the European Commission.

P R E A M B L E

Objectives

In 1973 the WHO Environmental Health Criteria Programme was initiated with the following objectives:

(i)   to assess information on the relationship between exposure to environmental pollutants and human health, and to provide guidelines for setting exposure limits;

(ii)   to identify new or potential pollutants;

(iii)   to identify gaps in knowledge concerning the health effects of pollutants;

(iv)   to promote the harmonization of toxicological and epidemiological methods in order to have internationally comparable results.

The first Environmental Health Criteria (EHC) monograph, on mercury, was published in 1976 and since that time an ever-increasing number of assessments of chemicals and of physical effects have been produced. In addition, many EHC monographs have been devoted to evaluating toxicological methodology, e.g., for genetic, neurotoxic, teratogenic and nephrotoxic effects. Other publications have been concerned with epidemiological guidelines, evaluation of short-term tests for carcinogens, biomarkers, effects on the elderly and so forth.

Since its inauguration the EHC Programme has widened its scope, and the importance of environmental effects, in addition to health effects, has been increasingly emphasized in the total evaluation of chemicals.

The original impetus for the Programme came from World Health Assembly resolutions and the recommendations of the 1972 UN Conference on the Human Environment. Subsequently the work became an integral part of the International Programme on Chemical Safety (IPCS), a cooperative programme of UNEP, ILO and WHO. In this manner, with the strong support of the new partners, the importance of occupational health and environmental effects was fully recognized. The EHC monographs have become widely established, used and recognized throughout the world.

The recommendations of the 1992 UN Conference on Environment and Development and the subsequent establishment of the Intergovernmental Forum on Chemical Safety with the priorities for action in the six programme areas of Chapter 19, Agenda 21, all lend further weight to the need for EHC assessments of the risks of chemicals.

Scope

The criteria monographs are intended to provide critical reviews on the effect on human health and the environment of chemicals and of combinations of chemicals and physical and biological agents. As such, they include and review studies that are of direct relevance for the evaluation. However, they do not describe *every* study carried out. Worldwide data are used and are quoted from original studies, not from abstracts or reviews. Both published and unpublished reports are considered and it is incumbent on the authors to assess all the articles cited in the references. Preference is always given to published data. Unpublished data are only used when relevant published data are absent or when they are pivotal to the risk assessment. A detailed policy statement is available that describes the procedures used for unpublished proprietary data so that this information can be used in the evaluation without compromising its confidential nature (WHO (1990) Revised Guidelines for the Preparation of Environmental Health Criteria Monographs. PCS/90.69, Geneva, World Health Organization).

In the evaluation of human health risks, sound human data, whenever available, are preferred to animal data. Animal and *in vitro* studies provide support and are used mainly to supply evidence missing from human studies. It is mandatory that research on human subjects is conducted in full accord with ethical principles, including the provisions of the Helsinki Declaration.

The EHC monographs are intended to assist national and international authorities in making risk assessments and subsequent risk management decisions. They represent a thorough evaluation of risks and are not, in any sense, recommendations for regulation or standard setting. These latter are the exclusive purview of national and regional governments.

Content

The layout of EHC monographs for chemicals is outlined below.

* Summary - a review of the salient facts and the risk evaluation of the chemical
* Identity - physical and chemical properties, analytical methods
* Sources of exposure
* Environmental transport, distribution and transformation
* Environmental levels and human exposure
* Kinetics and metabolism in laboratory animals and humans
* Effects on laboratory mammals and *in vitro* test systems
* Effects on humans
* Effects on other organisms in the laboratory and field
* Evaluation of human health risks and effects on the environment
* Conclusions and recommendations for protection of human health and the environment
* Further research
* Previous evaluations by international bodies, e.g., IARC, JECFA, JMPR

Selection of chemicals

Since the inception of the EHC Programme, the IPCS has organized meetings of scientists to establish lists of priority chemicals for subsequent evaluation. Such meetings have been held in: Ispra, Italy, 1980; Oxford, United Kingdom, 1984; Berlin, Germany, 1987; and North Carolina, USA, 1995. The selection of chemicals has been based on the following criteria: the existence of scientific evidence that the substance presents a hazard to human health and/or the environment; the possible use, persistence, accumulation or degradation of the substance shows that there may be significant human or environmental exposure; the size and nature of populations at risk (both human and other species) and risks for environment; international concern, i.e. the substance is of major interest to several countries; adequate data on the hazards are available.

If an EHC monograph is proposed for a chemical not on the priority list, the IPCS Secretariat consults with the Cooperating Organizations and all the Participating Institutions before embarking on the preparation of the monograph.

Procedures

The order of procedures that result in the publication of an EHC monograph is shown in the flow chart. A designated staff member of IPCS, responsible for the scientific quality of the document, serves as Responsible Officer (RO). The IPCS Editor is responsible for layout and language. The first draft, prepared by consultants or, more usually, staff from an IPCS Participating Institution, is based initially on data provided from the International Register of Potentially Toxic Chemicals, and reference data bases such as Medline and Toxline.

The draft document, when received by the RO, may require an initial review by a small panel of experts to determine its scientific quality and objectivity. Once the RO finds the document acceptable as a first draft, it is distributed, in its unedited form, to well over 150 EHC contact points throughout the world who are asked to comment on its completeness and accuracy and, where necessary, provide additional material. The contact points, usually designated by governments, may be Participating Institutions, IPCS Focal Points, or individual scientists known for their particular expertise. Generally some four months are allowed before the comments are considered by the RO and author(s). A second draft incorporating comments received and approved by the Director, IPCS, is then distributed to Task Group members, who carry out the peer review, at least six weeks before their meeting.

The Task Group members serve as individual scientists, not as representatives of any organization, government or industry. Their function is to evaluate the accuracy, significance and relevance of the information in the document and to assess the health and environmental risks from exposure to the chemical. A summary and recommendations for further research and improved safety aspects are also required. The composition of the Task Group is dictated by the range of expertise required for the subject of the meeting and by the need for a balanced geographical distribution.

EHC PREPARATION FLOW CHART

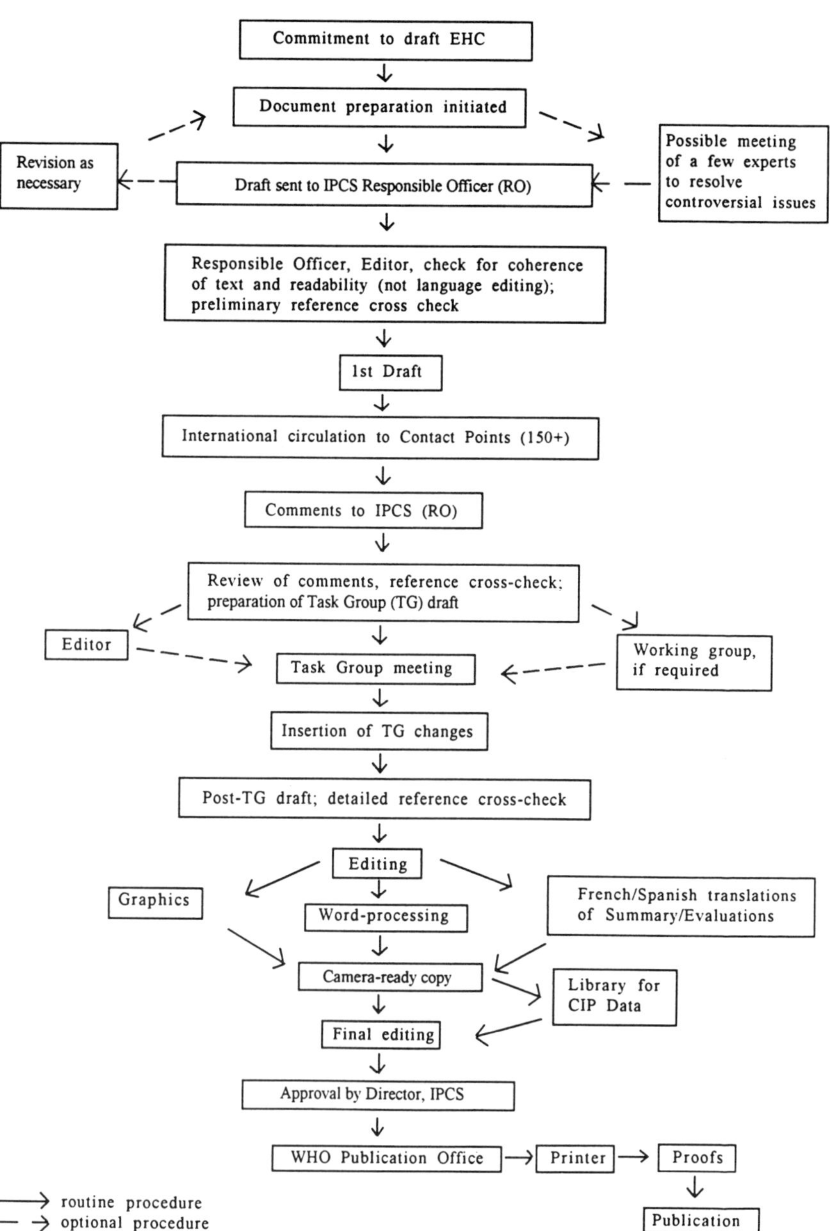

The three cooperating organizations of the IPCS recognize the important role played by nongovernmental organizations. Representatives from relevant national and international associations may be invited to join the Task Group as observers. While observers may provide a valuable contribution to the process, they can only speak at the invitation of the Chairperson. Observers do not participate in the final evaluation of the chemical; this is the sole responsibility of the Task Group members. When the Task Group considers it to be appropriate, it may meet *in camera*.

All individuals who as authors, consultants or advisers participate in the preparation of the EHC monograph must, in addition to serving in their personal capacity as scientists, inform the RO if at any time a conflict of interest, whether actual or potential, could be perceived in their work. They are required to sign a conflict of interest statement. Such a procedure ensures the transparency and probity of the process.

When the Task Group has completed its review and the RO is satisfied as to the scientific correctness and completeness of the document, it then goes for language editing, reference checking, and preparation of camera-ready copy. After approval by the Director, IPCS, the monograph is submitted to the WHO Office of Publications for printing. At this time a copy of the final draft is sent to the Chairperson and Rapporteur of the Task Group to check for any errors.

It is accepted that the following criteria should initiate the updating of an EHC monograph: new data are available that would substantially change the evaluation; there is public concern for health or environmental effects of the agent because of greater exposure; an appreciable time period has elapsed since the last evaluation.

All Participating Institutions are informed, through the EHC progress report, of the authors and institutions proposed for the drafting of the documents. A comprehensive file of all comments received on drafts of each EHC monograph is maintained and is available on request. The Chairpersons of Task Groups are briefed before each meeting on their role and responsibility in ensuring that these rules are followed.

WHO TASK GROUP ON ENVIRONMENTAL HEALTH CRITERIA FOR ALUMINIUM

Members

Dr T.M. Florence, Centre for Environmental Health Sciences, Oyster Bay, New South Wales, Australia

Dr M. Golub, California Regional Primate Research Center, University of California, Davis, California, USA

Mr P. Howe, Institute of Terrestrial Ecology, Monks Wood, Abbots Ripton, Huntingdon, Cambridgeshire, United Kingdom (*Co-Rapporteur*)

Professor D.R. McLachlan (*Retired from*: Centre for Research in Neurogenerative Diseases, University of Toronto, Toronto, Ontario, Canada

Dr M. Moore, National Health and Medical Research Council, National Research Centre for Environmental Toxicology, Coopers Plains, Brisbane, Australia (*Chairman*)

Dr T.V. O'Donnell, University of Otago, Wellington South, New Zealand (*Vice-Chairman*)

Professor B. Rosseland, Norwegian Institute of Water Research (NIVA), Oslo, Norway

Dr B. Simon, Fraunhofer Institute, Hanover, Germany (*Co-Rapporteur*)

Dr B. Sjogren, Department of Occupational Medicine, Swedish National Institute for Working Life, Solna, Sweden

Dr L. Smith, Disease Control Service, Public Health Branch, Ontario Ministry of Health, North York, Ontario, Canada

Dr E. Storey, Royal Melbourne Hospital, Department of Pathology, University of Melbourne, Parkville, Victoria, Australia

Dr H. Temmink, Department of Toxicology, Agricultural University, Wageningen, The Netherlands (*Vice-Chairman*)

Dr M.K. Ward, Department of Renal Medicine, Royal Victoria
Infirmary, Newcastle-upon-Tyne, United Kingdom

Dr M. Wilhelm, Health Institute, University of Dusseldorf,
Dusseldorf, Germany

Professor H.M. Wisniewski, New York State Institute for Basic
Research in Developmental Disabilities, Staten Island, New
York, USA

Professor P. Yao, Chinese Academy of Preventive Medicine,
Institute of Occupational Medicine, Ministry of Health, Beijing,
China

Observers

Dr K. Bentley, Environmental Health Assessment and Criteria,
Human Services and Health, Woden, Australia

Dr O.C. Bøckman, Norsk Hydro, Porsgrunn Research Centre,
Porsgrunn, Norway

Dr J. Borak, Occupational and Environmental Health, Jonathan
Borak & Co., New Haven, Connecticut, USA

Dr I. Calder, Occupational and Environmental Health, South
Australian Health Commission, Adelaide, Australia

Dr J.N. Fisher, ALCOA of Australia Ltd, Point Henry Works,
Geelong, Victoria, Australia

Mr D. Hughes, Environment, Mount Isa Mine Holdings, Brisbane,
Australia

Dr P. Imray, Environmental Health Branch, Queensland Health,
Brisbane, Australia

Ms M.E. Meek, Environmental Health Directorate, Health Canada,
Tunney's Pasture, Ottawa, Ontario, Canada

Dr N. Priest, AEA Technology, Harwell, Didcot, Oxfordshire,
United Kingdom

Dr D. Wilcox, Medical Section, Health Services, Sydney Water, Sydney, Australia

Secretariat

Dr G.C. Becking, International Programme on Chemical Safety Inter-regional Research Unit, World Health Organization, Research Triangle Park, North Carolina, USA (*Secretary*)

Dr D. Johns, DPIE, Coal and Mineral Division, Canberra, Australia (*Temporary Adviser*)

Mr D. Wagner, Chemicals Safety Unit, Human Services and Health, Canberra, Australia (*Temporary Adviser*)

WHO TASK GROUP ON ENVIRONMENTAL HEALTH CRITERIA FOR ALUMINIUM

A WHO Task Group on Environmental Health Criteria for Aluminium met in Brisbane, Australia, from 24 to 28 April 1995. The meeting was sponsored by a consortium of Australian Commonwealth and State Governments through a national steering committee chaired by Dr K. Bentley, Director, Health and Environmental Policy, Department of Health and Family Services, Canberra. The meeting was hosted and organized by the NHMRC National Research Centre for Environmental Toxicology (NRCET), Dr M. Moore, Director, being responsible for the arrangements. Dr D. Lange, Chief Health Officer, welcomed participants on behalf of Queensland Health, and Professor L. Roy Webb, Vice-chancellor, Griffith University, welcomed them on behalf of NRCET. Dr G.C. Becking, IPCS, welcomed the participants on behalf of Dr M. Mercier, Director of the IPCS and the three cooperating organizations (UNEP/ILO/WHO). The Task Group reviewed and revised the draft criteria monograph and made an evaluation of the risks to human health and the environment from exposure to aluminium.

The first draft was prepared under the coordination of Dr G. Rosner, Fraunhofer Institute of Toxicology and Aerosol Research, Germany, and Mr P. Howe, Institute of Terrestrial Ecology, Monks Wood, United Kingdom. The draft reviewed by the Task Group, incorporating the comments received following review by the IPCS Contact Points, was prepared through the cooperative effort of the Fraunhofer Institute, Institute of Terrestrial Ecology and the Secretariat.

Dr G.C. Becking (IPCS Central Unit, Inter-regional Research Unit) and Dr P.G. Jenkins (IPCS Central Unit, Geneva) were responsible for the overall scientific content and technical editing, respectively, of this monograph.

The efforts of all who helped in the preparation and finalization of this publication are gratefully acknowledged.

ABBREVIATIONS

AD	Alzheimer's disease
AIBD	aluminium-induced bone disease
cAMP	cyclic adenosine monophosphate
CI	confidence interval
$1,25\text{-}(OH)_2\text{-}D_3$	$1,25$-dihydroxy-vitamin D_3
DOC	dissolved organic carbon
EDTA	ethylenediaminetetraacetic acid
i.p.	intraperitoneal
i.v.	intravenous
LOAEL	lowest-observed-adverse-effect level
LOEL	lowest-observed-effect level
LTP	long-term potentiation
NFT	neurofibrillary tangle
NIOSH	National Institute for Occupational Safety and Health (USA)
NOEC	no-observed-effect concentration
NOEL	no-observed-effect level
NTA	nitrilotriacetic acid
OR	odds ratio
PHF	paired helical filaments
Pt	platinum unit (1 unit equals the colour produced by lung chloroplatinate in 1 litre of water)
PTH	parathyroid hormone
s.c.	subcutaneous
WAIS	Weschler Adult Intelligence Scale

1. SUMMARY AND CONCLUSIONS

1.1 Identity, physical and chemical properties

Aluminium is a silvery-white, ductile and malleable metal. It belongs to group IIIA of the Periodic Table, and in compounds it is usually found as Al^{III}. It forms about 8% of the earth's crust and is one of the most reactive of the common metals. Exposure to water, oxygen or other oxidants leads to the formation of a superficial coating of aluminium oxide, which provides the metal with a high resistance to corrosion. Aluminium oxide is soluble in mineral acids and strong alkalis but insoluble in water, whereas aluminium chloride, nitrate and sulfate are water soluble. Aluminium halogenides, hydride and lower aluminium alkyls react violently with water.

Aluminium possesses high electrical and thermal conductivity, low density and great resistance to corrosion. It is often alloyed with other metals. Aluminium alloys are light, strong and readily machined into shapes.

1.2 Analytical methods

Various analytical methods have been developed to determine aluminium in biological and environmental samples. Graphite furnace - atomic-absorption spectrometry (GF-AAS) and inductively coupled plasma - atomic-emission spectrometry (ICP-AES) are the most frequently used methods. Contamination of the samples with aluminium from air, vessels or reagents during sampling and preparation is the main source of analytical error. Depending on sample pretreatment, separation and concentration procedures, detection limits are 1.9-4 µg/litre in biological fluids and 0.005-0.5 µg/g dry weight in tissues using GF-AAS, and 5 $\mu g/m^3$ in air and 3 µg/litre in water using ICP-AES.

1.3 Sources of human and environmental exposure

Aluminium is released to the environment both by natural processes and from anthropogenic sources. It is highly concentrated in soil-derived dusts from such activities as mining and agriculture, and in particulate matter from coal combustion. Aluminium silicates (clays), a major component of soils, contribute to the aluminium levels of dust. Natural processes far outweigh direct anthropogenic contributions to the environment. Mobilization of aluminium through human actions is mostly indirect and occurs as a result of emission of acidifying substances. In general, decreasing pH results in an increase in mobility and bioavailability for monomeric forms of aluminium. The most important raw material for the production of aluminium is bauxite, which contains up to 55% alumina (aluminium oxide). World bauxite production was 106 million tonnes in 1992. Aluminium metal has a wide variety of uses, including structural materials in construction, automobiles and aircraft, and the production of metal alloys. Aluminium compounds and materials also have a wide variety of uses, including production of glass, ceramics, rubber, wood preservatives, pharmaceuticals and waterproofing textiles. Natural aluminium minerals, especially bentonite and zeolite, are used in water purification, sugar refining, brewing and paper industries.

1.4 Environmental transport, distribution and transformation

Aluminium occurs ubiquitously in the environment in the form of silicates, oxides and hydroxides, combined with other elements such as sodium and fluorine and as complexes with organic matter. It is not found as a free metal because of its reactivity. It has only one oxidation state (+3) in nature; therefore, its transport and distribution in the environment depend only upon its coordination chemistry and the chemical-physical characteristics of the local environmental system. At pH values greater than 5.5, naturally occurring aluminium compounds exist predominantly in an undissolved form such as gibbsite ($Al(OH)_3$) or as aluminosilicates, except in the presence of high amounts of dissolved organic material, which binds with aluminium and can lead to increased concentrations of dissolved aluminium in streams and lakes. Several factors influence aluminium mobility and subsequent transport within the environment. These include chemical speciation, hydrological flow paths, soil-water interactions, and the composition of the underlying geological materials. The solubility of aluminium in equilibrium with solid phase $Al(OH)_3$ is highly dependent on pH and on complexing agents such as fluoride, silicate, phosphate and organic matter. The chemistry of inorganic aluminium in acid soil and stream water can be considered in terms of mineral solubility, ion exchange and water mixing processes.

Upon acidification of soils, aluminium can be released into solution for transport to streams. Mobilization of aluminium by acid precipitation results in more aluminium being available for plant uptake.

1.5 Environmental levels and human exposure

Aluminium is a major constituent of a number of atmospheric components particularly in soil-derived dusts (both from natural sources and human activity) and particulates from coal combustion. In urban areas aluminium levels in street dust range from 3.7 to 11.6 µg/kg. Airborne aluminium levels vary from 0.5 ng/m^3 over Antarctica to more than 1000 ng/m^3 in industrialized areas.

Surface freshwater and soil water aluminium concentrations can vary substantially, being dependent on physico-chemical and geological factors. Aluminium can be suspended or dissolved. It can be bound with organic or inorganic ligands, or it can exist as a free aluminium ion. In natural waters aluminium exists in both monomeric and polymeric forms. Aluminium speciation is determined by pH and the concentrations of dissolved organic carbon (DOC), fluoride, sulfate, phosphate and suspended particulates. Dissolved aluminium concentrations for water in the circumneutral pH range are usually quite low, ranging from 1.0 to 50 µg/litre. This rises to 500-1000 µg/litre in more acidic water. At the extreme acidity of water affected by acid mine drainage, dissolved aluminium concentrations of up to 90 mg/litre have been measured.

Non-occupational human exposure to aluminium in the environment is primarily through ingestion of food and water. Of these, food is the principal contributor. The daily intake of aluminium from food and beverages in adults ranges between 2.5 and 13 mg. This is between 90 and 95% of total intake. Drinking-water may contribute around 0.4 mg daily at present international guideline values, but is more likely to be around 0.2 mg/day. Pulmonary exposure may contribute up to 0.04 mg/day. In some circumstances, such as occupational exposure and antacid use, the levels of exposure will be much greater. For example, > 500 mg of aluminium may be consumed in two average-sized antacid tablets. There are some difficulties in assessing uptake from these exposures because of analytical and sampling difficulties. Isotopic investigations with Al^{26} indicate that one of the most bioavailable forms of aluminium is the citrate and that there could be as much as 1% absorption when aluminium is in this form. However, humans would absorb only 3% of their total daily uptake of aluminium from drinking-water, a relatively minor source compared to food.

1.6 Kinetics and metabolism

1.6.1 Humans

Aluminium and its compounds appear to be poorly absorbed in humans, although the rate and extent of absorption have not been adequately studied. Concentrations of aluminium in blood and urine have been used as a readily available measure of aluminium uptake, increased urine levels having been observed among aluminium welders and aluminium flake-powder producers.

The mechanism of gastrointestinal absorption of aluminium has not yet been fully elucidated. Variability results from the chemical properties of the element and the formation of various chemical species, which is dependent upon the pH, ionic strength, presence of competing elements (silicon), and the presence of complexing agents within the gastrointestinal tract (e.g., citrate).

The biological behaviour and gastrointestinal absorption of aluminium in humans ingesting aluminium compounds has been studied by using the radioactive isotope Al^{26}. Significant intersubject variability has been demonstrated. Measured fractional uptakes of 5×10^{-3} for aluminium as citrate, 1.04×10^{-4} for aluminium hydroxide and 1.36×10^{-3} for the hydroxide given with citrate were reported. A study of the fractional uptake of aluminium from drinking-water showed an uptake fraction of 2.35×10^{-3}. It was concluded that members of the general population consuming 1.5 litres/day of drinking-water containing 100 µg aluminium/litre would absorb about 3% of their total daily intake of aluminium from this source depending upon the levels found in food and the frequency of antacid use.

The proportion of plasma Al^{3+} normally bound to protein in humans may be as high as 70-90% in haemodialysis patients with moderately increased plasma aluminium. The highest levels of aluminium may be found in the lungs, where it may be present as inhaled insoluble particles.

The urine is the most important route of aluminium excretion. After peroral administration of a single dose of aluminium, 83% was excreted in urine after 13 days and 1.8% in the faeces. The half-life of urinary concentration among welders exposed for more than 10 years was 6 months or longer. Among retired workers exposed to aluminium flake powders, the calculated half-lives were between 0.7 and 8 years.

1.6.2 Animals

Absorption via the gastrointestinal tract is usually less than 1%. The main factors influencing absorption are solubility, pH and chemical species. Organic complexing compounds, notably citrate, increase absorption. The aluminium absorption may interact with calcium and iron transport systems. Dermal and inhalation absorption has not been studied in detail. Aluminium is distributed in most organs within the body with accumulation occurring mainly in bone at high dose levels. To a limited but as yet undetermined extent, aluminium passes the blood-brain barrier and is also distributed to the fetus. Aluminium is eliminated effectively by urine. Plasma half-life is about 1 h in rodents.

1.7 Effects on laboratory mammals and *in vitro* test systems

The acute toxicity of metallic aluminium and aluminium compounds is low, the reported oral LD_{50} values being in the range of several hundred to 1000 mg aluminium/kg body weight per day. However, the LC_{50} values for inhalation have not been identified.

In short-term studies in which an adequate range of end-points was examined following exposure of rats, mice or dogs to various aluminium compounds (sodium aluminium phosphate, aluminium hydroxide, aluminium nitrate) in the diet or drinking-water, only minimal effects (decreases in body weight gain generally associated with decreases in food consumption or mild histopathological effects) have been observed at the highest administered doses (70 to 300 mg aluminium/kg body weight per day). Systemic effects following parenteral administration also included kidney dysfunction.

Adequate inhalation studies were not identified. Following intratracheal administration of aluminium oxide, particle-associated fibrosis was observed, similar to that found in other studies on silica and coal dust.

No overt fetotoxicity was noted, nor were general reproductive parameters noted after gavage treatment of rats with 13, 26 or 52 mg aluminium/kg body weight per day (as aluminium nitrate). However, a dose-dependent delay in the growth of offspring was noted with females administered 13 mg/kg and in male offspring at 26 mg/kg. The lowest-observed-adverse-effect level (LOAEL) for developmental effects (decreased ossification, increased incidence of vertebral and sternebrae terata and reduced fetal weight) was 13 mg/kg (aluminium nitrate). These effects were not observed at much higher doses of aluminium hydroxide. There were reductions in postnatal growth at 13 mg/kg (aluminium nitrate), although maternal toxicity was not examined. In studies on brain development, grip strength was impaired in offspring of dams fed 100 mg aluminium/kg body weight as aluminium lactate in the diet, in the absence of maternal toxicity.

There is no indication that aluminium is carcinogenic. It can form complexes with DNA and cross-link chromosomal proteins and DNA, but it has not been shown to be mutagenic in bacteria or induce mutation or transformation in mammalian cells *in vitro*. Chromosomal aberrations have been observed in bone marrow cells of exposed mice and rats.

There is considerable evidence that aluminium is neurotoxic in experimental animals, although there is considerable variation among species. In susceptible species, toxicity following parenteral administration is characterized by progressive neurological impairment, resulting in death with status epilepticus (LD_{50} = 6 µg Al/g dry weight of brain). Morphologically, the progressive encephalopathy is associated with neurofibrillary pathology in large and medium size neurons predominantly in the spinal cord, brainstem and selected areas of the hippocampus. These tangles are morphologically and biochemically different from those that occur in Alzheimer's disease (AD). Behavioural impairment has been observed in the absence of overt encephalopathy or neurohistopathology in experimental animals exposed to soluble aluminium salts (e.g., lactate, chloride) in the diet or drinking-water at doses of 50 mg aluminium/kg body weight per day or more.

Osteomalacia, as it presents in man, is observed consistently in larger species (e.g., dogs and pigs) exposed to aluminium; a similar condition is observed in rodents. These effects appear to occur in all species, including humans, at aluminium levels of 100 to 200 μg/g bone ash.

1.8 Effects on humans

No acute pathogenic effects in the general population have been described after exposure to aluminium.

In England, a population of about 20 000 individuals was exposed for at least 5 days to increased levels of aluminium sulfate, accidentally placed in a drinking-water facility. Case reports of nausea, vomiting, diarrhoea, mouth ulcers, skin ulcers, skin rashes and arthritic pain were noted. It was concluded that the symptoms were mostly mild and short-lived. No lasting effects on health could be attributed to the known exposures from aluminium in the drinking-water.

It has been hypothesized that aluminium in the drinking-water is a risk factor for the development or acceleration of AD as well as for impaired cognitive function in the elderly. It has also been suggested that stamped fine aluminium powder and fume may be risk factors for impaired cognitive function and pulmonary disease in certain occupations.

Some 20 epidemiological studies have been carried out to test the hypothesis that aluminium in drinking-water is a risk factor for AD, and two studies have evaluated the association between aluminiun in drinking-water and impaired cognitive function. Study designs ranged from ecological to case control. Eight studies in populations in Norway, Canada, France, Switzerland and England were considered of sufficiently high quality to meet the general criteria for exposure and outcome assessment and the adjustment for at least some confounding variables. Of the six studies that examined the relationship between aluminium in drinking-water and dementia or AD, three found a positive relationship but three did not. However, each of the studies had some deficiencies in the study design (e.g., ecological exposure assessment, failure to consider aluminium exposure from all sources and to control for important confounders such as education, socioeconomic status and family history, the use of surrogate outcome measures for AD, and selection bias). In general, the relative risks determined were less than 2, with large confidence intervals, when the total aluminium concentration in drinking-water was 100 µg/litre or higher. Based on current knowledge on the pathogenesis of AD and the totality of evidence from these epidemiological studies, it was concluded that the present epidemiological evidence does not support a causal association between AD and aluminium in drinking-water.

In addition to the epidemiological studies that examined the relationship between AD and aluminium in drinking-water, two studies examined cognitive dysfunction and AD in elderly populations in relation to the levels of aluminium in drinking-water. The results were again conflicting. One study of 800 male octogenarians consuming drinking-water with aluminium concentrations up to 98 µg/litre found no relationship. The second study used "any evidence of mental impairment" as an outcome measure and found a relative risk of 1.72 at aluminium concentrations greater than 85 µg/litre in 250 males. Such data are insufficient to show that aluminium is a cause of cognitive impairment in the elderly.

Reports of impaired cognitive function related to aluminium exposure are conflicting. Most studies are on small populations, and the methodology used in these studies is open to question with respect to magnitude of effect reported, exposure assessment and confounding factors. In a comparative study of cognitive impairment in miners exposed to a powder containing 85% finely ground aluminium and 15% aluminium oxide (as prophylaxis against silica) and unexposed miners, the cognitive test scores and the proportion impaired in at least one test indicated a disadvantage for the exposed miners. A positive exposure-related trend of increased risk was noted.

In all occupational studies reported, the magnitude of effects found, presence of confounding factors, problems with exposure assessment and the probability of mixed exposures all make the data insufficient to conclude that aluminium is a cause of cognitive impairment in workers exposed occupationally to aluminium.

Neurological syndromes including impairment of cognitive function, motor dysfunction and peripheral neuropathy have been reported in limited studies of workers exposed to aluminium fume. A small population of aluminium welders who were compared with iron welders were reported to show a small decrement in repetitive motor function. When a questionnaire methodology was used in another study, an increase in neuropsychiatric symptoms was reported.

Iatrogenic exposure in patients with chronic renal failure, exposed to aluminium-containing dialysis fluids and pharmaceutical products, may cause encephalopathy, vitamin-D-resistant osteomalacia and microcytic anaemia. These clinical syndromes can be prevented by reduction in exposure to aluminium.

Premature infants, even where kidney impairment is not severe enough to cause raised blood creatinine levels, may develop increased tissue loading of aluminium, particularly in bone, when exposed to iatrogenic sources of aluminium. Where there is kidney failure, seizures and encephalopathy may occur.

Although human exposure to aluminium is widespread, in only a few cases has hypersensitivity been reported following exposure to some aluminium compounds after dermal application or parenteral administration.

Pulmonary fibrosis was reported in some workers exposed to very fine stamped aluminium powder in the manufacture of explosives and fireworks. Nearly all cases involved exposure to aluminium particles coated with mineral oil. That process is no longer used. Other cases of pulmonary fibrosis have related to mineral exposures to other agents such as silica and asbestos and cannot be attributed solely to aluminium.

Irritant-induced asthma has been associated with inhalation of aluminium sulfate, aluminium fluoride, potassium aluminium tetrafluoride and with the complex environment of the potrooms during aluminium production.

There is insufficient information to allow for classification of the cancer risk from human exposures to aluminium and its compounds. Animal studies do not indicate that aluminium or aluminium compounds are carcinogenic.

1.9 Effects on other organisms in the laboratory and field

Aquatic unicellular algae showed increased toxic effect at low pH, where bioavailability of aluminium is increased. They are more sensitive than other microorganisms, the majority of 19 lake species showing complete growth inhibition at 200 µg/litre total aluminium (pH 5.5). Selection of aluminium-tolerant strains is possible; green algae capable of growing in the presence of 48 mg/litre at pH 4.6 have been isolated.

For aquatic invertebrates, LC_{50} values range from 0.48 mg/litre (polychaete) to 59.6 mg/litre (daphnid). For fish, 96-h LC_{50} values range from 0.095 mg/litre (American flagfish) to 235 mg/litre (mosquito fish). However, care must be taken when interpreting the results because of the significant effects of pH on the availability of aluminium. The wide range of LC_{50} values probably reflects variable availability. The addition of chelating agents, such as NTA and EDTA, reduces the acute toxicity of aluminium to fish.

Responses to aluminium by macroinvertebrates are variable. In the normal pH range aluminium toxicity increases with decreasing pH; however, in very acidic waters aluminium can reduce the effects of acid stress. Some invertebrates are very resistant to acid stress and can be very numerous in acidic waters. Increased drift rate of invertebrates has been reported in streams suffering either pH or pH/aluminium stress; this is a common response to a variety of stressors. Lake invertebrates generally survived field exposure to aluminium but suffered as a result of phosphate reduction in oligotrophic conditions induced by precipitation with aluminium.

Short- and long-term toxicity tests on fish have been carried out under a variety of conditions and, most importantly, at a range of pH values. The data show that significant effects have been observed at monomeric inorganic aluminium levels as low as 25 µg/litre. However, the complex relationship between acidity and aluminium bioavailability makes interpretation of the toxicity data more difficult. At very low pH (not normally found in natural waters) the hydrogen ion concentration appears to be the toxic factor, with the addition of aluminium tending to reduce toxicity. In the pH range 4.5 to 6.0 aluminium in equilibrium exerts its maximum toxic effect. Toxicity has also been shown to increase with increasing pH levels in the alkaline pH region. The mechanism of aluminium toxicity to fish has been attributed to the inability of fish to maintain their osmoregulatory balance, as well as respiratory problems associated with precipitation of aluminium on the gill mucus. The former effect is associated with lower pH levels. These laboratory findings have been confirmed by field studies especially in areas under acid stress.

Amphibian eggs and larvae are affected by acidity and aluminium, with interaction between the two factors. Reduced hatching, delayed hatching, delayed metamorphosis, metamorphosis at small size, and mortality have been reported in various species and at aluminium concentrations below 1 mg/litre.

Exposure of roots of terrestrial plants to aluminium can cause diminished root growth, reduced uptake of plant nutrients and stunted plant development. Tolerance to aluminium has been demonstrated both in the laboratory and the field.

1.10 Conclusions

1.10.1 *General population*

Hazards to neurological development and brain function from exposure to aluminium have been identified through animal studies. However, aluminium has not been demonstrated to pose a health risk to healthy, non-occupationally exposed humans.

There is no evidence to support a primary causative role of aluminium in Alzheimer's disease (AD), and aluminium does not induce AD pathology *in vivo* in any species, including humans.

The hypothesis that exposure of the elderly population in some regions to elevated levels of aluminium in drinking-water may exacerbate or accelerate AD lacks adequate supporting data.

The data in support of the hypothesis that particular exposures, either occupational or via drinking-water, may be associated with non-specific impaired cognitive function are also inadequate.

There is insufficient health-related evidence to justify revisions to existing WHO Guidelines for aluminium exposure in healthy, non-occupationally exposed humans. As an example, there is an inadequate scientific basis for setting a health-based standard for aluminium in drinking-water.

1.10.2 Subpopulations at special risk

In people of all ages with impaired renal function, aluminium accumulation has been shown to cause the clinical syndrome of encephalopathy, vitamin-D-resistant osteomalacia and microcytic anaemia. The sources of aluminium are haemodialysis fluid and aluminium-containing pharmaceutical agents (e.g., phosphate binders). Intestinal absorption can be exacerbated by the use of citrate-containing products. Patients with renal failure are thus at risk of neurotoxicity from aluminium.

Iatrogenic aluminium exposure poses a hazard to patients with chronic renal failure. Premature infants have higher body burdens of aluminium than other infants. Every effort should be made to limit such exposure in these groups.

1.10.3 Occupationally exposed populations

Workers having long-term, high-level exposure to fine aluminium particulates may be at increased risk of adverse health effects. However, there are insufficient data from which to develop with any degree of certainty occupational exposure limits with regards to the adverse effects of aluminium.

Exposure to stamped pyrotechnic aluminium powder most often coated with mineral oil lubricants has caused pulmonary fibrosis (aluminosis), whereas exposure to other forms of aluminium has not been proven to cause pulmonary fibrosis. Most reported cases had exposure to other potentially fibrogenic agents.

Irritant-induced asthma has been associated with inhalation of aluminium sulfate, aluminium fluoride or potassium aluminium tetrafluoride, and with the complex environment within the potrooms during aluminium production.

1.10.4 *Environmental effects*

Aluminium-bearing solid phases in the environment are relatively insoluble, particularly at circumneutral pH values, resulting in low concentrations of dissolved aluminium in most natural water.

In acidic or poorly buffered environments subjected to strong acidifying inputs, concentrations of aluminium can increase to levels resulting in adverse effects on both aquatic organisms and terrestrial plants. However, there exist large species, strain and life history stage differences in sensitivity to this metal.

The detrimental biological effects from elevated concentrations of inorganic monomeric aluminium can be mitigated in the presence of organic acids, fluorides, silicate and high levels of calcium and magnesium.

There is a substantial reduction in species richness associated with the mobilization of the more toxic forms of aluminium in acid-stressed waters. This loss of species diversity is observed at all trophic levels.

2. IDENTITY, PHYSICAL AND CHEMICAL PROPERTIES, ANALYTICAL METHODS

The element aluminium (Al) was first obtained in an impure form by Oersted in 1825, and pure aluminium was prepared by Woehler two years later. The name aluminium is derived from alum, which the ancient Greeks used as an astringent in medicine (Lide, 1991).

Aluminium is the most abundant metallic element and constitutes 8.13% of the earth's crust. Owing to its high reactivity, it is always found combined with other elements and does not occur in its pure state. Combined with oxygen, silicon, the alkali and alkaline-earth metals, and fluorine, and as hydroxides, sulfates and phosphates, aluminium appears in a wide variety of minerals (Frank et al., 1985; Hudson et al., 1985; Lide, 1991).

Some aluminium compounds, synonyms and molecular formulae are listed in Table 1. The most abundant natural aluminium ores are shown in Table 2.

2.1 Identity

Pure aluminium is a silvery-white, malleable, ductile metal with the atomic number of 13 and the relative atomic mass of 26.98. With few exceptions aluminium is found in chemical compounds as Al^{III}. Aluminium occurs naturally as ^{27}Al; eight radioactive isotopes are known, of which ^{26}Al is the most stable with a half-life of 7.4×10^5 years (Frank et al., 1985).

2.2 Physical and chemical properties

2.2.1 Aluminium metal

Elemental aluminium possesses many desirable characteristics and is therefore widely used in commerce (Sax & Lewis, 1987; Lide, 1991). Aluminium crystallizes in a face-centered cubic lattice that is stable from 4 K to melting point; the coordination number is 12, it is light and malleable, and thus is easily formed into a variety of shapes (Frank et al., 1985).

Table 1. Chemical names, synonyms and molecular formulae of elemental aluminium and aluminium compounds[a]

Chemical name	CAS registry number	Synonyms	Formula
Aluminium	7429-90-5	Aluminium, metana	Al
Aluminium chloride	7446-70-0	Aluminium trichloride	$AlCl_3$
Aluminium chlorohydrate	1327-41-9 11097-68-0 84861-98-3	Aluminium chlorohydroxide, aluminium chloride, basic, chlorhydrol, polyaluminium chloride[b]	$AlCl(OH)_5$ $Al_2Cl(OH)_5·2H_2O$
Aluminium fluoride	7784-18-1	Aluminium trifluoride	AlF_3
Aluminium lactate	18917-91-4	Aluctyl	$Al(C_3H_5O_3)_3$
Aluminium oxide[c]	1302-74-5	α-Alumina, corundum	Al_2O_3
Aluminium oxide hydroxide[c]	14457-84-2	Diaspore	α-AlO(OH) or α-$Al_2O_3·H_2O$
Aluminium oxide hydroxide[c]	1318-23-6	Boehmite	γ-AlO(OH) or γ-$Al_2O_3·H_2O$
Aluminium oxide, trihydrate[c]	20257-20-9	Bayerite, α-aluminium trihydroxide	α- $Al(OH)_3$ or α-$Al_2O_3·3H_2O$
Aluminium oxide, trihydrate[c]	13840-05-6	Nordstrandite, β-aluminium trihydroxide	β-$Al(OH)_3$ or β-$Al_2O_3·3H_2O$
Aluminium oxide, trihydrate[c]	14762-49-3	Gibbsite, hydrargillite, γ-aluminium trihydroxide	γ-$Al(OH)_3$ or γ-$Al_2O_3·3H_2O$

Table 1 (contd).

Chemical name	CAS registry number	Synonyms	Formula
Nitric acid, aluminium salt	13473-90-0	Aluminium trinitrate, aluminium nitrate	$Al(NO_3)_3$
Phosphoric acid, aluminium salt	7784-30-7	Aluminium orthophosphate	$AlPO_4$
Sodium aluminate	1302-42-7		$NaAlO_2$, $Na_2O\cdot Al_2O_3$ or $Na_2Al_2O_4$
Sulfuric acid, aluminium salt	10043-01-3	Alum, aluminium trisulfate, cake alum	$Al_2(SO_4)_3$
Trimethylaluminium[b]	75-24-1		$Al(CH_3)_3$
2-Propanol, aluminium salt[b]	555-31-7	Aluminium isopropoxide, aluminium isopropylate	$Al(OCH(CH_3)_2)_3$
2-Butanol, aluminium salt[b]	2269-22-9	Aluminium sec-butoxide, aluminium butylate	$Al(OC_4H_9)_3$

[a]   adapted from ATSDR (1992)
[b]   Zietz (1985)
[c]   Hudson et al. (1985)

Table 2. CAS chemical names and registry numbers, synonyms, trade names, content and molecular formula of aluminium ores[a]

Chemical name	CAS registry number	Synonyms and trade names	Composition	Formula
Aluminium magnesium silicate	-	Magnesium aluminium silicate	48.8% O 21.4% Si 20.6% Al 9.3% Mg	$MgAl_2(SiO_4)_2$
Aluminium silicate, hydrate	-	Kaolinite	40% Al_2O_3[b] 46% SiO_2 14% H_2O	$Al_2Si_2O_5(OH)_4$ or $Al_2O_3 \cdot SiO_2 . H_2O$
Aluminium silicofluoride	-	Topaz	71.2% F 17.6% Si 11.2% Al	$2Al_2O_3 \cdot 2Al(F,OH)_3 . 3SiO_2$
Ammonium aluminium sulfate, hydrate	7784-26-1	Ammonium alum, ammonium aluminium sulfate	-	$NH_4Al(SO_4)_2 . 12H_2O$ or $Al_2O_3 \cdot (NH_4)_2O \cdot 24HOH$
Bauxite	1318-16-7	-	30-75% Al_2O_3 3-25% Fe_2O_3 9-31% H_2O 2-9% SiO_2 1-3% TiO_2	-

Table 2 (contd).

Chemical name	CAS registry number	Synonyms and trade names	Composition	Formula
Potassium aluminium sulfate, hydrate	7784-24-9	Potash alum, potassium aluminium sulfate	37% Al_2O_3 11% K_2O 39% SO_3 13% H_2O	$K(AlO)_3(SO_4)_2.12H_2O$ or $Al_2(SO_4)_3.K_2SO_4\cdot24HOH$
Sodium aluminium fluoride	15096-52-3	Cryolite, greenland spar, isestone	-	Na_3AlF_6 or $3NaF\cdot AlF_3$
Sodium aluminium sulfate, hydrate	7784-28-3	Sodium alum, sodium aluminium sulfate	-	$NaAl(SO_4)_2\cdot12H_2O$ or $Al_2(SO_4)_2.Na_2SO_4.24HOH$
Sodium calcium silicoaluminate	-	Anorthosite, soda-lime feldspar	26-35% Al_2O_3 [b] 46-59% SiO_2 8-18% CaO 1-7% Na_2O	$Na_2O\cdot Al_2O_3\cdot6SiO_2$ & $CaO\cdot Al_2O_3\cdot2SiO_2$

[a]   From: Sax & Lewis (1987)
[b]   US Bureau of Mines (1967)

Owing to the high charge/radius ratio of Al^{3+} in aqueous solutions, the ion proteolyses part of the water envelope and forms hydroxo complexes. It can also complex with electron-rich species, such as fluoride and chloride. The chemical properties of aluminium resemble those of beryllium and silicon. Because of its amphoteric character, it reacts with mineral acids and strong alkalis (Sax & Lewis, 1987). Although aluminium is one of the most reactive of the common metals used commercially, it has excellent resistance to corrosion. Exposed to oxygen, water or other oxidants, a continuous film of aluminium oxide (Al_2O_3) grows rapidly on the nascent aluminium surface, providing the metal with a high resistance to corrosion. The oxide film dissolves in alkaline solutions with evolution of hydrogen and formation of soluble alkali-metal aluminates (Sax & Lewis, 1987).

The oxide film on the solid metal is resistant to some acids (e.g., nitric acid), and prevents further chemical attack on the metal. However, the protective oxide film dissolves in some acids (e.g., hydrochloric or hot sulfuric acids) and also in alkaline solutions, exposing the metal to further reactions. At elevated temperatures, aluminium metal reacts with water (above 180 °C), producing $Al(OH)_3$ and H_2, and with many metal oxides producing Al_2O_3 and the metal. This reaction is used to produce certain metals, for example, manganese and alloys (e.g., ferro-titanium).

Finely divided aluminium dust can ignite and cause explosions (Wade & Banister, 1973; Frank et al., 1985).

Many applications of aluminium and its alloys are based upon its inherent properties of high electrical and thermal conductivity, low density, and great resistance to corrosion. Pure aluminium is soft and lacks strength, but it can be alloyed with small amounts of Cu, Mg, Si, Mn and other elements to impart greater strength and a variety of other useful properties. Aluminium alloys are light, strong and readily worked into a variety of shapes (Frank et al., 1985; Lide, 1991).

2.2.2 *Aluminium compounds*

The aluminium compounds of the greatest industrial importance are aluminium oxide, aluminium sulfate and aluminium silicate. Some physical and chemical data of aluminium and selected aluminium compounds are summarized in Table 3.

Table 3. Physical and chemical properties of aluminium and some of its compounds[a]

Chemical name	Relative atomic/ molecular mass	Melting point (°C)	Boiling point (°C)	Relative density (g/cm^3)[b]	Crystalline form	Solubility[d]
Aluminium	26.98	660	2450[c]	2.708	silver-white cubic	sol alkali, HCl, H_2SO_4; insol H_2O, HNO_3[e]
α-Aluminium hydroxide (bayerite)	77.99	300 (-H_2O)		2.420	monoclinic, powder	sol acid; insol H_2O, alcohol[e]
Aluminium nitrate	213.00	74	135 (decomposes)	-	rhombic delinq.	sol H_2O, alkali, acetone, HNO_3
Aluminium oxide	101.94	2072	2980	3.965 (25)	hexagonal	very sl sol benzene; insol H_2O
γ-Aluminium oxide hydroxide (boehmite)	59.99	-	-	3.440	orthorhomic	sol acid; sl sol alkali; insol H_2O, alcohol[e]

Table 3 (contd).

Aluminium phosphate	121.95	1500	-	2.566	rhombic platelets	sol acid, alkali; insol H$_2$O
Aluminium sulfate, anhydrate	342.14	700 (decomposes)	-	2.710	powder	sol H$_2$O, dil acid; sl sol alkali
Aluminium sulfate, hydrate	666.41	87 (decomposes)	-	1.690 (17)	monoclinic	sol H$_2$O, dil. acid; sl sol alkali
Aluminium isopropoxide[e]	204.25	119	141	1.035 (20)	crystals	sol alcohol, benzene, chloroform

[a] Compiled from ATSDR (1992)
[b] Temperature is given in parentheses
[c] Sax & Lewis (1987)
[d] Sol = soluble; insol = insoluble; sl = slightly
[e] Lide (1991)

Aluminium oxide is a white powder that is found as balls or lump of various mesh sizes. Owing to its amphoteric character, it is soluble in mineral acids and strong alkali. Aluminium oxide is found in different modifications. The hexagonally closest-packed α-modification "corundum" (α-Al_2O_3) is the most stable oxide. Emery is an abrasive containing corundum, and ruby and sapphire are impure crystalline varieties of gem quality (Hudson et al., 1985). Formation of aluminium oxide by dehydration of the hydroxides produces a series of alumina types still containing a small proportion of hydroxyl groups and retaining some chemical reactivity. All oxides produced at low temperatures are collectively referred to as transitional oxides. Those formed by dehydration below 600 °C are known as γ-aluminas or activated aluminas, while the aluminas formed by dehydration at higher temperatures (900-1000 °C), the δ-aluminas, are nearly anhydrous Al_2O_3 (Wade & Banister, 1973). At 1400 °C all transitional alumina converts to α-alumina (Hudson et al., 1985). The structural and compositional differences among various forms of alumina are associated with differing particulate size, particulate surface area, surface reactivity and catalytic activity.

Various forms of aluminium hydroxides are known. The best defined forms are the trihydroxides ($Al(OH)_3$) and the oxide-hydroxides ($AlO(OH)$). Besides these well-defined crystalline forms, several other hydroxides have been described in the literature (Wefers & Bell, 1972). The aluminium hydroxides found abundantly in nature are gibbsite ($Al(OH)_3$), diaspore β-($AlO(OH)$), and boehmite α-($AlO(OH)$). They all convert to aluminium oxide when heated (Hudson et al., 1985).

Aluminium sulfate can exist with varying proportions of water, the common form being $Al_2(SO_4)_3 \cdot 18H_2O$. It is almost insoluble in anhydrous alcohol, but readily soluble in water. Above 770 °C decomposition to aluminium oxide is observed. Aluminium sulfate is mainly used in water treatment, dyeing, leather tanning and in the production of other aluminium compounds. Alums are crystalline double salts composed of aluminium, sulfate and a monovalent cation, such as potassium, sodium or ammonium, and have the general formula $M^+Al^{3+}(SO_4)_2 \cdot 12H_2O$. In aqueous solution, alums show all the chemical properties that their components show separately (Helmboldt et al., 1985).

Clays are aluminium silicates. They have cation-exchange capacity and the amounts and types of clay minerals in a soil largely determine its physical properties and suitability for agriculture (Wild, 1988).

Aluminium halogenides, hydrides and lower aluminium alkyls react violently with molecular oxygen, and are spontaneously inflammable in air and explosive with water. Industrially these compounds are used as co-catalysts for organometallic and organic synthesis, and as intermediates in various production processes (Stokinger, 1987; Budavari, 1989).

Further compounds of industrial interest are aluminium antimonide (AlSb) and selenide (AlSe), which are employed in the semiconductor technology industry (Budavari, 1989). Aluminium phosphide (AlP) is used as a rodenticide and pesticide, but it is not discussed in this monograph since its biocidal activity is due to the phosphide moiety and not to the aluminium.

2.3 Analytical methods

Various methods for sampling, sample preparation and determination of aluminium in biological and environmental samples have been developed and described. An overview of standard methods is given in Table 4.

2.3.1 *Sampling and sample preparation*

Because of the ubiquitous distribution of aluminium in nature, care must be taken during sampling and sample preparation to avoid contamination. Most analytical errors are due to contamination of the sample with aluminium from air, vessels and reagents during sampling and preparation for analysis. To prevent aluminium contamination, the use of aluminium-free polyethylene, polypropylene, teflon or quartz materials is recommended. Containers and laboratory materials have to be washed with warm, dilute nitric acid and subsequently rinsed with de-ionized water prior to use (Andersen, 1987).

Table 4. Analytical methods for aluminium and aluminium compounds[a]

Medium	Sample preparation	Analytical method	Detection limit	Recovery	Reference
Environmental samples					
Air	Sample collection on cellulose filter, ashing with HNO_3	FAAS	500 µg/m^3 (100-litre sample)	n.g.	NIOSH (1984)
	Sample collection on cellulose filter, ashing with HNO_3	ICP-AES	5 µg/m^3 (500-litre sample)	n.g.	NIOSH (1984)
Water	Reaction with sulfonitrazo DAF	Spectrophotometry	4 µg/litre	n.g.	Ermolenko & Dedkov (1988)
	Reaction with Chromazurol S	Spectrophotometry	0.0005 µg/0.5 ml-sample	n.g.	Schwedt (1989)
	Reaction with alizarin S	Spectrophotometry	10 µg/litre; 50 µg/litre (after digestion)	n.g.	DIN (1993)
	Digestion with HNO_3 and H_2O_2	ICP-AES	100 µg/litre	n.g.	DIN (1993)
	Filtration, digestion with HNO_3, reaction with 8-hydroxyquinoline	Spectrophotometry ICP-AES	6-13 µg/litre range 3 µg/litre limit detection	98-100%	van Benschoten & Edzwald (1990)
Soil	Extraction with H_2O, filtration, high-performance size exclusion chromatography	GF-AAS		n.g.	Gardinier et al. (1987)

Table 4 (contd).

Sample	Preparation	Method	Detection limit/range	Recovery	Reference
Soil	Extraction with H_2O, filtration, gel chromatography, reaction with Chromazurol	Spectrophotometry	0.005 µg (absolute)	n.g.	Dunemann & Schwedt (1984)
Fly ash	Vacuum dried	NAA		n.g.	Fleming & Lindstrom (1987)
Rock, soil, paint, citrus leaves	Dried, digestion with HNO_3/HCl	ICP-AES	1-5 µg/litre	> 57%	Que Hee & Boyle (1988)
Biological samples					
Serum	Centrifugation, dilution with $Mg(NO_3)_2$	GF-AAS	14.3-150 µg/litre (analytical range)	97-102%	Bettinelli et al. (1985)
Plasma, serum	Centrifugation, dilution with water	GF-AAS	4 µg/litre	90-102%	Gardinier et al. (1981)
Whole blood, plasma, serum	Dilution with Triton X-100	GF-AAS	1.9 µg/litre (serum), 1.8 µg/litre (plasma), 2.3 µg/litre (blood)	n.g.	van der Voet et al. (1985)

Table 4 (contd).

Medium	Sample preparation	Analytical method	Detection limit	Recovery	Reference
Biological tissue, urine	Wet-digestion, complexation with Tiron, anion-exchange chromatography	NAA	2.1 µg/litre (liver) 0.18 µg/ml (urine)	n.g.	Blotcky et al. (1992)
Urine, blood	Dilution with water	ICP-AES	6 µg/litre	n.g.	Sanz-Medel et al. (1987)
	Dilution with water	ICP-AES	0.3 µg/litre	n.g.	Mauras & Allain (1985)
Biological tissues	Freeze dry, grind	NAA		n.g.	Yukawa et al. (1980)
	Dried, digestion with HNO_3, dilution with water	GF-AAS	0.5 µg/g dry tissue	80-117%	Bouman et al. (1986)
	Dried, digestion with HNO_3, cation-exchange chromatography	AMS	10^6 atoms ^{26}Al	n.g.	Kobayashi et al. (1990)
	Digestion, high-performance ion-exchange chromatography, reaction with Tiron	Spectrophotometry	7 µg/litre	87-94%	Dean (1989)

Table 4 (contd).

Hair	Washed with 2-propanol, digestion with HNO_3	GF-AAS	0.65 µg/g dry weight	84-105%	Chappuis et al. (1988)
Body fluids	Dilution with HNO_3/HCl	ICP-AES	1-5 µg/litre	> 57%	Que Hee & Boyle (1988)
Haemodialysis concentrates	Dilution with HNO_3 and Triton X-100	GF-AAS (Zeeman-corrected)	3 µg/litre	93-108%	Andersen (1987)
Haemodialysis fluids	Reaction with ferron in CTAB	Phosphorimetry	5.4 µg/litre	n.g.	De La Campa et al. (1988)

[a] AMS = accelerator mass spectrometry; CTAB = cetyltriammonium bromide; EDTA = ethylenediaminetetraacetic acid; FAAS = flame atomic-absorption spectrophotometry; ferron = 7-iodo-8-quinolinol-5-sulfonic acid; GF-AAS = graphite furnace - atomic-absorption spectrophotometry; ICP-AES = inductively coupled plasma - atomic-emission spectrophotometry; NAA = neutron activation analysis; n.g. = not given; Tiron = 4,5-dihydroxy-1,3-benzenedisulfonic acid

Air is sampled with high volume samplers using low-ash cellulose or cellulose ester filters for particulate aluminium (NIOSH, 1984). Biological samples need to be preserved by cooling, freezing or lyophilization. Preservation with 10% formalin is not recommended because of a high risk of aluminium contamination (Bouman et al., 1986).

Homogeneity of the samples is an absolute prerequisite for accurate analysis. To prepare samples for analysis, inorganic samples are usually dissolved in nitric acid or extracted with water. Solutions are filtered with a membrane filter and the particulate residue is analysed separately (Dunemann & Schwedt, 1984).

Water (DIN, 1993) and urine should be acidified with HNO_3 or HCl to pH < 2 to prevent adsorption effects and the precipitation of salts. This ensures that aluminium remains in solution. Water samples for speciation analysis should be stored, without acidification, in high-density polyethylene bottles (Berden et al., 1994; Fairman et al., 1994). Prior to analysis biological tissues must be homogenized and separated or extracted. Blood and urine samples may be separated by centrifugation and diluted, or, if appropriate, analysed directly without pretreatment.

Free aluminium may be determined directly from the samples or the sample extracts. To determine insoluble aluminium compounds and organically bound species, the samples (organic matter, air-filters, water, soil, etc.) need to be subjected to wet ashing (digestion) or dry ashing. Wet ashing, i.e. heating with nitric acid under reflux, is suitable for most organic and biological samples. The residues are dissolved in acids before analysis (NIOSH, 1984; Kobayashi et al., 1990; DIN, 1993). After digestion, differentiation between free metal species and kinetically labile and stable complexes is not possible.

2.3.2 Separation and concentration

A fractionation procedure for aluminium species in water using an 0.22 μm size filter has been proposed by van Benschoten & Edzwald (1990). Total reactive aluminium is determined in the unfiltered, acidified sample. Dissolved monomeric aluminium is analysed in the unfiltered sample without acidification. Analysis of total dissolved aluminium is performed after filtration and acidification of the sample. Dissolved organically bound aluminium is analysed after separation of the filtered sample on a column of cation exchange resin. The eluate is acidified and analysed colorimetrically. For the determination of dissolved organic monomeric aluminium, samples are passed through a cation exchange column and are analysed with no acidification.

In order to carry out long-term characterization of the highly acute toxicity during the initial phase of aluminium polymerization in "mixing zones" (Rosseland et al., 1992), *in situ* fractionation techniques such as ultrafiltration (Lydersen et al., 1987) are recommended (see section 9.1.2.3).

For the extraction of aluminium bound to fulvic acids, soil samples may be extracted with copper chloride solution (Gardinier et al., 1987). The clean-up of aqueous extracts of soil samples can be performed by gel chromatography (Dunemann & Schwedt, 1984) or by size exclusion chromatography. These methods are very mild and thus suitable for the determination of labile aluminium species (Gardinier et al., 1987).

Water samples may be concentrated by careful evaporation (DIN, 1993). Macro quantities of aluminium can be separated from small amounts of interfering elements by precipitation of aluminium as its hydroxide or phosphate. Chelating agents, such as EDTA, 8-hydroxyquinoline, and 2,2′-dihydroxyazobenzene, can be used to extract aluminium into an organic solvent (Alderman & Gitelman, 1980).

Biological materials contain a variety of compounds that can severely interfere with aluminium determinations. Hence, chromatographic methods are often employed for sample purification. Biological tissue samples may be cleaned-up by cation-exchange chromatography after acid digestion (Dean, 1989; Kobayashi et al., 1990). Blotcky et al. (1992) proposed the chelating of aluminium prior to anion-exchange chromatography. Precolumn derivatization coupled with reversed-phase high performance liquid chromatography (RP-HPLC) is an effective method for the separation of the chelates of different interfering metal ions (Nagaosa et al., 1991). Solvent extraction of aluminium chelate complexes, e.g., 2,4-pentanedione and 4-methyl-2-pentanone, has been described as a separation and pre-concentration step in the analysis of body fluids (Buratti et al., 1984).

2.3.3 *Detection and measurement*

Spectrophotometric methods for aluminium analysis are simple and quick, and are most often used for the determination of aluminium in water. Samples are treated with inorganic or organic reagents to form coloured soluble complexes that can be measured by absorption spectrometry. Disadvantages of these methods are the narrowness of the pH range of the reaction, the instability of the complexes, the low selectivity, and the low sensitivity (Bettinelli et al., 1985). The working range for the aluminium determination with chromazurol C is 25-1000 µg/litre (Schwedt, 1989), with alizarin S it is 10-500 µg/litre (DIN, 1993), and with Tiron it is 7-5000 µg/litre (Dean, 1989). Detection limits of 1 µg/litre can be achieved. Chromatographic separation of chelates of interfering metals increases the selectivity of spectrophotometric methods.

De La Campa et al. (1988) and García et al. (1991) reported a room temperature phosphorimetric method for aluminium analysis. Aluminium reacts with 7-iodo-8-quinolinol-5-sulfonic acid (ferron) in cetyltrimethylammonium bromide micelles to form a highly phosphorescent complex. The method is used to determine aluminium in water and dialysis fluids. The given detection limits are 5.4 µg/litre and 2 µg/litre, respectively.

Instrumental methods applied to the determination of aluminium include neutron activation, X-ray fluorescence, flame atomic-absorption spectrophotometry, inductively coupled plasma - atomic-emission spectrophotometry (ICP-AES) and graphite furnace - atomic-absorption spectrophotometry (GF-AAS). However, neither X-ray fluorescence nor flame absorption methods are sensitive enough to measure trace levels in biological samples (Bettinelli et al., 1985). The NIOSH procedure for aluminium analysis in air is applicable over a working range of 50-5000 µg per sample or 0.5-10 mg/m^3 for a 100-litre sample (NIOSH, 1984).

Neutron activation analysis produces excellent results but the methods are time consuming and the facilities are not always readily available. The method is used for determining aluminium in fly ash (Fleming & Lindstrom, 1987) and biological tissues (Yukawa et al., 1980; Blotcky et al., 1992). After digestion and concentration of the biological samples, a detection limit of 2.1 µg/g was found for bovine liver (Blotcky et al. 1992).

GF-AAS is the most frequently used technique to determine aluminium at low concentrations. Detection limits between 0.5 and 4 µg/litre or µg/g are achieved with the analysis of various environmental and biological samples (Gardinier et al., 1981; van der Voet et al., 1985; Bettinelli et al., 1985; Andersen, 1987). Most liquid samples can be injected directly after dilution into GF-AAS. Dilution is necessary because most biological fluids have high salt contents (in the order of 30%) (Andersen, 1987). To prevent precipitation of aluminium and the formation of carbon residues, EDTA or Triton X can serve as diluents. Ammonia may be added to convert aluminium to aluminate and thus avoid loss of aluminium as its chloride (Gardinier et al., 1981). Triton X-100 is used to reduce the viscosity of the samples, and $MgNO_3$ is added as a matrix modifier to improve the volatility of aluminium (Bettinelli et al., 1985).

ICP-AES is used for the determination of aluminium in various biological and environmental samples, allowing the simultaneous determination of different elements at low levels of interference (Mauras & Allain, 1985; Sanz-Medel et al., 1987). The NIOSH method for aluminium determination in air samples is recommended for a working range of 5-2000 $µg/m^3$ for a 500-litre sample (NIOSH, 1984). A detection limit of 1 µg/litre in biological and environmental samples has been reported by Que Hee & Boyle (1988). ICP can also be combined with a mass spectrometer to further increase the sensitivity of the method. As a multi-element detector for reversed-phase liquid chromatography, ICP-MS offers the ability to measure isotope ratios on eluting peaks and to remove troublesome matrices on-line (Thompson & Houk, 1986).

For [26]Al tracer experiments (Kobayashi et al. 1990), the application of accelerator mass spectrometry (AMS) has been described. The limit of detection is 10^6 atoms; thus the sensitivity of AMS is 10^5 times greater than that of γ-ray counting techniques.

Aluminium concentrations in human brain can be investigated by laser multipoint microprobe mass analysis (LAMMA) using focussed laser ionization with time-of-flight mass spectrometry (Stern et al., 1986). [27]Al nuclear magnetic resonance (NMR) may be used to ascertain the coordination of aluminium in soil solutions (Schierl, 1985). Aluminium in natural water samples has been determined using reversed-phase liquid chromatography of the 8-quinolinol complex using spectrophotometric detection. A detection limit of 2 µg/litre was reported (Nagaose et al., 1991).

2.3.4 *Speciation analysis of aluminium in water*

Speciation analysis aims to distinguish and determine quantitatively different groups of physico-chemical species present in a water sample. All speciation methods, with the exception of potentiometric techniques and direct spectroscopic methods (e.g., NMR), will alter the speciation of the sample during measurement. This may not be a disadvantage, particularly if, as is usual, the speciation analysis is being carried out in order to estimate the toxicity of the sample to aquatic biota. Toxicity itself is a dynamic process, and the interaction of aluminium species in water with a biomembrane (e.g., a fish gill) will change the aluminium species distribution in the solution close to the biomembrane. The best speciation probe is one that reacts with aluminium in a water sample to a similar extent and at a similar rate to the reaction of a biomembrane with the aluminium in the samples.

Speciation analysis of aluminium in a water sample is usually carried out after first filtering the sample through a 0.45 µm membrane filter to remove particulate matter. The filtrate can then be analysed for groups of species by several different techniques, including kinetic spectrophotometry (Parker & Bertsch, 1992a,b), ion exchange (Driscoll, 1984) and ion chromatography (Jones, 1991). Combinations of methods such as sample acidification, kinetic spectrophotometry and ion exchange are frequently used to determine a variety of species (Driscoll, 1984; Courtijn et al., 1990; van Benschoten & Edzwald, 1990). These speciation schemes provide information on various speciation groups, including total dissolved aluminium, acid-soluble aluminium, total monomeric aluminium, reactive monomeric aluminium, non-reactive monomeric aluminium, aluminium fluoride complexes, organic monomeric aluminium and inorganic monomeric aluminium. The terms "reactive" and "labile", as applied to aluminium species, are operationally defined and refer to species that react rapidly with an analytical probe such as a cation exchange resin or a chromogenic reagent.

The aluminium species that are most toxic to aquatic organisms are believed to reside in the reactive monomeric inorganic aluminium fraction and to consist principally of aluminium hydroxy complexes (Helliwell et al., 1983; Fairman et al., 1994; Parent & Cambell, 1994).

Although the fluoro complex is toxic, it is less so than the aluminium hydroxy complexes (Helliwell et al., 1983).

3. SOURCES OF HUMAN AND ENVIRONMENTAL EXPOSURE

3.1 Natural occurrence

Aluminium is released to the environment both by natural processes and from anthropogenic sources. Natural processes far outweigh the contribution of anthropogenic sources because aluminium is a major constituent of the earth's crust, making up about 8% of the earth's surface (Lantzy & Mackenzie, 1979). Anthropogenic releases are mostly indirect, for example, through emission of acidifying substances such as sulfur dioxide and nitrogen oxides to the atmosphere. These acidify rain and soil and contribute to dissolution of aluminium from the soil. The largest anthropogenic impact on aluminium movement in the environment is through enhanced wind and water erosion from cultivated land, notably when fallow. Aluminium is the third most abundant element. It does not occur naturally in the metallic, elemental state, but is widely distributed in the earth's crust in combination with oxygen, fluorine, silicon and other constituents. Aluminium occurs ubiquitously in silicates such as feldspars and micas, complexed with sodium and fluoride as cryolite, and in bauxite rock, which is composed of hydrous aluminium oxides, aluminium hydroxides and impurities such as free silica. In general, decreasing pH as a result of acid rain or the release of acid mine drainage results in increased mobility of the monomeric forms of aluminium (ATSDR, 1992). Chemical speciation in soil and water affecting the bioavailability of aluminium to organisms is discussed in chapter 4.

3.2 Anthropogenic sources

Direct anthropogenic releases of aluminium compounds are primarily to the atmosphere and are associated with industrial processes such as smelting. However, the use of aluminium and aluminium compounds in processing, packaging, storage of food products and as flocculants in the treatment of drinking-water may contribute to its presence in drinking-water and food stuffs (ATSDR, 1992).

3.2.1 Production levels and processes

The most important raw material for the production of aluminium is bauxite, which contains up to 55% alumina (aluminium oxide). The commercial deposits of bauxite are mainly gibbsite ($Al_2O_3.3H_2O$) and boehmite ($Al_2O_3.H_2O$). The bauxite is extracted by open-cast mining (Dinman, 1983).

The production of the metal comprises two basic steps: refining and reduction. Refining involves the production of alumina from bauxite by the Bayer process in which bauxite is digested at high temperature and pressure in a strong solution of caustic soda. The resultant hydrate is crystallized and calcined to the oxide. Reduction involves the reduction of alumina to virgin aluminium metal by the Hall-Heroult electrolytic process using carbon electrodes and a cryolite flux (Dinman, 1983).

World bauxite production was 106 million tonnes in 1992. A comparison of the quarterly average figures for 1993 and 1994 with this figure shows that production in major producing countries is remaining fairly constant (World Bureau of Metal Statistics, 1994). The total primary aluminium production for 1992 is summarized in Table 5. The amount of aluminium recovered from purchased or tolled scrap in 1992 was 14% of the total primary production figure. The total alumina production for 1992 is summarized in Table 6. The total alumina production figure includes 30 million tonnes for metallurgical uses and 3 million tonnes for non-metallurgical uses. The total figures for primary aluminium and alumina production have not changed greatly since 1988.

3.2.2 Uses

Aluminium metal has a wide variety of uses including structural material for construction, automobiles and aircraft, and the production of metal alloys. Other uses include die-cast motor parts, cooking utensils, decorations, road signs, fencing, beverage cans, food packaging, foil, corrosion-resistant chemical equipment, solid fuel rocket propellents and explosives, dental crowns, and denture materials. In the electrical industry aluminium is used for power lines, electrical conductors, insulated cables and wiring (ATSDR, 1992).

Table 5. Primary aluminium production in 1992 (from: IPAI, 1993)

Geographical area	Thousands of tonnes
Africa	617
North America	6016
Latin America	1949
East and South Asia	1379
Europe	3319
Oceania	1483
Total	14 763

Table 6. Alumina production in 1992 (from: IPAI, 1993)

Geographical area	Thousands of tonnes
Africa	604
North America	5812
Latin America	7627
East and South Asia	2360
Europe	5565
Oceania	11 803
Total	33 771

Aluminium compounds and materials also have a wide variety of uses, some of which are listed in Table 7. Aluminium powder is used in paints, protective coatings and fireworks. Natural aluminium minerals especially bentonite and zeolite are used in water purification, sugar refining, brewing and paper industries. Aluminium sulfate is used for water purification, as a mordant in dyeing, and in paper production. Other aluminium compounds are used as tanning agents in the leather industry, and as components of human and veterinary medicines, glues, disinfectants, and in toothpaste, styptic pencils, deodorants, antacids and food additives. Clays (aluminium silicates) are used as industrial raw materials (e.g., production of ceramics), and aluminates are constituents of cement. Alkyl aluminium products are used as catalysts for the production of low pressure polyethylene (ATSDR, 1992).

Table 7. Main uses of aluminium compounds[a]

Aluminium compounds	Uses
alums	hardening agent and setting accelerator for gypsum plaster, in tanning and dyeing, and (formerly) in styptic pencils
aluminas	in water treatment and as accelerator for concrete solidification (high alumina cements)
alkoxides	in varnishes, for textile impregnation, in cosmetics and as an intermediate in pharmaceutical production
borate	production of glass and ceramics
carbonate	antacid
chlorides	production of rubber, lubricants and wood preservatives, and in cosmetics as an astringent; the anhydrous product is used as a catalyst and raw material in the chemical and petrochemical industries; active ingredient in antiperspirants
hydroxide	stomach antacid, other pharmaceuticals
isopropoxide	used in the soap and paint industries; waterproofing textiles
phosphate	antacid
silicate	component of dental cement; antacid, food additives
sulfate	used in water purification as a flocculent, in paper production, as a mordant in dyeing, and as a starting material for the production of other aluminium compounds
trioxide	used as an absorbent, abrasive and refractory material
sodium aluminium phosphate	food additives

[a] From: Helmbolt et al. (1985); ATSDR (1992)

4. ENVIRONMENTAL TRANSPORT, DISTRIBUTION AND TRANSFORMATION

4.1 Transport and distribution between media

Aluminium occurs ubiquitously in silicates such as feldspars and micas, complexed with sodium and fluoride as cryolite, and in bauxite rock composed of hydrous aluminium oxides, aluminium hydroxides, and impurities such as free silica (ATSDR, 1992). Aluminium is not found as a free metal because of its reactivity. It has only one oxidation state (+3); therefore, its transport and distribution in the environment depend upon its coordination chemistry and the characteristics of the local environmental system. Aluminium partitions between solid and liquid phases by reacting and complexing with water molecules and electron-rich anions, such as chloride, fluoride, sulfate, nitrate, phosphate and negatively charged functional groups on humic materials and clay.

At a pH greater than 5.5, naturally occurring aluminium compounds exist predominantly in an undissolved form such as gibbsite ($Al(OH)_3$) or as aluminosilicates, except in the presence of high amounts of dissolved organic material such as fulvic acid, which binds with aluminium and can cause an increase in dissolved aluminium concentrations in streams and lakes (ATSDR, 1992). Several processes influence aluminium mobility and its subsequent transport within the environment; these include chemical speciation, hydrological flow paths, other spatial and temporal factors related to soil-water interactions, and the composition of the underlying geological materials (Grant et al., 1990). Watersheds with shallow, acidic soils and poorly buffered surface waters mobilize aluminium when exposed to acidic deposition (Driscoll et al., 1988).

4.1.1 Air

Aluminium enters the atmosphere as a major constituent of a number of atmospheric particulates, such as soil-derived dusts from erosion and particulates from coal combustion (Grant et al., 1990). Eisenreich (1980) studied the atmospheric loading of aluminium to Lake Michigan, USA. It was found that aluminium was generally associated with large particles (> 2 µm diameter) and that these were deposited near the source. The total atmospheric loading of aluminium to the lake was calculated to be 0.86 kg/ha per year. The more industrialized area south of the lake contributes 75% of this total loading. Cambray et al. (1975) calculated the dry deposition flux of aluminium to the North Sea to be 51 000 tonnes/year. Ottley & Harrison (1993) calculated the flux to be 7300 tonnes/year; they suggest that the lower estimate is due to more spatially appropriate and extensive air monitoring since 1975. Rahn (1981) calculated the input of aluminium from the atmosphere to the Arctic Ocean at 30 000 tonnes/year. The input was significantly less than those of oceanic and riverine inputs (140 000 and 110 000 tonnes/year, respectively).

Guieu et al. (1991) compared atmospheric inputs with river inputs of aluminium for the Golfe du Lion, France. Atmospheric inputs were found to be 11% of total inputs of aluminium. Rainwater was analysed for aluminium and only 19% was found in the dissolved fraction (< 0.4 μm). Losno et al. (1993) monitored rainwater and snow for aluminium and found large variations in the solubility of aluminium. The variations seem to be largely due to pH, lower pH values increasing the solubility of aluminium. Thermodynamic calculations reveal that, at pH values higher than 5, equilibrium with gibbsite or an insoluble trivalent alkaline form of aluminium acts to limit solubility, whereas, at lower pH values, aluminium could be in equilibrium with a hydroxysulfate salt.

4.1.2 Freshwater

4.1.2.1 Dissolved aluminium

In groundwater or surface water systems an equilibrium is formed that controls the extent to which aluminium dissolution can occur. The solubility of aluminium in equilibrium with solid phase $Al(OH)_3$ is highly pH-dependent. Aquo complex $Al(H_2O)_6^{3+}$ predominates at low pH values (e.g., pH < 4), but as the pH of the solution increases (e.g., pH 4-6) and/or the temperature rises, the positive charge of aluminium forces hydrolysis of a water ligand producing the $Al(OH)(H_2O)_5^{2+}$ ion. The degree of hydrolysis increases as the solution pH increases, resulting in a series of Al-OH complexes such as $Al(OH)^{2+}$, $Al(OH)_2^{+}$, $Al(OH)_4^{-}$ (Schecher & Driscoll, 1987). Fluoride ions, being similar in size to hydroxyl ions, will readily substitute in these complexes. At pH < 5.5, molar concentrations of aluminium in certain areas exceed concentrations of fluoride ions and form low ligand number complexes. The concentration of Al-F complexes under those conditions is limited by the total concentration of fluoride ions. At pH > 7.0, Al-OH complexes predominate in waters that are low in dissolved organic matter and silicate. Under acidic conditions sulfate also forms complexes with aluminium. Even though sulfate concentrations are typically higher than those of fluoride in surface waters, Al-SO$_4^{2-}$ complexes are significant only at high sulfate concentrations and low pH values (Courtijn et al., 1987).

The chemical speciation of aluminium in natural water regulates its mobility, bioavailability and toxicity. The concentration of aluminium in some natural water as a function of pH can be estimated by thermodynamic calculations. The actual geochemical mobility of aluminium is very complex and difficult to predict in areas affected by acid deposition, as non-equilibrium processes usually predominate during episodic events associated with aluminium release and transport (Bull & Hall, 1986; Lawrence et al., 1988; Seip et al., 1989).

The chemistry of inorganic aluminium in acid soil and stream water can be considered in terms of mineral solubility, ion exchange and water mixing processes (Neal et al., 1990). The minerals that determine stream water Al^{3+} activity in acidic and acid-sensitive systems are kaoline (Al$_2$Si$_2$O$_5$(OH)$_4$), various forms of aluminium hydroxide (Al(OH)$_3$), aluminium hydroxy sulfate (Al(OH)SO$_4$) and aluminium hydroxy silicate (Seip et al., 1984; Neal & Williams, 1988; Nealet al., 1990).

Goenaga & Williams (1988) found that the concentrations of Al-F and Al-SO$_4$ complexes in Welsh upland water were < 40 µg/litre and accounted for less than 20% of the inorganic aluminium at pH < 5.0. Organic complexes were significant (16 to 49 µg/litre) even in samples with a low total organic carbon content. Organic monomeric aluminium increased during high flows as total organic carbon (TOC) and free ionic aluminium concentrations increased. LaZerte (1984) analysed streams and lakes during spring snow melt in acidified catchments in Ontario, Canada (pH 4.1-6.9, and TOC 1-24 mg/litre). Very little polymeric and amorphous aluminium was found, and most of the inorganic monomeric fraction was in the fluoride complexes.

Neal (1988) found that Plynlimon (Wales) stream water was saturated or over-saturated with respect to some crystalline form of

Al(OH)$_3$, and saturated or under-saturated with respect to amorphous Al(OH)$_3$: the level of saturation became less as pH decreased. The solubility relationship for the kaolin mineral group is that at low pH the waters are saturated with respect to crystalline kaolin (kaolinite) and under-saturated with respect to poorly crystalline kaolin (low crystallinity hallyosite). At higher pH the waters become progressively more over-saturated with respect to crystalline forms and near to saturation with respect to poorly crystalline forms. It appears that at high pH the waters are in approximate equilibrium with amorphous Al(OH)$_3$ whilst at low pH values the waters are in equilibrium with an aluminium hydroxy sulfate phase (equilibrium constant 10-4.9).

Aluminium begins to polymerize when the pH of an acidic solution increases notably over pH 4.5. Polymerization implies that in the first step, two hydroxyls are shared by two aluminium atoms, e.g.,

$$2 \, Al(OH)(H_2O)_5^{2+} \rightarrow Al_2(OH)_2(H_2O)_8^{4+} + 2 \, H_2O$$

Polymerization gradually proceeds to larger structures, eventually leading to the formation of the Al$_{13}$ "polycation" (Hem & Robertson, 1967; Parker & Bertsch, 1992a,b). As polymers coalesce, they increase in relative molecular mass, eventually becoming large enough to precipitate aluminium hydroxide from solution. As the precipitate ages the solubility decreases (Chow, 1992). Tipping et al. (1988b) found that if precipitation occurs at pH 4 to 6 it involves the formation of aluminium (oxy)hydroxide and not aluminosilicates or basic aluminium sulfates. The solubility of the (oxy)hydroxide was highly temperature dependent and decreased in the presence of sulfate and more particularly humate. Lükewille & van Breemen (1992) analysed precipitates from stream bottoms in the Senne area of northern Germany and found them to consist of amorphous aluminium hydroxide, co-precipitated with minor amounts of sulfate, phosphate and silica.

Aluminium is predominantly cationic under acidic conditions and strongly binds with negatively charged organic functional groups such as fulvic acid and humic acid (Chow, 1992). Aluminium-humate complex formation has been modelled by several researchers. For example, Tipping et al. (1988a,c) developed a model using data collected from acidified streams in northern England and Scotland. This model describes the equilibria between humic acid substances, aluminium species, calcium ions and hydrogen ions under acidic conditions (pH < 6) (Tipping et al., 1989a). Tipping & Backes (1988) reported on two models of aluminium–humic acid complexation. Reasonable results were obtained only at pH 4.0 to 5.0. Plankey & Patterson (1987) used a fluorescence technique to study the complex formation kinetics of aluminium with a single metal-free fulvic acid isolated from an Adirondack mountain soil (USA). At pH 3.0 to 4.5 two types of aluminium binding sites were identified.

4.1.2.2 *Aluminium adsorbed on particles*

Goenaga et al. (1987) collected stream water from tributaries of Llyn Brianne reservoir, Wales. Analysis of the freshwater samples showed total aluminium and monomeric aluminium concentrations to be positively correlated with suspended solid content. The levels of total (acid digestible) aluminium that were detected in filtrates of freshwater samples were affected by the pore diameter of the membrane filter used. Between 13% and 50% of this form of aluminium initially present in the sample could be removed by a 0.4 µm pore diameter membrane, depending on the level of suspended solid originally present. Goenaga & Williams (1988) calculated the amount of aluminium adsorbed onto suspended solids by measuring monomeric aluminium before and after separation of suspended solids by filtration (0.015 µm pore diameter). Adsorbed aluminium was low (< 20 µg/litre) during dry weather periods; however, the adsorbed fraction was very significant (> 40 µg/litre) for samples with high suspended solids (> 20 mg/litre) collected from a Welsh upland area during a storm episode. Goenaga & Williams (1990) found that aluminium associated with particles > 0.015 µm was negligible (< 20 µg/litre) in spot samples with a suspended solid content of < 5 mg/litre but significant (< 200 µg/litre) for episode samples with high suspended solids (> 20 mg/litre); between 40% and 60% of the adsorbed aluminium was found to be associated with particles > 0.4 µm. Tipping et al. (1989b) studied the adsorption of aluminium in water from various acidified streams in northern England. The adsorption of aluminium by particles was found to increase with total aluminium, pH and particle concentration. Calculations using an adsorption equation, and taking competition by dissolved humic substances into account, suggest that adsorbed aluminium may commonly account for a significant proportion (> 10%) of total monomeric aluminium in such water.

4.1.2.3 *Aluminium in acidified waters*

Fisher et al. (1968) monitored aluminium concentrations in acidified streams of the Hubbard Brook Experimental Forest, New Hampshire, USA from 1964 to 1966. Annual loads of aluminium were calculated to be between 0.9 and 2.4 kg/ha for three streams. The acidic deposition at the Hubbard Brook ecosystem has induced a series of geochemical responses. Firstly, hydrogen ion acidity is neutralized by the dissolution of alumina primarily found in the soil zone. Secondly, hydrogen ion acidity and aluminium acidity are neutralized by the chemical weathering of silicate materials (Johnson et al., 1981). Hall et al. (1980) acidified a stream in the Hubbard Brook Experimental Forest. The pH of the control stream ranged from 5.7 to 6.4 and in the acidified stream from 3.9 to 4.5. Dissolved aluminium increased significantly in the acidified stream water by an average of 181%compared to the control stream. Lawrence et al. (1988) reported that at high elevations the increased stream flow was associated with reduced surface water acidity and decreased inorganic aluminium concentrations. At low elevations, increased stream flow was associated with increases in stream acidity and concentrations of inorganic aluminium. The contributions of flow from the more acidic upper region of the watershed during high-flow conditions appear to be the major hydrological influence on stream chemistry. In the acid-affected Experimental Forest system, acidity of low-order stream water was high due to elevated inputs of strong acids (sulfuric and nitric) relative to the releases of basic cations from soil. Concentrations of aluminium were also high and predominantly in labile (inorganic) monomeric form. For comparison, samples were collected from the Jamieson Creek watershed, British Columbia, Canada. For this watershed the low-order stream water was acidic due to low concentrations of basic cations coupled with the presence of organic acids. Concentrations of aluminium were relatively low and largely associated with organic solutes (Driscoll et al., 1988).

Large temporal and spatial variations in aluminium concentration occur in Welsh stream water due to hydrological and land use controls. The most acidic streams have the highest aluminium concentration. Variations in stream and soil water aluminium concentrations in the order semi-natural moorland < conifer forested moorland < recently harvested forest can be explained by ion exchange reactions related to changes in the anion concentrations passing through the system and weathering (Neal et al., 1990). Lawrence et al. (1986) found that observed altitude trends in stream aluminium chemistry may be related to spatial variations in vegetation type and mineral soil depth. Mobilization of aluminium was studied in streams at the Hubbard Brook Experimental Forest, New Hampshire, USA. At the highest altitudes maximum densities of spruce and fir vegetation occur, and aluminium appears to be mobilized by transformations involving dissolved organic matter. At mid-altitudes hardwood vegetation predominates and the mechanism of aluminium mobilization shifts to dissolution by strong acids within the mineral soil. At the lowest altitudes relatively thick mineral soil seems to limit aluminium mobility resulting in low concentrations in stream water. During 1983 and 1984 an experimental watershed at Hubbard Brook was commercially whole-tree harvested. Whole-tree harvesting resulted in a large increase in stream nitrate concentrations, followed by a decrease in pH and concomitant increase in inorganic aluminium (Lawrence et al., 1987). Ormerod et al. (1989) studied the spatial patterns in aluminium and pH data from 113 Welsh catchments of contrasting land use. It was found that pH declined and aluminium increased significantly with increasing forest cover. The percentage contribution of labile aluminium to the total filterable concentration ranged from 39% to 90%, the highest levels being associated with streams draining forest. Neal et al. (1992) found that felling conifers led to decreases in pH and increases in aluminium concentrations in streams and soils at Plynlimon, Wales, for the first 2 years. The major changes were found to occur during the winter storm flow periods. The trends were reversed after the first two years. The short-term effects (2-3 years) of forest harvesting on soil and stream water inorganic aluminium chemistry were predominantly controlled by the nitrogen dynamics of the site. A reduction in inorganic aluminium was observed concomitant with declines in nitrate and total inorganic anions. However, 4-5 years after harvesting, inorganic aluminium concentration in soil and stream water of Welsh and Cumbrian study sites was still greater than that expected in moorland catchments (Reynolds et al., 1992).

Bird et al. (1990) compared the effects of a winter "rain on snow" episode with a summer storm episode on the pH and dissolved aluminium levels in a moorland stream and a conifer forest stream. The pre-episode conditions were broadly similar in both streams. In winter, following the snow melt, both moorland and forest stream showed reduced pH accompanied by increases in dissolved aluminium concentrations as buffering capacity provided by the calcium was exceeded by anions such as sulfate. The timing of flow changes was similar, but flush of solutes to the moorland stream was more rapid. Both streams had a similar buffering capacity, but the changes in the forest stream were much greater (pH reduction of 2 units and dissolved aluminium levels exceeding 1 mg/litre), reflecting a greater flux of anions. The surface run-off and reduced buffering capacity from frozen soils led to the changes in both streams. During the summer episode, again the forest stream showed a greater reduction in pH and higher increase in dissolved aluminium; however, the concentrations of sulfate were much lower in both streams and less aluminium was mobilized.

Mach & Brezonik (1989) studied the biogeochemical cycling of aluminium in acidified and reference basins of Little Rock Lake, Wisconsin, USA. Background dissolved lake water aluminium concentrations were 7 µg/litre (0.4 µm pore-size). The acidified basin was acidified in a step-wise manner. Acidification to pH 5.1 resulted in a 45% elevation of dissolved aluminium levels (15.5 µg/litre) over reference basin levels (10.7 µg/litre). Analysis of suspended particulate matter collected from both basins revealed lower levels of particulate aluminium in the acidified basin, demonstrating that there is reduced affinity for particulate matter at the lower pH. Brezonik et al. (1990) studied the effects of acidification of Little Rock Lake on the dissolved concentrations of aluminium. Aluminium desorbed from sediments of the lake basin at pH 4 and below in laboratory studies. In littoral enclosures, dissolved aluminium was elevated above control levels at pH 4.5, and elevated levels were observed in pelagic enclosures at both pH 5.0 and 4.5. Dissolved aluminium levels remained constant in the acidified basin at pH 5.6 and 5.1 (16 µg/litre, while concentrations in the reference basin declined to 11 µg/litre during the study period. The authors stated that these levels of aluminium were low compared with other reported values because the lake was hydrologically isolated.

Cosby et al. (1985) presented a mathematical model (MAGIC; Model Acidification of Groundwater In Catchments) that uses quantitative descriptions of soil chemical processes to estimate the long-term chemical changes that occur in soil, soil water and surface waters of catchments in response to changes in atmospheric deposition. The model is based on soil base cation exchange, dissolution of aluminium hydroxide and solution of carbon dioxide. The model uses "average" or lumped representations of these spatially distributed catchment processes. The long-term responses of the model are controlled by sulfate adsorption and primary weathering of base cations in the catchment soils. The model was applied to the Shenandoah National Park, Virginia, USA, and indicated that the alkalinity of surface waters had been reduced by as much as 50% over the last 140 years.

Cosby et al. (1986) applied the MAGIC model to a sub-catchment in southwestern Scotland. Assuming that deposition rates are maintained in the future at 1984 levels, the model indicated that stream pH was likely to decline. Neal et al. (1986) reported that the model predicts increases in pH (reductions in acidity) with conifer deforestation. In the Welsh uplands the model simulates quite accurately the acidification of catchments (Whitehead et al., 1990). The model shows that atmospheric deposition is the primary cause of stream acidification with conifer afforestation enhancing stream acidity. Historical trends determined by the model indicate that acidification has been present since the turn of the century (Whitehead et al., 1988). Ormerod et al. (1990) compared the predicted effects of reduced acidic deposition and liming on stream acidification with actual treatments. The results indicate that liming and 90% reduction in sulfate deposition reduce concentrations of soluble aluminium to similar levels. However, calcium concentrations and pH were increased by liming to values that were high by comparison with conditions simulated under low acid deposition.

A dynamic model has been developed that reproduces major trends in chemical and hydrological behaviour in Norwegian catchments. Christophersen & Seip (1982) reported that a simple two-reservoir model incorporating a small number of physically realistic processes accounts for the major short-term variations in stream water chemistry during the snow-free season at a 0.41 km^2 catchment in coniferous forest on granite bedrock at Birkenes, Norway. The model incorporates both hydrolytic and sulfate sub-models, and a cation sub-model that includes hydrogen, aluminium, calcium and magnesium ions. Typical characteristics predicted by the model include positive correlations between hydrogen ions and aluminium concentrations and discharge, and negative correlations between these factors and the calcium and magnesium concentrations. Seip et al. (1989) attempted to model episodic changes in stream water chemistry of hydrogen and aluminium ions. However, only partial success was achieved. Trends were correct for hydrogen ions but there were discrepancies at peak heights. There were correct predictions for aluminium concentrations in the autumn but not in the spring.

4.1.3 Seawater

In contrast to fresh water, seawater (salinity > 32%) has a constant pH of approximately 8.2. Hydes (1977) found that bottom and suspended clay sediments probably act as a source of dissolved aluminium to seawater. However, removal below predictions of clay solubility is probably the result of biological activity.

Hydes & Liss (1977) reported that approximately 30% of the dissolved aluminium entering the Conwy Estuary, Wales, appears to be removed during mixing with seawater. The removal occurs during the early stages of mixing and is virtually complete by the time the salinity reaches 8%. The authors concluded that the most likely mechanism involves the trapping of aluminium adsorbed onto the surface of fine clay particles entering with the freshwater as the particles are irreversibly coagulated on mixing with saline water.

Mackenzie et al. (1978) measured the concentration of aluminium in a vertical hydrographic profile of the Mediterranean Sea. They found that the concentrations did not correspond to seasonal thermocline, nitrate minimum and an oxygen maximum, thus supporting the hypothesis that aluminium cycles in the oceans are associated with the activity of diatoms. Stoffyn (1979) stated that experimental evidence using the diatom *Skeletonema costatum* supports the hypothesis that the concentration and distribution of dissolved aluminium in ocean water is controlled by biological activity in the surface waters. However, Hydes (1979) reported that the distribution of dissolved aluminium in open ocean waters is probably controlled by the solution of aluminium from atmospherically derived particles and bottom sediments balanced against scavenging by siliceous shells of dead organisms. Chou & Wollast (1989) studied eight vertical profiles of dissolved aluminium in the Mediterranean Sea. They found that dissolved aluminium is depleted in surface waters as compared with deep waters. The high concentrations of aluminium in deep water may result from fluxes from pore water in sediments to the overlying water. These authors suggested that aluminium is possibly removed by biological processes in the euphotic zone.

4.1.4 Soil

In soil, aluminium is released into solution for transport to streams upon acidification. The chemistry of inorganic aluminium in acid soil and, in particular, the solubility controls are very similar to those given in section 4.1.2 for fresh water (Furrer, 1993). However, the extrapolation of stream water chemistry to soil is difficult because of the complexity of hydrological pathways and chemical reactivity during water mixing (Neal, 1988).

Water mixing processes may be important in determining the relationship between aluminium (inorganic) and hydrogen ions. Consequently there is a need to model how these species vary as a function of mixing so that comparisons can be made with field observation. In order to resolve the effects of mixing, a basic calculation is made to allow soil to mix and degas carbon dioxide in the stream. To do this it is assumed that pCO_2 in soil/groundwater and the stream is 25 and 2 times the atmospheric value, respectively, and that bicarbonate principally controls the acid buffering (Neal et al., 1990).

In soils, solid-phase aluminium occurs in the lattice structure of minerals, in inter-layer sites of expanding clay minerals, and in poorly ordered minerals (allophane and hydrous oxides) of variable composition. Natural acidification processes result in increasing solubility of aluminium. At moderately acidic levels (pH 5.5) aluminium appears as the exchangeable cation that dominates in the lower mineral horizons initially as poly-nuclear hydroxy ions but subsequently as the simple mono-nuclear ions. Aluminium ions displace calcium at permanent-charge exchange sites (Bache, 1980). The cation exchange system of acid soils provides a large reserve of ionic aluminium, which can be brought into solution when soluble salts percolate through soil. Ligands, such as fluoride and organic anions, which form aluminium complexes, combine with aluminium and maintain higher concentrations of aluminium than might be expected, especially at pH 5-7 (Bache, 1986). In soil the most soluble form of aluminium under acidic conditions is non-silicate organically bound aluminium, while the amorphous aluminium hydroxy forms are more soluble than the crystalline forms (ATSDR, 1992; Sjöström, 1994).

Bloom et al. (1979) found that hydrolysis of organically bound aluminium is a major source of buffering in the pH range 4 to 5 for dilute salt suspensions of acid soils. The exchange of aluminium ions from organic matter exchange sites controls the relationship between pH and Al^{3+} activity in acid soils that have a low amount of permanent-charge cation exchange capacity relative to the quantity of organic matter. Walker et al. (1990) studied the influence of organic matter on the solubility of aluminium in organic soil horizons from different geographical regions of North America. The equilibrium solubility of aluminium was dependent on pH and the degree to which soil organic matter was saturated with aluminium. Soluble aluminium increased with decreasing pH and increased with increasing surface-bound aluminium at each pH level. Temperature dependence and rate studies suggested that aluminium solubility was governed by an ion-exchange reaction between H^+ and aluminium and the organic matter.

Litaor (1987) studied the aluminium chemistry in an alpine watershed, Front Range, Colorado, USA. It was found that the aluminium solubility in the interstitial water is complex and controlled by organic solutes, H_4SiO_4 and pH. However, neither pH nor sulfate concentrations correlated with aluminium concentrations. The chemical equilibrium of aluminium was controlled by amorphous aluminosilicate.

The most important inorganic aluminium complexes are the mononuclear and to a lesser extent the polynuclear hydroxo species. The formation of these complexes is directly coupled to pH and also, to a lesser extent, to ionic strength. The hexa aqua-aluminium cation $(Al(H_2O)_6^{3+})$ predominates at low pH, whereas the mononuclear $(Al(OH)_2^+)$ and dihydroxo-mononuclear species $(Al(OH)_2^+)$ become important in the circumneutral pH range. The tetrahydroxo aluminium anion (aluminate, $Al(OH)_4^-$) is the predominant species at higher pH, and is responsible for the increasing solubility of aluminium above pH 6.2. Polynuclear aluminium complexes can be the predominant species in solution over a wide pH range, although, being formed under non-equilibrium conditions, they are difficult to predict (Grant et al., 1990). Dahlgren & Ugolini (1989) collected leachates from subalpine spodosol located in the Cascade Range, Washington, USA. The ability of organic acids to complex aluminium in these subalpine soils increases from pH 3.8 to 5.0. Walker et al. (1988) found that adsorption of aluminium by aluminosilicate clay minerals, such as montmorillonite, kaolinite and vermiculite, is controlled by a simple electrostatic cation exchange involving outer sphere complexes. Adsorption to vermiculite may also be controlled by internal ion diffusion. Equilibrium constants (K_a) for the formation of an adsorbed aluminium clay complex were high (~105) for the three minerals, suggesting that they play a significant role in controlling aluminium concentrations in soil solutions.

Blume & Brümmer (1991) studied the influence of soil acidity on aluminium binding in sandy soils with a low humus content (< 2%). Binding was found to decrease steadily from very strong at pH 5.5-7.0 to very weak at pH 2.5. The binding of aluminium was found to be increased by increasing the organic matter content. In loam or clay soils binding was increased compared with sandy soils at all levels of pH.

Driscoll et al. (1989) studied the chemistry and transfer of aluminium in a forested watershed of the Adirondack region, New York, USA. The drainage waters from the watershed were highly acidic due to elevated inputs of both sulfuric and nitric acids compared with the release of basic cations. The conditions facilitated the mobilization of aluminium. Alumino-organic solutes were mainly released from the soil organic horizon with inorganic monomeric aluminium derived predominantly from the mineral soil and to a lesser extent from the soil organic horizon. Inorganic monomeric aluminium predominated in the drainage water. The deposition of organic monomeric aluminium in the stream bed coincided with the dissolved organic content retention whilst the deposition of inorganic monomeric aluminium appeared to be facilitated by nitrate retention.

Nilsson & Bergkvist (1983) studied soil acidification and aluminium chemistry in three adjacent catchments on the Swedish west coast. The concentration of organic aluminium was linearly correlated with concentrations of carbon. The percentage of organic species in the dissolved aluminium decreased with increasing depth from > 90% in the upper layers to < 10% below 55 cm. The average concentration of total aluminium increased with increasing depth from 3.3 to 9.8 µmole/litre at 5 cm to 95.3 to 115 µmole/litre below 55 cm.

Atmospheric acid inputs have a strong impact on the aluminium chemistry of acidic sandy soils with low concentrations of basic cations. The base saturation of such soils is low and the rate of basic cation weathering does not increase with rate of acid input. Any additional acidic deposition is neutralized by aluminium. Dissolution of aluminium is the major acid sink in such soils, neutralizing 30% to 95% of the total acid load (Mulder et al., 1989).

Bergkvist (1987) studied the leaching of aluminium in a brown forest soil and a podzol with adjacent stands of spruce, beech and an open regeneration area in South Sweden using lysimeter techniques. The leaching of aluminium was greatest from the podzol. The solubility of aluminium increased suddenly within a small pH range (4.5-4.0) in the B horizon (15 to 55 cm). The concentration of aluminium in soil solution increased from 2 to 10 mg/litre when the pH decreased from 4.4 to 4.2. Berggren et al. (1990) reported that forest soils of south Sweden are losing base cations, such as aluminium, owing to increased leaching rates following soil acidification. The processes controlling the mobilization of aluminium in podzols and cambisols of southern Sweden were investigated by Berggren (1992). Podzols in spruce and beech stands had a high release of organic compounds from the upper 5 to 7 cm (O/Ah horizons), which resulted in high organic complexation of aluminium in soil solution at a depth of 15 cm (E horizon). Organic complexes were mainly adsorbed or precipitated at 20 to 40 cm (upper Bh horizon) and the overall transport of aluminium at 50 cm was governed by a pH-dependent dissolution of solid-phase aluminium. In the cambisols inorganic aluminium predominated at both 15 cm and 50 cm with solubility being closely related to solution pH. The results indicate that the relatively large organically bound solid-phase aluminium pools in both soil types give rise to the measured solution aluminium activities. The authors also found that aluminium in solution efficiently competed for exchange sites and played an important role in the mobilization of cadmium in these soils.

In laboratory studies simulating snow melt leaching of forest soils, nitric acid leached more aluminium than did sulfuric acid from soil columns representative of high elevation forest soils and watersheds thought to be sensitive to acidification by acid precipitation. Increasing the nitric acid concentration 100-fold (pH 5 to 3) increased the total aluminium concentration in the leachate from 0.70 to 0.85 mmol/litre, while increasing the sulfuric acid had no effect. Similar experiments with albic and ochric mineral soil horizons revealed no difference between the acids and no effect of increasing acid concentrations (James & Riha, 1989).

The acidity produced by soil nitrification is buffered by exchange with base cations. In acidified soils aluminium will be dissolved or the pH of the soil will decrease. Aluminium release from soil is also dependent on the sulfate supply and the capacity of the soil to provide aluminium hydroxides. The molar ratio between aluminium and nitrate is important in evaluating the effects of nitrification. During dry summers the release of aluminium ions may be entirely controlled by the acidification caused by nitrification (Gundersen & Rasmussen, 1990).

4.1.5 Vegetation and wildlife

Mobilization of aluminium by acid rain results in more aluminium being available to plants (ATSDR, 1992).

Henriksen et al. (1988a) found during acidification experiments in Norwegian streams that the buffering capacity was 20 times higher than that associated with the water alone and a reduction of the pH to 5 resulted in large releases of aluminium (up to 2500 µg/litre). The source of the buffering and the reservoir of aluminium was hypothesized to be dense growths of liverwort. A second experiment confirmed that liverworts are involved in the ion exchange of base cations and aluminium during acid episodes.

Vogt et al. (1987) studied the aluminium concentrations of above- and below-ground tissues of a white fir (*Abies amabilis*) stand in the Cascade mountains, Washington, USA. It was found that 97% of the total detrital cycling of aluminium was below ground. When compared with the other elements analysed, aluminium showed the highest proportion of total annual element pool circulated (82%). The large root biomasses of these stands allows large amounts of aluminium to be accumulated and immobilized. The high root turnover observed for these stands appears to be due to the root senescence occurring in response to high aluminium accumulation. However, there is little impact on short-term elemental cycling because the roots decay very slowly (99% decay = 456 years).

4.2 Biotransformation

4.2.1 Biodegradation and abiotic degradation

Elemental aluminium does not degrade in the environment. In the trivalent oxidation state, it can complex with electron-rich species (ATSDR, 1992).

4.2.1 Bioaccumulation

4.2.2.1 Plants

Plants differ in their ability to take up aluminium; some accumulate aluminium whereas others are able to immobilize it at the root surface (Roy et al., 1988). Exposure to aluminium in nutrient solution leads to accumulation, especially in the roots (Lee, 1972; Boxman et al., 1991).

Aluminium taken up by roots is mainly found in the mucilage layer on the root tip surface (Horst et al., 1982) and in the walls of the epidermis and cortex cells (Huett & Menary, 1980). In the cell wall pectins, aluminium ions compete with calcium ions for the same absorption sites (Wagatsuma, 1983). Some aluminium is taken up in the cytoplasm and bound to nucleic acids and acid-soluble phosphates (Wagatsuma, 1983). Aluminium is translocated only to a small extent to shoots.

The concentrations of aluminium in leaf tissue of a variety of plants growing on limestone soils in Sweden (pH around 8) were found to be similar to those in plants growing on an acid silicate (granite; pH 4.1-4.9) site, although the aluminium concentration in the topsoil solution was at least one order of magnitude lower in the limestone than in the acid silicate soils (Tyler, 1994).

4.2.2.2 Invertebrates

Ryther et al. (1979) cultured soft shell clams (*Mya arenaria*), hard shell clams (*Mercenaria mercenaria*), American oysters (*Crassostrea virginica*) and sand worms (*Nereis virens*) in tanks containing fly ash from a coal-burning power station. The fly ash contained a wide range of elements including aluminium at 105.8 g/kg. After a period of 4 months the sand worms and the edible parts of the clams and oyster were analysed. Aluminium concentrations were 9645 mg/kg (dry weight) for the sand worms and 8218, 268 and 1373 mg/kg for soft shell clams, hard shell clams and oysters, respectively.

Crayfish (*Orconectes virilis*) from a lake with an average total aluminium concentration of 36 µg/litre were placed in caged tubes spiked with 40 µg/litre total aluminium and transferred to a lake with background levels of 8 µg/litre total aluminium. Half of the tubes were acidified to pH 5.3 and the others remained at pH 6.7. None of the crayfish accumulated aluminium. Controls had lower aluminium concentrations in the hepatopancreas and abdominal muscle after 25 to 27 days. Crayfish under acidified conditions retained aluminium in the hepatopancreas and not in the muscle whereas those at pH 6.7 retained aluminium in the muscle and not the hepatopancreas. The same authors also carried out a laboratory experiment with crayfish obtained from the original lake. Crayfish were maintained in a solution of 500 µg/litre for 14 days. No tissues showed an increase in aluminium levels. However, crayfish transferred back to the original lake water for 16 days retained aluminium only in the carapace and gills (Malley et al., 1987).

Havas (1985) exposed water fleas (*Daphnia magna*) to total aluminium concentrations of 0.02, 0.32 and 1.02 mg/litre for 24 h. Bioconcentration was related to pH, the highest concentration factors occurring at pH 6.5 and the lowest at pH 4.5; there was no effect of increasing the calcium concentration from 2.5 to 12.5 mg/litre. Mean bioaccumulation factors ranged from 11 000 to 18 000 at pH 6.5, 3000 to 9000 at pH 5.0, and 1200 to 4300 at pH 4.5.

Frick & Herrmann (1990) studied the accumulation of aluminium by nymphs of the mayfly (*Heptagenia sulphurea*) exposed to concentrations of 0.2 and 2 mg inorganic monomeric aluminium/litre at pH 4.5 for up to 4 weeks. The highest mean concentrations found in mayflies were 1.24 and 2.34 mg/g aluminium (dry weight) for the higher treatment groups, which did not undergo moulting. The major part of the aluminium was deposited on/in the exuviae of the nymphs, as aluminium determinations revealed a 70% decrease in content after moulting.

4.2.2.3   *Fish*

Cleveland et al. (1986) exposed brook trout (*Salvelinus fontinalis*) eggs, larvae and juveniles to 300 µg/litre total aluminium at three pH levels. At 30 days post-hatch for larvae and for an exposure period of 30 days for juveniles (37 to 67 days), significantly more aluminium was accumulated at pH 5.28 than at either pH 7.24 or 4.44. Aluminium levels at pH 5.28 were 398 and 112 mg/kg for the larvae and juveniles, respectively. At pH 7.24 residues were 12 and 33 mg/kg, and at pH 4.44, 71 and 17 mg/kg, respectively. Cleveland et al. (1991) maintained brook trout in water containing 200 µg/litre total aluminium at pH values of 5.0, 6.0 and 7.2 for 56 days. Estimated steady state bioconcentration factors for aluminium, which were inversely related to pH, were 215 at pH 5.3, 123 at pH 6.1 and 36 at pH 7.2. The estimated time to 90% steady state was 1.5 days at pH 5.3, 4.2 days at pH 6.1 and 1.7 days at pH 7.2. Elimination during the 28-day depuration phase was more rapid at pH 5.3 than at pH 6.1 or 7.2. Karlsson-Norrgren et al. (1986b) found that brown trout (*Salmo trutta*) accumulated significantly more aluminium in gill tissue at pH 5.5 than at pH 7.0 (60-160 µg/kg and 10-40 µg/kg dry weight, respectively) when exposed to 200-500 µg total aluminium/litre. Skogheim et al. (1984) found a gill aluminium accumulation of 70 to 341 µg/g fresh weight in dying Atlantic salmon (*Salmo salar*) during an episodic fish kill in the river Ogna, Norway, at pH 5.4-5.5 and total aluminium and labile aluminium concentrations of 160 and 130 µg/litre, respectively.

Segner et al. (1988) exposed young brown trout (*Salmo trutta*) to total aluminium (230 µg/litre) at pH 5.0 in high calcium water at a temperature of 12 °C for 5 days. Whole body aluminium concentrations were 230 mg/kg dry weight in aluminium-exposed fish, as compared to 75 mg/kg (pH 5.0) and 44 mg/kg (pH 7.2) for fish in aluminium-free water.

Wicklund Glynn et al. (1992) exposed minnows (*Phoxinus phoxinus*) to acidic water (pH 5.0) with and without total aluminium (150 µg/litre) at varying calcium (0, 0.07 and 2 mmol/litre) and humus (5 and 25 Pt) concentrations for 15 days. Aluminium concentrations in the gills were highest in the lower calcium level groups with or without humus. In the absence of calcium the median aluminium level in the gills was 109 mg/kg wet weight, and at 2 mmol/litre calcium the aluminium level was 50 mg/kg.

4.2.2.4 Birds

Carrière et al. (1986) fed ring doves (*Streptopelia risoria*) on a diet containing 0.1% aluminium sulfate with reduced calcium and phosphorus (0.9% Ca; 0.5% P) for a period of 4 months. Analysis of the tissues of breeding adult doves revealed that there was no accumulation of aluminium in kidney, brain or male femurae; however, the femurae of female doves showed a significant increase from a mean of 7.42 mg/kg dry weight in controls to 15.87 mg/kg in treated birds. Juvenile doves fed on diets containing 500, 1000 and 1500 mg/kg aluminium sulfate did not accumulate aluminium in leg and wing bones but did show a significant tendency to accumulate in the sternum.

Sparling (1991) fed black ducks (*Anas rubripes*) and mallard (*Anas platyrhynchos*) on a diet containing 200, 1000 or 5000 mg aluminium/kg with varying amounts of calcium (3600 and 15 100 mg/kg) and phosphorus (6200, 13 500 and 21 500 mg/kg) for a period of 10 weeks. All of the diets produced a dose-related and significant increase in the aluminium content of the femur. Black ducks maintained on normal calcium and phosphorus levels showed femur aluminium concentrations of 5.42, 13.6 and 19.5 mg/kg after 10 weeks at the three dose levels, respectively. Mallard femurs contained aluminium levels of 9.49, 12.1 and 18 mg/kg, respectively.

5. ENVIRONMENTAL LEVELS AND HUMAN EXPOSURE

5.1 Environmental levels

Aluminium is ubiquitous in the environment and its chemistry is controlled by pH, mineralogical composition, and the quantity and qualitative nature of the organic constituents present. It is, therefore, difficult to provide generalized estimates of natural background concentrations (Grant et al., 1990). Aluminium is released to the environment by both natural processes and anthropogenic sources. It is a major constituent of the earth's crust, and natural mobilization of aluminium far outweighs the direct contribution from anthropogenic sources (Lantzy & Mackenzie, 1979). The concentrations of aluminium in the different environmental compartments are dependent on its speciation and mobilization (see section 4.1). Jones & Bennett (1985) summarized the data on aluminium concentrations in the environment and produced a list of representative values as follows: urban air 1000 ng/m^3 (160-7000 ng/m^3), rural air 200 ng/m^3 (150-325 ng/m^3), agricultural soil 70 000 mg/kg (10 000-300 000 mg/kg), fresh water (dissolved) 50 µg/litre (1-2250 µg/litre), ocean (dissolved) 2 µg/litre (1-5 µg/litre), and terrestrial plants 100 mg/kg (50-600 mg/kg).

5.1.1 Air

Aluminium is a major constituent of a number of atmospheric components, being highly concentrated in soil-derived dusts and in particulates from coal combustion (Grant et al., 1990). The sources of soil-derived dust are both natural (Sorenson et al., 1974) and from human activity such as mining and agriculture (Eisenreich, 1980). Leharne et al. (1992) monitored street dust from the inner London area, United Kingdom, and found aluminium levels ranging from 3.7 to 11.6 µg/kg. The largest sources of particle-borne aluminium are the flux of dust from soil and rock materials in the earth's crust and from volcanic eruptions (Lee & von Lehmden, 1973; Sorenson et al., 1974; Lantzy & Mackenzie, 1979). Atmospheric aluminium concentrations show widespread temporal and spatial variations. The concentrations of aluminium in air are summarized in Table 8 and range from 0.5 ng/m^3 over Antarctica to > 1000 ng/m^3 in industrialized areas.

Table 8. Concentrations of aluminium in air

Area	Year	Particle size (μm)[a]	Aluminium concentration (ng/m^3)	Reference
Antarctic	1970	NR	0.57 (0.32-0.81)	Zoller et al. (1974)
Arctic (Barrow, Alaska)	1976-1978	NR	25	Rahn (1981)
Hawaii	1967	> 0.15	2-40	Hoffman et al. (1969)
Atlantic Ocean		NR	8-370	Duce et al. (1975)
		NR	95 (41-160)	Windom (1981)
Atlantic Ocean near coast of USA		NR	102-184	Windom (1981)
North Sea	1988-1989	NR	294.5 (21-887)	Chester & Bradshaw (1991)
	1988-1989	NR	197 (17-903)	Ottley & Harrison (1993)
	1985-1986	NR	210 (64-600)	Kersten et al. (1988)
Baltic Sea	1985	NR	218 (47-800)	Häsänen et al. (1990)
Kiel Bight, Germany	1981-1983	NR	394 (68-720)	Schneider (1987)
USA cities & industrial areas	1975-1977	< 3.5	48-1983	Stevens et al. (1978)
	1975-1977	> 3.5	331-8678	Stevens et al. (1978)
Buffalo, New York, USA	1968-1969	NR	1000-8000	Pillay & Thomas (1971)
Southern Arizona (urban)	1974	NR	5700	Moyers et al. (1977)
Southern Arizona (rural)	1974	NR	1200	Moyers et al. (1977)

Table 8 (contd).

Area	Year	Particle size (μm)[a]	Aluminium concentration (ng/m³)	Reference
Charleston, West Virginia	1976	< 3.5	74	Lewis & Macias (1980)
	1976	> 3.5	1100	Lewis & Macias (1980)
UK (non-urban sites)	1972-1973	NR	27-640 ng/kg	Cawse (1974)
Birkenes, S. Norway	1978-1979	NR	80	Amundsen et al. (1992)
	1985-1986	NR	73	Amundsen et al. (1992)

[a] NR = not reported

Amundsen et al. (1992) analysed air samples from Birkenes, southern Norway, for aluminium and found concentrations to be highest in the spring period from March to May. The authors concluded that this was due to soil dust from wind erosion and agricultural activities because soils in Europe are likely to be dry during this period. Windom (1981) measured aluminium concentrations of 28 000 ng/m³ during a dust storm.

Aluminium was found to be concentrated up to 2650 ng/m³ in the Baltimore harbour tunnel, a two-fold increase on the air intake levels (Ondov et al., 1982).

5.1.2 *Precipitation*

Aluminium has been measured in atmospheric precipitation in the USA at concentrations of up to 1200 μg/litre (Feth et al., 1964; Fisher et al., 1968; Norton, 1971).

Feth et al. (1964) analysed snow samples from the northern Sierra Nevada, USA, in 1959. Aluminium was detected in 7 out of 8 samples at a mean concentration of 30 μg/litre. Ecker et al. (1990) measured aluminium in wet-deposited snow at several sites in Japan, both urban and rural. Mean aluminium concentrations ranged from 9.6 to

25.8 µg/litre. Average aluminium concentrations of freshly deposited snow at Shiramine (a mountain site) were 2.4 µg/litre in the insoluble fraction (> 0.45 µm) and 15.0 µg/litre in the soluble fraction (< 0.45 µm).

Rainwater collected in southern central Florida, USA, between 1967 and 1969 contained aluminium concentrations ranging from not detectable to 900 µg/litre (Dantzman & Breland, 1969). Guieu et al. (1991) monitored rainfall at 45 sites in the south of France and found mean aluminium concentrations of 487 µg/litre and 55 µg/litre in the particulate (> 0.4 µm) and dissolved fractions (< 0.4 µm), respectively. Cawse (1974) measured aluminium in rainfall and dry deposition from seven non-urban United Kingdom sites in 1972 and 1973. Aluminium concentrations ranged from 56 to 14 800 µg/litre for rainfall and from 3.9 to 42 µg/cm^2 per year for dry deposition. Aluminium concentrations in rainfall, total and dry deposition were measured for Bagauda, Nigeria, in 1976. Aluminium concentrations were 1700 µg/litre for rainfall and 220 and 145 µg/cm^2 per year for total and dry deposition, respectively (Beavington & Cawse, 1979).

5.1.3 Water

5.1.3.1 Freshwater

Surface freshwater aluminium concentrations can vary significantly, being dependent on the various physicochemical and mineralogical factors described in section 4.1. Aluminium can occur in a number of different forms in freshwater. It can be suspended or dissolved. It can be bound with organic or inorganic ligands, or it can exist as a free aluminium ion. It can exist as a monomer in natural water, but tends to polymerize with time (see section 2.3.4). Aluminium speciation is determined by pH, dissolved organic carbon (DOC), fluoride, sulfate, phosphate, silicate and suspended particulate matter. Dissolved aluminium concentrations for water in the circumneutral pH range are usually quite low, ranging from 1.0 to 50 µg/litre, and rise to 500 to 1000 µg/litre in more acidic waters. At the extreme acidity of waters affected by acid mine drainage, dissolved aluminium concentrations of up to 90 mg/litre can be measured (Filipek et al., 1987). Aluminium can also be leached from landfill containing coal combustion ash and aluminium smelting wastes (Sorenson et al., 1974). The concentrations of aluminium in freshwater are summarized in Table 9.

Table 9. Concentrations of aluminium in freshwater

Area	Year	pH	Particle size (μm)	Aluminium concentration (μg/litre)	Detection limit (μg/litre)	Reference
Lake Gardsjon catchment, Sweden	1981	4.0-6.4	< 0.45	300-2500		Lee (1985)
Swedish lakes	1980	5.7-8.8		69 (10-243)	10	Borg (1987)
Loch Ard Forest and	1979-1980	4.63	< 1.0	400		Caines et al. (1985)
Galloway streams, Scotland		6.62	< 1.0	25		Caines et al. (1985)
Llyn Brianne catchment, Wales	1984-1985	4.6-5.3	< 0.45	120-430		Goenaga & Williams (1990)
	1984-1985	4.87		42 μEq/litre		Whitehead et al. (1988)
	1984-1985	5.2		18 μEq/litre		Whitehead et al. (1988)
	1984-1985	6.9		7 μEq/litre		Whitehead et al. (1988)
Rivers Esk and Duddon, Cumbria, UK						
(moderate flow)	1983-1984	4.3-7.2		20-940		Bull & Hall (1986)
(low flow)	1983-1984	4.8-7.5		5-245		Bull & Hall (1986)

Table 9 (contd).

Shield lakes, Ontario and Quebec	1982	4.4-7.1		46-372		Stokes et al. (1985)
Zaire river	1976	6.8	< 0.45	28-44		van Bennekom & Jager (1978)
Niger river	1976	6.7	< 0.45	3-6		van Bennekom & Jager (1978)
Reservoirs, Madras, India	1991			14 (5-210)	2	Pitchai et al. (1992)
Orange river, Vioolsdrif, South Africa	1958-1959	6.4-8.1		36-1080		de Villiers (1962)
River Yodo, Japan	1981-1990			10-1150		Yagi et al. (1992)

Table 9 (contd).

Area	Year	pH	Particle size (µm)	Aluminium concentration (µg/litre)	Detection limit (µg/litre)	Reference
Vosges mountain streams, France	1990	6.96		64		Mersch et al. (1993)
	1990	4.64-5.74		185-351		Mersch et al. (1993)
Boglakes, NE Belgium	1984-1986	3.4-3.9	< 0.4	150-3770	20	Courtijn et al. (1987)
	1984-1985	3.4-3.9	> 0.4	3200-65 000		Courtijn et al. (1987)
	1984-1986	6.0	< 0.4	< 20	20	Courtijn et al. (1987)
	1984-1985	6.0	> 0.4	78 100-145 100		Courtijn et al. (1987)
Stream water, California, USA			< 0.45	15	7	Silvey (1967)
St Lawrence river, USA	1974-1976	7.6-8.0	< 0.4	64		Yeats & Bewers (1982)
	1974-1976	7.6-8.0	> 0.4	964		Yeats & Bewers (1982)
South central Florida, streams	1969			200-300		Dantzman & Breland (1969)
Highway drains, Louisiana	1990			412 (250-1270)		Madigosky et al. (1992)
Northern California streams	1972			5-10		Jones et al. (1974)

Aluminium occurs ubiquitously in natural waters. Aluminium levels in surface waters can be increased by intense urban and industrial activity (Eisenreich, 1980). Kopp & Kroner (1970) monitored rivers and lakes in the USA from 1962 to 1967 and detected aluminium in 31% of samples. Mean dissolved aluminium levels ranged from 11 to 333 µg/litre, the highest levels of 2760 µg/litre being measured in the Missouri river. Aluminium was found to be predominantly in the suspended sediment fraction (> 0.45) with a mean concentration of 3860 µg/litre (compared with the dissolved phase at 74 µg/litre).

Filipek et al. (1987) reported that weathering of sulfide ores exposed to the atmosphere in inactive mines and tailings dumps released large quantities of sulfuric acid and metals such as aluminium (up to 90 mg/litre). Boult et al. (1994) measured aluminium in the Afon Goch, Anglesey, Wales, a stream polluted by mine drainage. Sampling sites with pH 2.40, 5.99 and 6.49 gave mean soluble aluminium concentrations (< 0.45 µm) of 55.56, 1.14 and 0.12 mg/litre, respectively; mean aluminium concentrations in the particulate phase (> 0.45 µm) were 0.31, 2.15 and 0.69 mg/litre, respectively. Koga (1967) sampled water discharged from Wairakei drill holes in 1965. Total aluminium concentrations in filtered water ranged from 0.023 to 0.05 mg/litre. Zelenov (1965) found elevated levels (4913 mg/litre) of aluminium in water of a volcanic crater lake in Indonesia.

The concentrations of dissolved aluminium in water vary with pH levels and the humic-derived acid content of the water (ATSDR, 1992). Watt et al. (1983) compared Nova Scotian river water samples from 1954-1955 with those from 1980-1981 and found that significant decreases in the pH corresponded to significant increases in dissolved aluminium. High aluminium concentrations occur in surface waters when the pH is less than 5 (Sorenson et al., 1974; Filipek et al., 1987). In general, aluminium levels in surface waters at pH levels above 5.5 will be less than 0.1 mg/litre (Sorenson et al., 1974). However, even at neutral pHs, higher aluminium levels have been detected where the humic acid content is high (ATSDR, 1992).

In the Thousand Lake Survey in Norway (Henriksen et al., 1988b), 90% of the lakes with pH below 5.4 had a concentration of inorganic monomeric aluminium above 60 µg/litre. Lakes with a pH of 4.6-4.8 and 4.8-5.0 had concentrations of 146-170 and 101-135 µg/litre, respectively.

Generally, the data indicate that total aluminium concentrations in surface waters are elevated during periods of high flow, following episodic storm events, and/or during spring snow melt. Many studies also reported corresponding increases in the labile or inorganic aluminium fraction during these periods (LaZerte, 1984; Bull & Hall, 1986; Henriksen et al., 1988c; Lawrence et al., 1988).

Jones et al. (1974) monitored streams in Northern California and found that samples collected during low flow periods contained aluminium concentrations of between 1 and 3 µg/litre, whereas those collected during moderate flow periods contained 10 µg/litre. Values of aluminium that were higher than expected were associated with storm run-off.

Caines et al. (1985) monitored streams in the Loch Ard Forest and Galloway areas of Scotland during 1978, 1979 and 1980. The concentrations of aluminium were found to be very closely dependent on the hydrogen ion concentrations in the stream water. The maximum concentration of aluminium in a stream with an average pH of 6.62 was 25 µg/litre, compared with almost 400 µg/litre in a stream with an average pH of 4.63. The seasonal variation that occurred in the most acid stream had a maximum of 394 µg/litre in February, which declined rapidly to 35 µg/litre in May, during 1980. The authors stated that the sharp decrease coincided with a period of low rainfall which resulted in a rise in stream pH and greatly reduced leaching of aluminium from the catchment.

Bull & Hall (1986) measured aluminium in the rivers Esk and Duddon, Cumbria, United Kingdom, and their tributaries. The findings showed a relationship between inorganic aluminium and pH, while organic aluminium was generally low in these rivers. In general, lower pHs and higher aluminium concentrations occurred at higher river flow rates.

Ecker et al. (1990) monitored aluminium in the first and last meltwater run-off from snowfields at Shiramine, a mountainous area in Japan. Average aluminium concentrations were non-detectable and 445.6 µg/litre in the insoluble fraction (> 0 45 µm) of the first and last run-offs, respectively, and 25.0 and 19.9 µg/litre, respectively, in the soluble fraction (< 0.45 µm).

5.1.3.2 Seawater

The concentrations of aluminium in seawater are summarized in Table 10. The concentration of aluminium is dependent on the salinity of the water. Concentrations in open seawater are typically around 1 to 2 µg/litre in the dissolved fraction (< 0.45 µm). Bruland (1983) stated that the concentration of aluminium in surface seawater in the open ocean reflects atmospheric input and scavenging processes; the concentration is low at high latitudes in the North Atlantic because of a low atmospheric input and a higher scavenging rate resulting from intensified biological activity in these waters. Aluminium is higher in surface waters of mid-latitudes due to the higher atmospheric input and lower scavenging rate in these oligotrophic waters.

5.1.4 Soil and sediment

Aluminium partitions from water to sediment and particulate matter especially at circumneutral pH. The concentrations of aluminium in sediment are summarized in Table 11. Mean aluminium concentrations range from 20 000 to 80 000 mg/kg. Subramanian et al. (1988) measured heavy metals in the bed sediments and particulate matter of the Ganges Estuary, India. Average aluminium concentrations were 56 526 mg/kg for bed sediments and 70 222 mg/kg for suspended sediments. Sanin et al. (1992) measured elements in the sediments of the river Goksu and the Tasucu Delta, Turkey. Mean aluminium concentrations ranged from 20 700 to 26 800 mg/kg for the river and from 30 150 to 42 875 mg/kg for the delta. Benninger & Wells (1993) sampled sediment from the Neuse river estuary, North Carolina, USA, between 1982 and 1990. Aluminium concentrations ranged from 2.1 to 4.9 mmol/g, equivalent to 10.7% to 25.0% aluminium oxide. Fileman et al. (1991) found a mean aluminium level of 2490 mg/kg in suspended particulate material from the Dogger Bank region of the central North Sea.

Aluminium is one of the most abundant elements in soil and concentrations vary widely. Shacklette & Boerngen (1984) collated the aluminium concentrations measured by the US Geological Survey; levels ranged from 700 to 100 000 mg/kg with an average of 72 000 mg/kg. Beavington & Cawse (1979) analysed soil from Baguada, Nigeria, and found aluminium levels of 24 000 µg/g (dry weight).

Table 10. Concentrations of aluminium in seawater

Area	Year	Depth (m)	Salinity (%)	Particle size (µm)	Aluminium concentration (µg/litre)	Reference
Open Atlantic Ocean	1980-1982				15.2 and 25.4 nmol/kg	Kremling (1985)
North-East Atlantic Ocean	1982 1982	< 150 > 1000	35-37 35-37		16-32 nmol/litre 6-11 nmol/litre	Hydes (1983)
Atlantic Ocean near Carribean islands	1974 1977-1978	300-1100 0-2730	 33-37		0.3-4.26 0.51-2.41	Alberts et al. (1976) Stoffyn & Mackenzie (1982)
Atlantic Ocean near USA coast	1951-1952				0-10	Simons et al. (1953)

Table 10 (contd).

Area	Year	Depth (m)	Salinity (%)	Particle size (μm)	Aluminium concentration (μg/litre)	Reference
Gulf of Mexico	1951-1952			> 0.45	2.0 (0.2-10.2) 2-5	Feely et al. (1971) Simons et al. (1953)
Pacific Ocean near USA coast		0.3		< 0.45 > 0.45 < 0.45	1 0.2-27 9.8 (3.7-166)	Sackett & Arrhenius (1962) Sackett & Arrhenius (1962) Silvey (1967)
Weddel Sea, Antarctica				< 0.45 > 0.45	1 4-120	Sackett & Arrhenius (1962) Sackett & Arrhenius (1962)
North Sea	1988	6	34-35	< 0.4	10.2-49.2 nmol/litre	Hydes & Kremling (1993)
Mediterranean Sea	1976-1977	0-1500	35-38		1.0-4.8	Stoffyn & Mackenzie (1982)

Table 11. Concentrations of aluminium in sediment

Area	Year[a]	Aluminium concentration (mg/kg)	Reference
River Goksu, Turkey	NR	20 800 to 26 600	Sanin et al. (1992)
Tasucu Delta, Turkey	NR	30 150 to 42 875	Sanin et al. (1992)
Tadenac Lake, Ontario	1979	31 000 to 64 800	Wren et al. (1983)
Turkey Lakes, Ontario	1981-1982	31 000 to 56 300	Johnson et al. (1986)
Hamilton, Ontario (urban run-off)	1986-1987	25 941 to 68 870	Irvine et al. (1992)
Fontana Lake, North Carolina	1978	36 400 to 84 600	Abernathy et al. (1984)

[a] NR = not reported

Aluminium is found in soil interstitial water at levels similar to those reported for freshwater. Litaor (1987) measured a mean aluminium concentration of 24.8 µmole/litre for the interstitial water (pH 6.0) of soil from the Green Lakes Valley Front Range in Colorado, USA.

5.1.5 *Terrestrial and aquatic organisms*

Mason & MacDonald (1988) monitored aluminium levels in aquatic moss (*Fontinalis squamosa*) from the River Mawddach catchment, Wales (polluted with drainage water from disused mines) in 1984 and 1985. Mean aluminium concentrations ranged from 1970 to 26 800 mg/kg (dry weight). Mersch et al. (1993) transplanted aquatic moss (*Amblystegium riparium*) from a non-acidified stream to streams with pH values ranging from 4.64 to 5.74. The moss accumulated aluminium, those exposed to acidified streams containing aluminium ranging from 10 390 to 12 700 µg/g (dry weight) and those in a control stream (pH 6.96) containing 7750 µg/g. Caines et al.

(1985) collected aquatic liverworts (*Nardia compressa* and *Scapania undulata*) from streams in the Loch Ard and Galloway areas of Scotland. Mean liverwort aluminium concentrations were 3148, 6166 and 8532 mg/kg (dry weight) from streams containing 195, 71 and 24 µg/litre, respectively. Bioconcentration of aluminium occurred in all streams; however, increased hydrogen ion concentrations were associated with decreased liverwort aluminium concentrations. Albers & Camardese (1993a) monitored aquatic plants from acidified and non-acidified constructed wetlands. Aluminium concentrations for bur-reed (*Sparganium americnum*) and bladderwort (*Utricularia* spp.) were 167 and 533 µg/g (dry weight), respectively, for acidified wetlands and 104 and 487 µg/g for non-acidified wetlands. Duckweed (*Lemna* spp.) and green algae (*Oedogonium* spp.) contained 998 µg aluminium/g at the non-acidified sites; acidified wetlands did not contain duckweed or green algae. Bur-reed (Sparganium spp.), bladderwort and pondweed collected from sites in Maryland and Maine contained aluminium concentrations of 74.6, 1740 and 296 µg/g, respectively. The accumulation of aluminium by these aquatic plants correlated poorly with the water concentration (Albers & Camardese, 1993b).

Leinonen (1989) collected leaves of *Vaccinium myrtillus* from untreated forest, clear-cut untilled forest and clear-cut tilled land in Kuru, southern Finland in 1987. Aluminium levels were significantly higher in the tilled area, with levels of approximately 140 mg/kg dry weight in untilled areas and 185 mg/kg in the tilled area. Moomaw et al. (1959) collected a wide selection of Hawaiian plant species from highly leached latosol soils of low pH and high aluminium content. Aluminium concentrations ranged from 59 to 16 000 mg/kg dry weight. Thirteen of the 23 species contained aluminium levels in excess of 1000 mg/kg; the highest levels were found in the pteridophyte *Polypodium phymatoides* and the dicotyledon *Melastoma malahathricum*. Beavington & Cawse (1979) analysed sorghum grain from Bagauda, Nigeria, and found aluminium levels of 90 µg/g dry weight.

Wyttenbach et al. (1985) collected needles of *Picea abies* from around the city of Winterthur, Switzerland. The washed needles were analysed for a wide range of elements including aluminium. The mean aluminium content of the needles was 19 mg/kg (10-64 mg/kg). It was found that washing the needles had removed more than 80% of the aluminium residue. Landolt et al. (1989) sampled spruce needles from locations throughout Switzerland in 1983 to study the distribution of elements. The mean aluminium concentration was found to be 61.4 mg/kg with a range of 12.88 to 344.5 mg/kg. Häsänen & Huttunen (1989) measured the aluminium content of the annual rings of pine trees (*Pinus sylvestris*). The mean concentration for the period 1920 to 1980 was 4.2 mg/kg (3.4-5.1 mg/kg). In the areas associated with higher sulfur deposition there had been increases in aluminium uptake since 1950.

Malley et al. (1987) collected crayfish (*Orconectes virilis*) from a lake in northwestern Ontario containing a total aluminium concentration of 36 µg/litre. Mean aluminium concentrations in the crayfish were highest in the gut tissue (774 mg/kg) and there were levels of 65.2, 84.4 and 50.4 mg/kg in the carapace, green gland and ovary, respectively. Madigosky et al. (1991) monitored red swamp crayfish (*Procambarus clarkii*) from roadside drainage ditches in Louisiana, USA. Aluminium concentrations ranged from 1.75 to 981.50 mg/kg dry weight in the order abdominal muscle < hepatopancreas < exoskeleton < alimentary canal tissue. The crayfish contained significantly higher levels of aluminium than those found in control crayfish sampled from a commercial crayfish farm. Madigosky et al. (1992) collected crayfish during 1990 from a site near to a Louisiana highway intersection. Aluminium concentrations were 2409 and 2342 mg/kg for intestinal tissue and contents, respectively, while concentrations of 527 and 27 388 mg/kg were found for stomach tissue and contents, respectively. It was found that purging the crayfish in 1.5% sodium chloride for 6 h did not significantly reduce aluminium in the gut tissue. However, there was an increase in the water concentration of aluminium probably caused by its release from exterior tissue sites.

Albers & Camardese (1993a) collected aquatic insects from both acidified and non-acidified constructed wetlands; aluminium concentrations were 94.3 and 158 µg/g (dry weight) for the two types of wetland, respectively. Albers & Camardese (1993b) analysed aquatic insects from sites in Maryland (224 µg/g) and in Maine (102 µg/g). The same authors analysed crayfish and snails from sites in Maryland and Maine in 1987. Whole body aluminium concentrations were found to be 66 to 542 µg/g (dry weight) and 27 to 398 µg/g for the two species, respectively.

Brumbaugh & Kane (1985) collected smallmouth bass (*Micropterus dolomieui*) from the Chatuge reservoir on the border between Georgia and North Carolina, USA. The reservoir receives run-off from poorly buffered, forested watersheds, and the average pH of the reservoir was 6.3. Mean aluminium concentrations were 58 µg/g wet weight for gills and 3.0, 2.5, 1.5 and < 1.0 µg/g for the carcass, gut, liver, and kidney, respectively. Fish collected from the vicinity of a liquid waste site in North Carolina, USA contained mean aluminium levels ranging from 10.9 to 18.2 mg/kg (wet weight - based on whole gutted fish) (Loehle & Paller, 1990). Buergel & Soltero (1983) analysed plankton and fish (*Oncorhynchus mykiss*) from a lake in Washington State, USA, that had been treated with aluminium sulfate to reduce high phosphorus concentrations. Total and dissolved aluminium in the lake water ranged from 0.16 to 0.75 mg/litre, and from 0.09 to 0.42 mg/litre, respectively. Aluminium concentrations in plankton ranged from 6.53 to 49.81 mg/kg, while those in various fish tissues ranged from 0.07 to 6.25 mg/kg with the highest levels concentrated in the gills. The aluminium concentrations measured in the fish were not significantly different from those analysed in fish from untreated lakes. Berg & Burns (1985) compared the aluminium concentrations in fish tissues from a lake receiving water treatment plant sludge containing aluminium hydroxide with a control lake. Both lakes had pH values in the range 7.0 to 8.0. Dissolved aluminium was 0.1 mg/litre in the treated lake and < 0.1 mg/litre in the control lake. Aluminium was found in all tissues of all fish analysed. Liver, kidney and gill samples from channel catfish (*Ictalurus punctatus*) taken from the polluted lake contained significantly more aluminium than those from the control lake. For catfish brain and muscle, and for all tissues from largemouth bass (*Micropterus salmoides*) and gizzard shad (*Dorosoma cepedianum*) there were no significant differences. Aluminium concentrations ranged from 60.8 to 1808.9 mg/kg; the highest concentrations were found in the liver and brain.

Karlsson-Norrgren et al. (1986a) collected and analysed brown trout (*Salmo trutta*) from two fish farms within acid-susceptible areas in Sweden using lime-treated waters. Preliming, the water had a pH of 4.6 to 4.7, with total and labile aluminium concentrations of 390-516 and 270-300 µg/litre, respectively. The post-liming water quality (to the hatchery) was 208-261 µg/litre as total aluminium and 12-80 µg/litre as labile aluminium. Trout from a third non-acidified location (pH 6.9; total aluminium levels in water 35 µg/litre) were also analysed. Aluminium concentrations ranged from 89.3 mg/kg (wet weight) for gills to 0.8 mg/kg for muscle in fish from acid-susceptible areas. Fish from the control area contained aluminium ranging from 2.6 mg/kg in the intestine to 0.6 mg/kg in muscle, while levels in the gills were 1.9 mg/kg.

Hellou et al. (1992a) analysed muscle samples from the bluefin tuna (*Thunnus thynnus*) collected off the cost of Newfoundland, Canada, in 1990. Aluminium concentrations ranged from 0.4 to 1.9 µg/g dry weight with a mean value of 1.0 µg/g. Hellou et al. (1992b) found aluminium concentrations of < 1 to 8 µg/g dry weight in muscle, liver and ovaries of cod (*Gadus morhua*) sampled from several sites off the coast of Newfoundland during 1990 and 1991.

Wren et al. (1983) analysed fish, bird and mammal muscle from Tadenac Lake (a Precambrian Shield lake), Ontario, Canada, and its surrounding area. The lake had a pH of 7.1 and contained 47 400 mg aluminium/kg in the sediment. Mean aluminium concentrations ranged from 1.7 to 2.8 mg/kg (wet weight) for fish and from 2.5 to 5.2 mg/kg for birds and mammals.

5.2 Occupational exposure

The levels of aluminium to which workers are exposed vary greatly according to the type of industry and whether adequate industrial hygiene practices are adhered to. Most studies have dealt with inhalation of aluminium-containing dust particles rather than aluminium *per se*. Some, however, have utilized urinary aluminium determinations as an indicator of exposure (Sjögren et al., 1983; Gitelman et al., 1995). Utilizing such a technique for exposure is essential, since it is rare for a worker to be exposed solely to aluminium but rather to a mixture of aluminium-containing dusts and chemicals.

Occupational exposure limits for aluminium fumes and dust have been developed in many countries. Time-weighted averages of 5 mg/m^3 (respirable dust) and 10 mg/m^3 (total dust) have generally been accepted. However, an occupational exposure limit of 1 mg/m^3 calculated as aluminium has been proposed in Sweden regarding aluminium-containing respirable fumes (Sjögren & Ekinder, 1992).

Given the minimal amount of data on actual aluminium levels in workplace air, it is difficult to estimate a daily exposure from the occupational setting. Based on a recent publication, aluminium process and production workers are generally exposed to less than 1 mg per 8-h shift, assuming 10 m³ inhaled per shift (Gitelman et al., 1995). It should be noted that, in some occupations and under less than optimal industrial hygiene practices, occupational exposures to aluminium could be higher. Welders performing metal-inert gas welding have been exposed to 4 mg/m³ (calculated as aluminium) and these particles are generally less than 1 µm (Sjögren & Ulfvarson, 1985; Sjögren et al., 1985). Assuming 10 m³ inhaled per shift, this implies an exposure of 40 mg per shift.

Occupational exposures have been reported as total dust or particulate matter: e.g., potroom workers, 1.67 mg/m³ (Kongerud & Samuelsen, 1991); production of abrasives, 0.2 to 44.6 mg aluminium oxide/m³ (Jederlinic et al., 1990); MIG welders, 10 mg/m³; TIG welders, 1 mg/m³; respirable particles with a mean aluminium content of 39% (Ulfvarson, 1981; Sjögren et al., 1985) and aluminium soldering of aluminium cables, 1.1 mg/m³ respirable dust decreasing to 0.7 mg/m³ after installation of a vacuum collection system (Hjortsbert, 1994).

5.3 General population exposures

5.3.1 Air

Pulmonary exposure to aluminium is determined by air concentration, particulate size and ventilatory volume. Air concentrations vary between low levels in rural settings (20-500 ng/m³) and higher levels in urban settings (1000-6000 ng/m³) (see Table 8). Particles larger than 5-10 µm diameter tend to be removed from inhaled air and penetrate poorly into the lungs. Humans living in an urban area with ambient aluminium concentrations of about 2000 ng/m³, particle size < 5 µm and a ventilatory volume of 20 m³/day would be exposed to 40 µg aluminium/day by inhalation.

5.3.2 Food and beverages

Since aluminium is a major component of the earth's crust, it is naturally present in varying amounts in most food-stuffs consumed. The actual concentration in food and beverages from various countries will vary widely depending upon the food product, the type of processing used and, in particular, the levels of aluminium-containing food additives permitted and the geographical area in which food crops are grown. In general, the foods highest in aluminium are those than contain aluminium additives (e.g., grain products (flour), processed dairy products, infant formulae, etc.). Foods naturally high in aluminium include baked potato (skin on), spinach, prune juice and tea (Pennington & Schoen, 1995).

The preparation and storage of food in aluminium vessels, foil or cans, may increase the aluminium content, particularly in the case of foods that are acidic, salty or alkaline (Greger et al., 1985b; Nagy & Nikdel, 1986; Baxter et al., 1988). Preparing acidic foods such as tomatoes and rhubarb in aluminium pans was found to lead to a significant increase in the level of aluminium in the food (0.5 mg/kg wet weight raw tomatoes to 3.3 mg/kg wet weight cooked), whereas only a slight increase was noted in similarly prepared rice or potatoes (Greger et al., 1985b). Although individual foodstuffs may leach aluminium from the vessel, there are indications that aluminium from cookware represents only a small fraction of the total dietary intake (Kupchella & Syty, 1980; Savory et al., 1987).

The total intake of aluminium from food and beverages (excluding drinking-water) in several countries is given in Table 12. All estimates are less than 15 mg/day, with the lower values probably reflecting a lower use of aluminium additives in the preparation of cereal grain products (bread, etc.) (UK MAFF, 1993).

5.3.3 *Drinking-water*

Aluminium levels in drinking-water, whether distributed through household plumbing or as bottled water, vary according to the natural levels found in the source and whether aluminium flocculants were used during the purification process. An international drinking-water guideline for aluminium was based on aesthetic rather than health grounds (WHO, 1993).

Results from extensive monitoring of drinking-water supplies have been obtained from Germany (Wilhelm & Idel, 1995), Ontario Canada (OMEE, 1995), and the United Kingdom (UK MAFF, 1993).

Table 12. Estimated average dietary intake of aluminium in various countries

Country	Method of sampling[a]	Estimated intake of aluminium (mg/day)	Reference
Australia	MB	2.4 (male) 1.9 (female)	NFA (1993)
Canada	MB	0.08-0.69[b] (infants)	Dabeka & McKenzie (1992)
Finland	TD	6.7	Varo & Koivistoinen (1980)
Germany	MB MB DD	11.0 (males) 8.0 (females) 0.78 (5-8 years old)	Treptow & Askar (1987) Wilhelm et al. (1995)
Japan	TD	4.5	Teraoka et al. (1981)
Netherlands	DD	3.1 (mean male and female)	Ellen et al. (1990)
Sweden	DD	13.0 (female)	Jorhem & Haegglund (1992)
Switzerland	DD	4.4	Knutti & Zimmerli (1985)
UK	TD TD	0.03-0.05 (4-month infant)[c] 0.27-0.53 (4-month infant)[d] 3.9	UK MAFF (1993)
USA	TD	0.7 (6-11 month old infant) 6.5 (6 years old) 11.5 (14-16 year old male) 7.1 (adult female) 8.2 (adult male)	Pennington & Schoen (1995)

[a] MB = Market basket survey; TD = Total diet study; DD = Duplicate diet study
[b] Range represents intake of an infant (0-1 month old) fed cow's milk to that for an infant (1-3 month old) fed exclusively soya-based formulae
[c] Range for infants fed cow's milk-based formulae
[d] Range for infants fed soya-based formulae

In Germany, levels of aluminium in public water supplies averaged (median) 10 µg/litre in the western region while 2.7% of public supplies in the eastern region exceeded 200 µg/litre. It was estimated that 500 000 people were exposed to these high levels. Aluminium levels of up to 10 000 µg/litre were reported in drinking-water from private wells in areas where the soil had low buffering capacity and was subjected to high acidic stress (Mühlenberg, 1990; Wilhelm & Idel, 1995).

In a province-wide survey of the aluminium content of public water supplies in Ontario, Canada, approximately 75% of all average levels in 1993 and 1994 were less than 100 µg/litre, the present operational guideline for Ontario (OMEE, 1995). The range of average values was 40 to 851 µg/litre.

A large monitoring programme in 1991 by the water companies in the United Kingdom (75 305 samples) reported that only 553 (0.7%) exceeded the United Kingdom aluminium standard of 200 µg/litre (UK MAFF, 1993). Drinking-water would add about 400 µg aluminium to the daily intake, assuming a consumption of 2 litres water daily at the aesthetic guideline value of 200 µg/litre (WHO, 1993). From the monitoring data discussed above and normal intakes of water, a more realistic intake would be at or below 200 µg/day from monitored municipal supplies.

5.3.4 Miscellaneous exposures

The use of antacids and buffered analgesics may result in large intakes of aluminium, far in excess of that normally consumed in food (Shore & Wyatt, 1983; Lione, 1983; Schenck et al., 1989). It has been estimated that daily doses of aluminium in antacids and buffered analgesics range from 840 to 5000 mg and 130 to 730 mg per day, respectively (Lione, 1983). These are approximately two to three orders of magnitude greater than normal dietary intakes (see Table 12) and well in excess of the recommended provisional tolerable weekly intake (PTWI) of 420 mg for a 60-kg adult (FAO/WHO, 1989).

Aluminium compounds are widely used in the preparation of cosmetics, particularly in antiperspirants (Sorenson et al., 1974). However, there are no reliable data supporting dermal absorption from such products.

5.3.5 Total human intake of aluminium from all environmental pathways

In calculating total human exposures one must be aware of the quality of the sampling and analytical procedures, particularly when using data from earlier studies. Total intake of aluminium must consider all routes of exposure, i.e. inhalation, oral and dermal.

For humans, non-occupationally exposed to aluminium, oral intake of aluminium represents the major route of exposure. As shown in Table 12 the total daily intake of aluminium in adults ranges from 2.5 to 13 mg/day, depending upon the country of origin as well as the age and sex of the subject. The variation reflects different dietary habits as well as the level of additives used in food processing. For infants (under 6 months) daily intakes range from 0.27 to 0.53 mg/day for those consuming soya-based formulae and 0.03 to 0.05 mg/day for infants consuming cow's milk formulae (UK MAFF, 1993). Similar values were reported from Canada (respectively, 0.08 and 0.69) (Dabeka & McKenzie, 1990). Aluminium intake from breast milk has been calculated to be < 0.04 mg/day (UK MAFF, 1993).

In conclusion, the total intake of aluminium by the general population varies between 2.5 and 13 mg/day. In most countries over 95% of this comes from food and less than 1% from airborne aluminium. As noted in section 5.3.4, these intakes can be increased greatly (10 to 100 times) through the use of aluminium-containing antacids and buffered analgesics. Total daily exposure to aluminium from all sources, other than medicines, and for all age groups has been shown to be less than the PTWI of 1 mg/kg per day (WHO, 1993).

5.3.6 Aluminium uptake

In view of the fact that over 95% of the normal daily intake of aluminium comes from food and water, uptake from the gastrointestinal tract will play a major role in determining tissue levels of the metal. The ratio of intake to uptake will be a major determinant in the risk of orally ingested aluminium to humans. Factors affecting gastrointestinal absorption of aluminium are discussed in section 6.1.2.

Recent studies of the bioavailability and uptake of aluminium in human volunteers have employed the radioactive isotope ^{26}Al, which may be detected at very low masses, i.e. 5×10^{-15} g using accelerator mass spectrometry (AMS). The first of these was a study by Day et al. (1991), who measured the uptake of aluminium in one volunteer following the ingestion of 1.1 µg of the isotope in sodium citrate. For this study aluminium uptake was assessed by extrapolation from a single measurement of ^{26}Al in blood plasma 6 h after administration. The fraction of absorbed aluminium was estimated to be 1%. Later, the same technique was employed by Day et al. (1994) to estimate aluminium uptake from orange juice (with or without added silicate) in control subjects and Down's syndrome patients. For the normal subjects uptake factors ranging from 0.04 to 1.5×10^{-4} were calculated. The addition of silica reduced the uptake by a factor of about 7. In the Down's syndrome patients, many of whom develop AD, uptake was approximately 5 times higher than in controls (4.7×10^{-4} compared with 0.91×10^{-4}).

Most recently, human bioavailability studies have been undertaken by Priest (1994) using a more vigorous methodology, employing the collection of blood samples and total excreta for a period of up to a week after a single administration of the aluminium compound. The results obtained showed significant intersubject variability in the extent and timing of aluminium absorption and indicated that the method employed by Day et al. (1994) was of limited utility. Two main studies were undertaken. The first was a study of the uptake of aluminium, as aluminium citrate, aluminium hydroxide and aluminium hydroxide in the presence of citrate, from the gut following the administration of 100 mg aluminium by gastric tube (Priest, 1994). The measured fractional uptakes were as follows: 5×10^{-3} for aluminium as citrate; 1.04×10^{-4} for aluminium hydroxide; 1.36×10^{-3} for hydroxide in the presence of sodium citrate. This study demonstrated the greater bioavailability of the citrate complex and the ability of citrate to enhance the uptake of aluminium taken in another chemical form. The second study measured the fractional uptake of aluminium from drinking-water using a similar technique, but different volunteers (Priest et al., 1995a,b,c). The measured uptake fraction was 2.2×10^{-4}. It was concluded that members of the public, drinking 1.5 litres per day of water containing 100 µg aluminium/litre, would absorb from this source about 3% of their total daily aluminium uptake. This result suggests that drinking-water, under most circumstances, is likely to be a minor source of aluminium for humans.

6. KINETICS AND METABOLISM IN LABORATORY ANIMALS

Investigations into the kinetics of aluminium include estimation of typical toxicokinetic parameters as well as issues specifically related to the chemistry of aluminium and its compounds. Many studies have been performed at high-dose levels. Since there are indications that the toxicokinetics of aluminium are dose-dependent, these results should be interpreted cautiously with respect to their relevance to humans (Wilhelm et al., 1990). In addition, owing to large variations in experimental protocols employed, many data-sets are not comparable, making the interpretation of these data very difficult.

6.1 Absorption

6.1.1 Animal studies

6.1.1.1 Inhalation exposure

Reports of systematic studies of the pulmonary absorption of aluminium in experimental animals have not been identified. However, aluminium has been detected in organs other than the lung following some inhalation experiments.

In rats and guinea-pigs exposed for 24 months to 0.25-25 mg/m^3 aluminium chlorohydrate, aluminium was present primarily in the lungs. The only other organs with significant concentrations of aluminium were the peribronchial lymph nodes in guinea-pigs and the adrenal glands in rats (Stone et al., 1979).

In New Zealand rabbits exposed to 0.56 mg aluminium/m^3 for 5 months, there was a 2.5 fold increase in the aluminium content of the brain (10.1 mg/kg dry weight) compared to control (4.1 mg/kg dry weight) animals, while the concentration of aluminium in serum was only slightly increased (Röllin et al., 1991a).

6.1.1.2 Oral administration

The gastrointestinal tract is the most important port of entry. In addition, inhaled aluminium aerosols that are cleared from the surface of the mucous membranes of the respiratory tract by action of the mucociliary escalator are swallowed and thus may be absorbed from the gastrointestinal tract.

Based on available data, absorption via the gastrointestinal tract in experimental animals is generally less than 1%. However, estimates of the proportion absorbed vary considerably, in part, as a result of the different conditions of exposure (i.e., use of citrate versus hydroxide salts, etc.) to various compounds (see Table 13). Values from balance studies are probably overestimates, since the amount of aluminium retained in the gut was probably calculated as absorbed aluminium. The rather high value obtained by Gupta et al. (1986) has not been confirmed. Some studies on aluminium uptake after oral administration of various compounds are summarized in Table 14 and Table 15, where uptake has been measured by blood aluminium levels or tissue levels.

Results from studies on isolated intestinal organ systems support the findings of low absorption rates of aluminium from the gastrointestinal tract (Jäger et al., 1991). Also, although not directly applicable to the human situation, experiments where aluminium salts have been given to rats and mice by interperitoneal injection further support the low amount of aluminium absorbed from the gastro-intestinal tract (Leblondel & Allain, 1980; Muller et al., 1992; Greger & Powers, 1992). For example, blood aluminium levels in rats given 10 mg aluminium chloride/kg body weight per day for 11 days were about 15 times greater than controls (20 µg/litre compared to 300 µg/litre) (Muller et al., 1992). In contrast, in rats fed 0.1% aluminium chloride in the diet for up to 25 days there was only a 22% increase in blood aluminium levels (0.91 mg/litre compared to 1.11 mg/litre) (Mayor et al., 1977).

The mechanism of intestinal absorption of aluminium is fairly complex and not yet fully elucidated (van der Voet, 1992). This complexity results from the very particular chemical properties of the element, i.e. (1) great variability of solubility at different pH values, amphoteric character, and formation of various chemical species depending on the pH, the ionic strength and the presence of complexing agents in the intestine (Martin, 1992), and (2) the complex organisation of the mammalian digestive tract where the chyme passes through a sequence of chemical environments differing in pH, presence of secretory products, etc. In addition, the different parts of

Table 13. Gastrointestinal absorption of aluminium compounds[a]

Species	Dose	Form	f (%)[b]	Method[c]	Remarks	References
Rat	8.1 mg/kg	$AlCl_3$	27	3		Gupta et al. (1986)
Rat	1; 12 mg Al/kg	lactate	0.18	2		Wilhelm et al. (1992)
Rat	1; 12 mg Al/kg	lactate	0.02	3		Wilhelm et al. (1992)
Rat	35 mg Al/kg	sucralfate, lactate	0.015	2		Froment et al. (1989a)
Rat	35 mg Al/kg	$AlCl_3$	0.037	2		Froment et al. (1989a)
Rat	1.20 mmol Al/kg	lactate	0.037	2		Froment et al. (1989a)
Rat	3.8 ng ^{26}Al and 63 ng ^{27}Al in citrate and citrate-free solutions		0.02 0.02	2 2		Jouhanneau et al. (1993)
Rat	1; 12 mg Al/kg	lactate	0.18	2		Wilhelm et al. (1992)
Rat	1; 12 mg Al/kg	lactate	0.02	3		Wilhelm et al. (1992)

Table 13 (contd).

Species	Dose	Compound	f	Method	Effect	Reference
Rat	35 mg Al/kg	sucralfate	0.015	2		Froment et al. (1989a,b)
Rat	35 mg Al/kg	$Al(OH)_3$	0.015	2		Froment et al. (1989a,b)
Rat	35 mg Al/kg	$AlCl_3$	0.037	2		Froment et al. (1989a,b)
Rabbit	10.8, 540 mg Al/kg	lactate	0.70-1.9	3	no significant influence of dose	Yokel & McNamara (1985)
Rabbit	2.5-10 mmol/kg	various	0.3-2.2	3	absorption: soluble>insoluble; minor differences between organic and inorganic forms; best bioavailability, citrate; minor influence of renal impairment	Yokel & McNamara (1989)
Sheep	1-2 g/day	$Al_2(SO_4)_3$; Al-citrate; $AlCl_3$	2-15	1	order of absorption: $Al_2(SO_4)_3$>Al citrate>$AlCl_3$	Allen & Fontenot (1984)

[a] Modified from: Wilhelm et al. (1990)

[b] f = mass Al absorbed + mass Al ingested

[c] 1 = balance study; 2 = estimation based on urinary excretion; 3 = comparison of areas under plasma aluminium concentration after oral and intravenous application

Table 14. Tissue aluminium concentrations in experimental animals administered aluminium compounds orally[a]

Species	Treatment	Bone	Brain	Reference
Mouse (BALB/c, 5-10/group)	$AlCl_3$, gavage 200 mg/kg per day 300 mg/kg per day	n.d.	n.d.	Cranmer et al. (1986)
Mouse (Swiss, 6/group)	Al lactate, 25 mg Al/kg (= control), 500 mg Al/kg diet 1000 mg Al/kg diet	(5.3 mg/kg w.w.) 5.0 mg/kg w.w. 6.5 mg/kg w.w.	35.3 mg/kg w.w. 38.3 mg/kg w.w. 108.7 mg/kg w.w.	Golub et al. (1989)
Rat (8 Wistar)	2835 mg Al/kg in feed, (as $Al_2(SO_4)_3$), 24 days	femur (702 mg/kg w.w.) 912 mg/kg w.w.	(7.1 mg/kg w.w.) 10.8 mg/kg w.w.	Ondreicka et al. (1966)
Rat (juvenile, male SD, 8/group)	aluminium in water (1) control (2) 0.32 g Al/litre, 29 days (3) low Ca^{2+} + Al	n.d.	n.d.	Cann et al. (1979)

Table 14 (contd).

Species	Treatment			Reference
Rat (male SD, 8/group)	100 mg Al/kg b.w. 6 d/w; by gavage $Al(OH)_3$ (9 weeks); Al citrate (4 weeks); citric acid (4 weeks)	cortex: (0.013 mg/kg w.w.) 0.013 mg/kg w.w. 0.057 mg/kg w.w. 0.028 mg/kg w.w.	(0.36 mg/kg w.w.) 0.41 mg/kg w.w. × 40 increased × 20 increased	Slanina et al. (1984)
Rat (male SD, 7/group)	gavage; 3 d/w; 11 week $Al(OH)_3$ Al citrate $Al(OH)_3$ + citrate	(0.016 mg/kg w.w.) 0.012 mg/kg w.w. 0.048 mg/kg w.w. 0.092 mg/kg w.w.	(0.22 mg/kg w.w.) 0.89 mg/kg w.w. 10.7 mg/kg w.w. 26.6 mg/kg w.w.	Slanina et al. (1985)
Rat (weanling, male SD, 6/group)	270 mg Al/kg diet, 18 days $Al(OH)_3$ Al palmitate Al lactate $AlPO_4$	(0.0 mg/kg w.w.) 2.2 mg/kg w.w. 0.6 mg/kg w.w. 1.6 mg/kg w.w. 1.3 mg/kg w.w.	tibia: (1.9 mg/kg w.w.) 15.6 mg/kg w.w. 15.0 mg/kg w.w. 13.0 mg/kg w.w. 14.5 mg/kg w.w.	Greger et al. (1985a)
Rat (weanling, male SD, 9/group)	$Al(OH)_3$ in diet, 67 days 257 mg Al/kg diet 1075 mg Al/kg diet	n.d.	tibia: (4.04 mg/kg) 11.3 mg/kg (3.13 mg/kg) 10.4 mg/kg	Greger et al. (1986)
Rat (male SD, 10/group)	$Al(NO_3)_3$, in water, 4 w 375 mg/kg/d 750 mg/kg/d 1500 mg/kg/d	(1.4 mg/kg w.w.) 7.7 mg/kg w.w. 10.1 mg/kg w.w. 7.9 mg/kg w.w.	(5.75 mg/kg w.w.) 11.4 mg/kg w.w. 8.5 mg/kg w.w. 17.7 mg/kg w.w.	Gómez et al. (1986)

Table 14 (contd).

Species	Treatment	Bone	Brain	Reference
Rat (female SD, 10/group)	$Al(NO_3)_3$, oral, 100 d 360 mg/kg w.w. 720 mg/kg w.w. 3600 mg/kg w.w.	(17.15 mg/kg w.w.) 75.08 mg/kg w.w. 79.18 mg/kg w.w. 56.39 mg/kg w.w.	(< 0.5 mg/kg w.w.) 4.93 mg/kg w.w. 2.09 mg/kg w.w. 4.28 mg/kg w.w.	Domingo et al. (1987b)
Rat (SD, weanling 6/group)	$Al(OH)_3$, in feed, 10 d 50-60 mg/kg b.w.	femur: (6.8 mg/kg d.w.) 8.4 mg/kg d.w.	n.d.	Chan et al. (1988)
Rat (male, weanling SD)	$Al(OH)_3$, 28 d 13 mg Al/kg diet + 5 mmol/kg citrate 41 mg Al/kg diet + 5 mmol/kg citrate	tibia: 36 mmol/kg w.w. 36 mmol/kg w.w. 50 mmol/kg w.w. 69 mmol/kg w.w.	n.d.	Ecelbarger & Greger (1991)
Rat (18 male, weanling SD)	$Al(OH)_3$ in feed, 29 days 0.39 µmol Al/g diet aluminium + 4% citrate 100 µmol Al/g diet + 4% citrate	tibia: (28.9 mmol/kg w.w.) 52.6 mmol/kg w.w. 74.4 mmol/kg w.w. 79.6 mmol/kg w.w.	n.d.	Greger & Powers (1992)

Table 14 (contd).

Rabbit (female NZ, 8/group)	inhalation exposure 0.56 mg Al/m^3 as Al$_2$O$_3$ 8 h/d; 5 d/w; 5 months	(18.2 mg/kg d.w.) 22.2 mg/kg d.w.	(4.1 mg/kg d.w.) 10.1 mg/kg d.w.	Röllin et al. (1991a)
Rabbit (male NZ, 3-4/group)	50 g/kg AlCl$_3$, in feed 1 month ethanol aluminium + ethanol	(n.d.)	cortex, gray matter: (n.d.) 3.1 mg/kg d.w. 1.3 mg/kg d.w. 3.0 mg/kg d.w.	Thornton et al. (1983)
Dog	Al(OH)$_3$ in feed, 3 g/d; 5 months	n.d.	cerebral cortex: 0.77 mg/kg d.w. 2.4 mg/kg d.w.	Arieff et al. (1979)
Cattle (steer, 6/group)	AlCl$_3$ in feed, 84 d 300 mg/kg 600 mg/kg 1200 mg/kg	(n.d.)	(6.4 mg/kg w.w.) 7.6 mg/kg w.w. 5.5 mg/kg w.w. 7.7 mg/kg w.w.	Valdivia et al. (1978)

Values in parentheses are normal control values in unexposed animals; b.w. = body weight; d = day; d.w. = dry weight; n.d. = not detected; NZ = New Zealand; SD = Sprague-Dawley; w = week; w.w. = wet weight

Table 15. Blood aluminium concentrations in experimental animals exposed orally to aluminium compounds[a]

Species	Sample	Dose	Duration	Compound	Aluminium concentration (control value)	Reference
Rat (8 Wistar)	blood	2835 mg Al/kg feed	24 days	$Al_2(SO_4)_3$	(6.5 mg/kg w.w.) 10.8 mg/kg w.w.	Ondreicka et al. (1966)
Rat (male albino)	serum	150 mg Al/kg/d, gavage		$Al(OH)_3$	(0.24 mg/litre) 0.99 mg/litre	Berlyne et al. (1972)
Rat (male SD, 8/group)	serum	0.1% aluminium in feed		$AlCl_3$	(0.91 mg/litre) day 10: 1.12 mg/litre, day 25: 1.09 mg/litre	Mayor et al. (1977)
Rat (male SD, 7/group)	blood	3 d/w, gavage	11 weeks	$Al(OH)_3$ Al citrate $Al(OH)_3$ + citrate	(0.005 mg/kg w.w.) 0.009 mg/kg w.w. 0.014 mg/kg w.w. 0.039 mg/kg w.w.	Slanina et al. (1985)
Rat (male SD, 10/group)	blood	375 mg/kg/d 750 mg/kg/d 1500 mg/kg/d, in water		$Al(NO_3)_3$	(3.7 mg/kg w.w.) 3.1 mg/kg w.w. 2.5 mg/kg w.w. 3.0 mg/kg w.w.	Gómez et al. (1986)

Table 15 (contd).

Species	Sample	Dose	Duration	Compound	Concentration	Reference
Rat (female SD, 10/group)	blood	360 mg/kg w.w. 720 mg/kg w.w. 3600 mg/kg w.w., oral	100 days	$Al(NO_3)_3$	(< 0.5 mg/kg) < 0.5 mg/kg < 0.5 mg/kg < 0.5 mg/kg	Domingo et al. (1987b)
Rat (18 male, weanling SD)	serum	0.39 mmol Al/kg diet aluminium + 4% citrate 100 mmol Al/kg diet + 4% citrate, in feed	29 days	$Al(OH)_3$	(0.28 µmol/litre) 0.98 µmol/litre 1.15 µmol/litre 1.09 µmol/litre	Greger & Powers (1992)
Rat (weanling SD, 4/group)	serum	160 mg Al/kg d, gavage, 1,25-$(OH)_2$-D_3 1,25-$(OH)_2$-D_3 + $Al(OH)_3$ 1,25-$(OH)_2$-D_3 + Al citrate	10 days		(18.8 µg/litre) 24.3 µg/litre 29.5 µg/litre 16.3 µg/litre	Santos et al. (1987)
Rabbit (male NZ, 3-4/group)	serum	50 g/kg in feed	1 month	$AlCl_3$ Al+ethanol	(5 µg/litre) 14 µg/litre 24 µg/litre	Thornton et al. (1983)
Cattle (steer, 6/group)	blood	300 mg/kg 600 mg/kg 1200 mg/kg, in feed	84 days	$AlCl_3$	(0.103 mg/litre) 0.118 mg/litre 0.100 mg/litre 0.120 mg/litre	Valdivia et al. (1978)

[a] 1,25-$(OH)_2$-D_3 = 1,25-dihydroxy-vitamin D_3; d = day; NZ = New Zealand; SD = Sprague-Dawley; w = week; w.w. = wet weight

the intestine may be distinct with regard to their resorptive properties and may be influenced by variation in physiological conditions. There are indications that aluminium interacts with the gastrointestinal calcium transport system (Adler & Berlyne, 1985; Provan & Yokel, 1988) and with transferrin-mediated iron uptake (van der Voet & de Wolff, 1987; Jäger et al., 1991). There is consistent evidence that absorption of aluminium increases in the presence of citrate (Slanina et al., 1986; Froment et al., 1989a,b). There are some data suggesting that uptake increases after fasting (Walton et al., 1994).

6.1.1.3 Dermal

Aluminium absorption via the skin in animals has not been studied.

6.1.2 Studies in humans

6.1.2.1 Inhalation exposures

Studies dealing with the absorption of aluminium compounds in humans usually use the blood aluminium concentration or the urinary aluminium excretion as a marker of uptake (Schaller & Valentin, 1984; Ganrot, 1986). However, part of the aluminium-containing particulates deposited in the respiratory tract is cleared from the organ by mucociliary action and, when swallowed, enters the digestive tract. This means that after inhalation exposure to aluminium compounds not all aluminium appearing in the systemic circulation or in the urine necessarily arises solely from absorption in the respiratory tract.

"Insoluble" particulates may be slowly dissolved and thus enter the blood circulation. Owing to the chemical properties of aluminium, the absorption of aluminium metal or its compounds by the respiratory system depends on the aluminium species inhaled and the biological environment in the tissue compartment where they are deposited (Martin, 1992).

There is evidence from a number of reports that even aluminium compounds that are almost insoluble in water are bioavailable when introduced into the respiratory system. For example, increased urinary concentrations have been observed in aluminium welders and aluminium flake and powder producers after exposure to relatively insoluble particulate matter and metallic fumes and dusts. The levels of tissue aluminium after inhalation exposures are given in Table 16. When comparing the analytical results given in these tables, one has to keep in mind, however, that the analytical precision of the aluminium determination has been hampered by the potential for contamination during sampling and processing in view of the ubiquitous presence of the element (Steinegger et al., 1990). Analytical techniques for determination of aluminium have been improved considerably during recent years (see Chapter 2).

6.1.2.2 *Oral administration*

In view of the fact that over 95% of the normal daily intake of aluminium comes from food and water, uptake from the gastrointestinal tract will play a major role in determining tissue levels of the metal.

The mechanism of gastrointestinal absorption of aluminium is fairly complex and has not yet been fully elucidated (van der Voet, 1992). This complexity results from (1) the unique chemical properties of the element, particularly its amphoteric character, leading to marked variability in solubility at different pH values and the formation of various chemical species in the gut depending on the pH, the ionic strength and the presence of complexing agents (Martin, 1992), and (2) the complex organization of the mammalian digestive tract where the chyme passes through a sequence of chemical environments differing greatly in pH, presence of secretory products, etc. In addition, the different parts of the intestine may be distinct with regard to their absorptive and resorptive properties with respect to aluminium.

Aluminium species may be modified in the gut prior to absorption (Skalsky & Carchman, 1983; Ganrot, 1986; Martin, 1986, 1992). Quantitatively the intraluminal absorption depends upon the amount of the chemical species present in the gut lumen, in the blood, and in the interstitial fluid. Absorption is influenced by the presence of other complexing ligands (citrate, lactate, etc.) and competing ions (e.g., iron, silicon). Other factors proposed to influence absorption include: age; renal function; and iron and calcium status (Birchall, 1991; van der Voet, 1992; Edwardson, 1993).

To date, research concerning the intestinal absorption of aluminium in humans has been mainly guided by clinical problems and has used a variety of physiological states and chemical conditions.

Table 16. Blood and urine aluminium concentrations in humans after oral ingestion of aluminium compounds[a]

Subjects and treatment	Aluminium concentration in blood (µg/litre)	Aluminium concentration in urine (µg/litre)	Remarks	Reference
5 normal subjects, 2 patients with CRF; $Al(OH)_3$ antacids, 86-91 mmol/day	not specified	not specified	Al absorption normal: 0.3-3.6 mmol/day CRF: 3.3-9.1 mmol/day	Cam et al. (1976)
Normal subjects, $Al(OH)_3$, oral, 3.8 g Al/day for 3 days	not detected	(85.8 µg/day) increased by 4-10 times		Recker et al. (1977)
Normal subjects, 2.2 g Al for 3 days $Al(OH)_3$ $Al_2(CO_3)_3$ $Al(OH)_2$-aminoacetate $AlPO_4$	plasma: (6-7) 17 14 17 9	(8-16) 176-325 51-355 243-726 52-60	cumulative increase in excretion (µg) 730 ± 487 567 ± 437 1430 ± 1157 123 ± 77	Kaehny et al. (1977a)
Normal subjects CRF CRF + Al	6.2 (serum) 13.4 (serum) 34.1	not detected		Marsden et al. (1979)

Table 16 (contd).

Normal subjects, antacids taken orally, 23-313 mg/day for 18-30 days	plasma Al: 2-fold increase	urinary Al excretion: 2- to 6-fold increase	Al balance positive during Al administration	Gorsky et al. (1979)
Al-hydrocarbonate (Lithiagel), oral, 1.84 g Al/day; 5 days	(before Al: 8.35) 3-day Al: 15.9 5-day Al: 14.8 after 1 week Al: 8.0	(before Al: 6.35) 3-day Al: 430.8 5-day Al: 262.5 after 1 week Al: 12.2	serum aluminium in dialysed patients treated with Aludrox: 6-254 µg/litre	Mauras et al. (1982)
Al-supplemented diet control: 4.6 mg Al/day test: 125 mg Al/day	serum (before: 4) control: 4 test: 7	urinary excretion: control: 35-36 µg/day test: 105-129 µg/day	normalized to creatinine control: 20 mg/kg test: 57-72 mg/kg	Greger & Baier (1983a)
12 subjects (normal young) given 280 nM Mg + 190 nM Al/day for 4 weeks	serum Al placebo: 0.3-0.9 test: 0.8-1.1	placebo: 1.0-3.0 test: 3.6-20.2		Herzog et al. (1982)
CRF, on home dialysis on CAPD	(3.4 plasma) 37.7-68.7 33.9-45.0		no correlation with Al concentration in hair	Wilhelm et al. (1989)

[a] control values are given in parentheses
CAPD = continuous ambulatory peritoneal dialysis; CRF = chronic renal failure

93

Owing to the large variations in experimental conditions, many results are not comparable and interpretation of their relevance to the health population becomes very difficult or impossible.

Gastrointestinal absorption of aluminium in humans ingesting antacids or phosphate binders is well documented. Variable quantities of $Al(OH)_3$ or $Al_2(CO_3)_3$ given to volunteers or patients for different periods of time resulted in significant increases in plasma and/or urinary aluminium concentrations (Cam et al., 1976; Kaehny et al., 1977a; Recker et al., 1977; Gorsky et al., 1979; Mauras et al., 1982; Herzog et al., 1982; Greger & Baier, 1983a). Administration of the insoluble $AlPO_4$ did not significantly alter blood and urinary aluminium levels (Kaehny et al., 1977a). The results of these studies are summarized in Tables 16 and 17. It must be emphasized, however, where compounds are poorly bioavailable, the expected incremental increase in the plasma aluminium level after exposure may be lower than can be detected against normal plasma aluminium levels.

Recent studies of the bioavailability and uptake of aluminium in human volunteers have employed the radioactive isotope ^{26}Al, which may be detected at very low concentrations (5×10^{-15} g) using accelerator mass spectrometry (AMS). The first of these was a study by Day et al. (1991) who measured the uptake of aluminium in one volunteer following the ingestion of 1.1 µg of the isotope in sodium citrate. For this study aluminium uptake was assessed by extrapolation from a single measurement of ^{26}Al in blood plasma 6 h after administration. Day estimated the fraction of absorbed aluminium to be 1%. Later, the same technique was employed by Day et al. (1994) to estimate aluminium uptake from orange juice (with or without added silicate) in control subjects and patients with Down's syndrome. Results were expressed as the gastrointestinal absorption factor (F_1), defined as the ratio of mass of aluminium absorbed to mass of aluminium ingested. For the normal subjects uptake factors ranging from 0.04 to 1.5×10^{-4} were calculated. The addition of silica reduced the uptake by a factor of about 7. In the Down's syndrome patients uptake was apparently 5 times higher than in controls (4.7×10^{-4} compared to an average of 0.91×10^{-4} in controls).

Most recently, human bioavailability studies have been undertaken by Priest and his co-workers using a methodology employing the collection of blood samples and total excreta for a period of up to a week after a single administration of aluminium compound.

Table 17. Tissue aluminium concentrations (mg/kg) in humans exposed to aluminium compounds[a]

Subjects and treatment	Bone	Muscle	Kidney	Liver	Lung	Brain	Remarks	Reference
Normal adult	n.d.	1.55 d.w.	2.02 d.w.	2.4 d.w.	122.5 d.w.	1.4 d.w.	adrenal: 4.8 d.w. spleen: 3.7 d.w. duod.: 4.56 d.w. jejun.: 2.84 d.w. ileum: 9.86 d.w.	Tipton & Cook (1963)
Healthy human controls	hard water area: 73.4 w.w. soft water area: 60 w.w.	0.5 w.w.	whole kidney: 0.4 w.w. cortex: 0.4 w.w. medulla: 0.3 w.w.	2.6 w.w.	18.2 w.w.	whole brain: 0.5 w.w. frontal lobe: 0.05 w.w. basal ganglia: 0.07 w.w.		Hamilton et al. (1973)
Normal males Stonemason	< 15 d.w. n.d.	n.d. n.d.	11 d.w. 16 d.w.	19 d.w. 130 d.w.	230 d.w. 2000 d.w.	n.d.	spleen: (22 d.w.) 520 d.w. heart: (11 d.w.) 2.0 d.w. adrenal: (37 d.w.) n.d.	Teraoka (1981)
Ball-mill room worker in aluminium powder factory	30 w.w.	n.d.	n.d.	90 w.w.	upper lobe: 430 w.w. lower lobe: 340 w.w.	5 w.w.		McLaughlin et al. (1962)

Table 17 (contd).

Subjects and treatment	Bone	Muscle	Kidney	Liver	Lung	Brain	Remarks	Reference
Surgical and autopsy speci-men (hyperpara-thyroidism)	n.d.	no Al intake: 2.0 d.w. Al intake: 7.6 d.w.	n.d.	n.d.	n.d.	n.d.	no Al intake: PT: 13 d.w. thy: 3.5 d.w. Al intake: PT: 78 d.w. thy: 8.8 d.w.	Cann et al. (1979)
Normal controls: uraemia, non-dial: uraemia, dial: DES:	10.6 6.4 23.5 272.7	23.6 24.7 39.6 13.8	17.5 33.8 44.1 156.5	15.8 19.7 32.9 610.2	97.2 142.3 127.1 99.6	11.9 n.d. 12.1 66.1	spleen: 17.2 25.1 37.9 454.5	Flendrig et al. (1976)
DES normal control uraemia/dial uraemia/non-dial	cortical bone: (3.88) 46.83 8.4 trabecular bone: (2.39) 98.48 37.4	(1.22) DES: 23.6 non-DES: 10.24	n.d.	n.d.	n.d.	grey matter: (2.18) non-DES: 6.5 DES: 24.98	brain white matter: (2.00) non-DES: 3.81 DES: 5.59	Alfrey et al. (1976)[b]

Table 17 (contd).

Iliac bone (biopsy or autopsy spec.) control uraemia, non-dial dial dial + transpl	 5.7 ash 13.6 ash 151.8 ash 92 ash	n.d.	n.d.	n.d.	n.d.	n.d.	correlation of duration of dialysis and bone Al	Ellis et al. (1979)
Patients healthy controls uraemia, non-dial uraemia, dial DES	 3.3 d.w. 27 d.w. 115 d.w. 281 d.w.	 1.2 d.w. 2.6 d.w. 9.1 d.w. 15 d.w.	n.d.	 4.0 d.w. 25.5 d.w. 160 d.w. 301 d.w.	 56 d.w. 75 d.w. 89 d.w. 215 d.w.	grey matter: 2.2 d.w. 4.1 d.w. 8.5 d.w. 24.5 d.w.	spleen: 3.8 d.w. 35 d.w. 243 d.w. 493 d.w.	Alfrey (1980)
Uraemia + dial normal control osteomalacia osteitis fibrosa mixed lesions mild lesions	 2.4 d.w. 175 d.w. 46 d.w. 81 d.w. 67 d.w.	n.d.	n.d.	n.d.	n.d.	n.d.		Hodsman et al. (1982)
Normal, necropsy	n.d.	n.d.	n.d.	n.d.	n.d.	cortex: 0.23-2.7 d.w. white matter: 0.6-1.1 d.w.		Crapper et al. (1973)

Table 17 (contd).

Subjects and treatment	Bone	Muscle	Kidney	Liver	Lung	Brain	Remarks	Reference
Normal adult infant fetus	n.d.	n.d.	n.d.	n.d.	n.d.	1.9 d.w. 0.7 d.w. 0.7 d.w.		Crapper et al. (1976)
Normal controls	n.d.	n.d.	n.d.	n.d.	n.d.	2.5 d.w. 5.6 d.w. 2.4 d.w. 1.4 d.w. 2.9 d.w. 2.9 d.w. 2.6 d.w. 1.5 d.w. 4.1 d.w. 1.3 d.w.	whole brain hippocampus frontal cortex temporal cortex parietal cortex occipital cortex cerebellum corpus callosum mininges isolated neurons	McDermott et al. (1979)
Normal adult normal infant	n.d.	n.d.	n.d.	n.d.	n.d.	0.467 w.w. 0.298 d.w.		Markesbery et al. (1981)
Al welders (2) welding fumes	(0.6-5 d.w.) 18-29 d.w.	n.d.	n.d.	n.d.	n.d.	n.d.	also increased: blood and urinary Al concentration	Elinder et al. (1991)

Table 17 (contd).

	(median values)							
CRF, cumulative oral Al intake:							no correlation with Al concentration in hair:	Wilhelm et al. (1989)
0 kg	5.3						control: 2.6	
< 0.25 kg	47.5						dial: 1.6-5.5	
0.25 to 0.5 kg	56.7							
0.5 to 1.0 kg	62.6							
1.0 to 5.0 kg	133.4							
Controls (surgical specimens)	18.8 w.w.	n.d.	n.d.	n.d.	n.d.	n.d.	no differences between cortical and medullary bone; no correlation with age	Burnel et al. (1982)
CRF (biopsies; intake of variable amounts of Al)	6-130 w.w.							

[a] Normal control values are given in parentheses
  DES   = dialysis encephalopathy syndrome;   dial   = on haemodialysis;
  w.w.   = wet weight;   non-dial   = not on haemodialysis;
  d.w.   = dry weight;   transpl   = transplantation;
  n.d.   = no data;   PT   = parathyroid gland;
  ARF   = acute renal failure;   thy   = thyroid gland
  CRF   = chronic renal failure;
[b] All concentrations expressed as mg Al/kg fat-free solid

The results of these experiments showed significant intersubject variability in the extent and timing of aluminium absorption, indicating the shortcomings of the methods employed by Day et al. (1991, 1994). Two main studies were undertaken. The first was a study of the uptake from the gut of aluminium, as aluminium citrate, aluminium hydroxide, and aluminium hydroxide in the presence of citrate, following the administration of 100 mg aluminium by gastric tube (Priest, 1994). The absorption fractions obtained were as follows: 5×10^{-3} for aluminium as citrate; 1.04×10^{-4} for aluminium hydroxide; and 1.36×10^{-3} for hydroxide in the presence of sodium citrate. This study demonstrated the greater bioavailability of the citrate complex and the ability of citrate to enhance the uptake of aluminium taken in another chemical form. The second study measured the fractional uptake of aluminium from drinking-water using a similar technique, but different volunteers (Priest et al., 1995a). The measured uptake fraction was 2.2×10^{-4}. It was concluded that members of the public, drinking 1.5 litres/day of water containing 100 µg of aluminium/litre, would absorb about 3% of their total daily aluminium uptake from this source. This result suggests that drinking-water, under most circumstances, is likely to be a minor source of aluminium for humans.

6.1.2.3 Dermal exposure

There is no direct evidence that aluminium is absorbed through the intact skin of humans.

6.2 Distribution

6.2.1 Animal studies

After absorption aluminium is bound in the plasma primarily to transferrin and, to a lesser extent, also to albumin (Trapp, 1983; Bertholf et al., 1984; Martin, 1986). There are indications that aluminium binding to protein is dose-dependent, with low binding rates at unexposed plasma levels (Höhr et al., 1989; Wilhelm et al., 1990). Aluminium distribution depends on the animal species used, route of administration and the aluminium compound administered. Volumes of distribution for aluminium have been estimated only following parenteral administration (Wilhelm et al., 1990) and are thus not relevant to the exposure of the general population. After a single dose of aluminium lactate (1 mg/kg body weight) in rats, no tissue uptake could be detected, whereas at 12 000 mg/kg body weight the only significant increase in tissue aluminium occurred in bone (Wilhelm et al., 1992). In other oral studies summarized in Table 17, more or less significant increases in tissue levels after aluminium ingestion were found, these increases generally being dose-dependent. In animals receiving aluminium, increases in tissue levels were most marked in bone.

It has to be considered that at high-dose levels aluminium is toxic to the tissue of the gastrointestinal tract, thus inducing pathological changes that might be followed by increased uptake (Jäger et al., 1991). Gut tissue pathology has not been investigated in most distribution studies.

Two studies have reported on aluminium accumulation following administration in drinking-water. Fulton et al. (1989) administered 0, 0.1, 2.0 or 100 mg/litre Al(OH)$_3$ or AlCl$_3$ (equivalent to 0, 0.01, 0.2 or 5.5 mg Al/kg body weight per day) in drinking-water containing acetate or citrate at various pH levels to Sprague-Dawley rats (6 rats per group) for 10 weeks. In the highest-dose group, aluminium accumulated in intestinal cells but not in other tissues investigated. The effect was more pronounced when citrate was added and when water with an acidic pH was used.

In a recent study, Walton et al. (1995) administered to eight fasted adult rats by gavage 4 ml of aluminium-free drinking-water containing 1.0 µg ^{27}Al and 70 becquerel (0.1 µg) ^{26}Al. Two experimental animals had brain ^{26}Al/^{27}Al ratios similar to the two controls while the remaining six animals had ratios of ^{26}Al/^{27}Al in brain tissue that were substantially higher than background. However, the variation between animals was marked (148 ± 19 to 5220 ± 208).

Studies in mice (Golub et al., 1993), rats (Muller et al., 1992) and rabbits (Yokel, 1984) indicate that aluminium is not readily transferred from the dam to offspring via nursing.

Studies in mice (Golub et al., 1993) and rabbits (Yokel, 1985) indicate that aluminium compounds that are bioavailable and therefore available to the dam also reach the fetus. However, a study in rats reported elevated levels of aluminium in maternal tissue, but not in the fetus, after exposure to aluminium lactate in the diet during gestation (Muller et al., 1993). Limited data in mice (Cranmer et al., 1986) and rabbits (Yokel, 1985) show higher concentrations of aluminium in the placenta than in maternal or fetal tissues after administration of aluminium to dams.

6.2.2 Human studies

6.2.2.1 Transport in blood

The extent to which plasma aluminium is normally bound to proteins may be as high as 70 to 90% in haemodialysis patients with moderately increased plasma aluminium levels (25 to 200 µg/litre).

Studies using [26]Al (Day et al., 1994) have shown that one day after injection, 99% of aluminium in blood is present in the plasma fraction and 1% in the erythrocytes. By contrast, 880 days after injection, 14% was associated with the erythrocyte fraction, indicating the probable incorporation of aluminium into the erythrocytes during erythropoiesis. One day after injection, 80% of the plasma fraction was found to be associated with transferrin, 10% with albumin, 5% with low molecular weight proteins (5000-50 000 molecular weight) and about 4% with a lower molecular weight fraction. No details of the plasma speciation at 880 days were given. Priest et al. (1996) found that only about 50% of injected aluminium was recoverable from blood at 15 min after injection. It was suggested that aluminium may pass through blood vessel walls to establish an equilibrium between aluminium in blood and aluminium in the extravascular tissue fluids. In contrast, the same study showed that gallium remained in the blood. This and other observations suggested that gallium is an inappropriate surrogate for aluminium in bioavailability and kinetic studies (Priest et al., 1991).

6.2.2.2 Plasma aluminium concentrations in humans

The role of aluminium in the etiology of dialysis-related disorders such as encephalopathy, vitamin-D-resistant osteomalacia, and normochromic microcytic anaemia has drawn attention to the possible mechanisms of aluminium uptake through the parenteral and intestinal routes.

Normal human plasma or serum aluminium values reported vary largely, mainly due to methodological problems in the analytical technique and with sample contamination. Ganrot (1986) emphasized this in his extensive review.

As methods have improved, suggested reference values for plasma levels have been revised downwards, and it was suggested by Nieboer et al. (1995) that the actual value in normal subjects lies in the range of 0.04 to 0.07 µmol/litre (1.1 to 1.9 µg/litre).

Seasonal variations in serum aluminium concentrations in patients with moderate chronic renal failure were observed by Nordal et al. (1988), with peak levels occurring in the autumn. These variations were presumed to be related to an increased gastrointestinal absorption due to waterborne factors.

The data summarized in Tables 16 and 17 indicate that, as is the case with experimental animals, the aluminium concentrations in human blood and selected tissues are increased after ingestion or inhalation of aluminium compounds.

6.2.2.3 *Tissue aluminium concentrations in humans*

(a) *Normal concentrations*

The available data relating to the aluminium concentrations found in various human tissues are summarized in Table 17. It should be noted that the measurement of tissue concentrations is difficult. In particular, where the average concentrations for a tissue have been reconstructed, by extrapolation, from the analysis of small samples of the tissues concerned, they may be significantly affected by lack of homogeneity in the distribution of the metal in the organ and will also amplify errors due to sample contamination. In this respect the reconstruction of average bone concentrations is particularly difficult, given that small samples of bone collected from disparate skeletal sites will contain very different levels of aluminium as a result of the different amounts of bone surface to which the metal binds. Owing to the above difficulties it is commonly prudent to ignore measurements that indicate very high levels of aluminium in a particular tissue without additional biological data to explain the findings. This approach has been taken by a Canadian group (Nieboer et al., 1995), which based its conclusions on the lowest levels consistently reported for the tissues considered (bone and brain). It was concluded that normal levels of aluminium in bone are in the order of 1-3 µg/g (wet weight) and that background levels in brain tissue (mostly in the grey matter) are around 1-3 µg/g (dry weight) or < 0.5 µg/g (wet weight), based on the lowest levels consistently reported. The authors also showed that the bone and brain aluminium levels are significantly elevated in patients with renal failure who are treated with either aluminium-containing phosphate scavengers or who received total parenteral nutrition with aluminium-contaminated intravenous nutrient solutions.

With respect to other tissues, measurements suggest that the highest levels of aluminium are found in the lung (56-215 mg/kg dry weight) (Alfrey et al., 1980), presumably as inhaled, undissolved, aluminium-containing particles. Similarly, inhaled particles may relocate in the regional (hilar) lymph nodes and in the organs comprising the reticulo-endothelial system, i.e. liver, spleen and bone marrow. This may explain some or, in the case of the lymph nodes, most of the aluminium present in these organs. For example, Teraoka (1981) reported the levels of aluminium in the lungs and reticulo-endothelial organs of a stone mason dying from silicosis and cor pulmonale: lungs (2 g/kg dry weight); hilar lymph nodes (3.2 g/kg dry weight); spleen (520 mg/kg dry weight) and liver (130 mg/kg dry weight). Excluding particulate aluminium, it is likely that of all the extrapulmonary tissues only the skeleton contains significant levels of aluminium. This is the conclusion of Priest (1993), who based his conclusion on a theoretical consideration of ion size of Al^{3+}, supported by measurements of the distribution of the sources of ^{26}Al gamma-emission in a human volunteer at earlier times after injection (using the same techniques gallium uptake in the liver was estimated to be about 30%). The possibility that at later times liver levels build up would be consistent with rather high levels for this tissue (Flendrig et al., 1976) and with the observation of Day et al. (1994) that some aluminium is taken up by red blood cells - considering the role of the liver in the breakdown of old red blood cells.

(b)   *Concentrations after aluminium exposure*

Data on the tissue burden of aluminium-exposed humans are mostly derived from patients with chronic uraemia as well from occupationally exposed workers. In these patients, the aluminium intake may come from more than one source and is difficult to follow.

More than 40 years after exposure, the cerebrospinal fluid of an aluminium powder worker exposed heavily during 1944-1946 contained 250 µg aluminium/litre. Aluminium-associated pulmonary fibrosis (aluminosis) was diagnosed in 1946 (Sjögren et al., 1994a,b). The normal value for cerebrospinal fluid is less than 10 µg/litre.

In two heavily exposed aluminium welders, bone aluminium concentrations were 18 mg/kg dry weight and 29 mg/kg dry weight, clearly above the reference range for the investigators (0.6-5 mg/kg dry weight) (Elinder et al., 1991). In a worker producing fine aluminium powder, who developed encephalopathy and pulmonary fibrosis after 13.5 years of work, the aluminium concentration in lung and brain was increased 20-fold and in the liver 122-fold (McLaughlin et al., 1962).

In patients with impaired renal function, a wide range of tissue aluminium concentrations have been reported (bone, 8.4-281 mg/kg; muscle, 2-23.6 mg/kg; brain, 2.2-25 mg/kg; Table 16). This wide range reflects the variable exposure to aluminium-containing phosphate-binding pharmaceutical agents and the duration of haemodialysis. The increased tissue concentrations are associated with the clinical syndromes of encephalopathy, osteomalacia and microcytic anaemia. Channon et al. (1988) reported a positive correlation between the dose of aluminium-containing phosphate-binding pharmaceutical agent prescribed and bone aluminium content, but no correlation with the serum aluminium concentration for the 6 months preceding bone biopsy.

In a worker exposed to aluminium dust and powder in a ball-mill room for 13.5 years, the aluminium concentration in lung and brain was increased 20 times and that of the liver 122 times over the normal value (Table 16). Teraoka (1981) published data indicating that aluminium concentrations were increased in the lungs (2000 mg/kg dry weight), hilar lymph nodes (3200 mg/kg dry weight), spleen (520 mg/kg dry weight), and liver (130 mg/kg dry weight) in a stone-mason dying from silicosis. The average organ concentrations in normal unexposed control males were 230, 2000, 22 and 19 mg/kg, respectively (Table 16).

6.3 Elimination and excretion

6.3.1 Animal studies

In animals aluminium is eliminated effectively by urine.

Following single intravenous doses of up to 100 µg/kg body weight in rats, aluminium was quantitatively recovered from urine (Wilhelm et al., 1992). It is difficult to obtain an accurate half-life for low oral doses, since the rate of aluminium absorption is low. Data on plasma half-life and on renal clearance have been mainly obtained from parenteral administration generally using high doses of aluminium (Wilhelm et al., 1990). It seems that at doses comparable with human exposure the plasma half-life is less than 1 h.

Based on stop-flow experiments conducted in pigs, Monteagudo et al. (1988) concluded that aluminium excretion occurs in the distal tubule of the kidney and is situated close to the sites of maximal calcium and sodium ion reabsorption.

6.3.2 Human studies

6.3.2.1 Urinary excretion

The biokinetics of aluminium in man has been evaluated by Priest and his co-workers (Priest et al., 1991, 1995b, 1996; Talbot et al., 1995) using ^{26}Al injected into human volunteers. These authors described the pattern of urinary excretion of the isotope following its intravenous injection as citrate, the effect of excretion on body retention and the relationship between aluminium levels in blood and in urine/faeces. In a first study using a single volunteer (Priest et al., 1991, 1995b, 1996), the authors confirmed that aluminium is overwhelmingly excreted by the urinary route and that most blood aluminium is cleared to excretion. More than half of the ^{26}Al had left the blood within 15 min and the decline continued, leaving < 1% in the blood after 2 days. Total excretion up to 13 days was 83% (urine) and 1.8% (faeces), leaving 15% in the body. After 4 months more than 90% was excreted. With increasing time the rate of urinary excretion, as indicated by the fraction of retained aluminium (R_t), decreased with time (t) according to the power function:

$$R_t = 35.4\, t^{-0.32}\ (t \geq 1)$$

At 1178 days after injection about 4% remained in the body; an estimated 94% had been excreted by the urinary route and 2% in the faeces. Faecal excretion most likely represented aluminium that had entered the gastrointestinal tract in bile. The power function calculated for the fraction of aluminium excreted by the urinary route (U_t) at time (t) after intake was:

$$U_t = 0.47\ t^{-1.36}$$

The excretory clearance rate (ECR) from whole blood (in kg/day) during the first two weeks after injection was expressed as:

$$ECR = 42\ t^{-0.14}$$

In a second study (Talbot et al., 1995) of shorter duration, but using six male volunteers, inter-subject variability was examined. This showed significant inter-subject variation in the pattern of aluminium excretion. For example, after 5 days an average of 71.8% ± 7.3% (SD) of the injected activity had been excreted in urine (range 62.4-82.9%). Of this total, an average of 59.1% was excreted in the first day, 7.2% in day two, 2.6% in day three, 1.7% in day four and 1.1% in the fifth day. In the same period an average of 1.2% was excreted in the faeces. With respect to blood clearance to urine, the study showed a gradual decrease in the fraction of blood aluminium excreted per unit time, indicating a changing speciation of aluminium in the blood. Overall, the results of the study were wholly consistent with those generated in the single volunteer study, with the first volunteer showing aluminium biokinetics in the middle of the range of results generated by the multi-volunteer study.

Sjögren et al. (1985) studied previously unexposed volunteers and individuals previously exposed to welding fumes containing aluminium at their workplaces for different periods of time. All subjects were exposed to welding fumes containing aluminium during a working day for about 8 h. In previously unexposed individuals urinary aluminium concentration after exposure was increased but decreased to pre-exposure levels after a few days. The half-life of the first phase of excretion was approximately 8 h. In welders exposed for less than 2 years the urinary aluminium concentration decreased during the weekend, the half-life being about 9 days. In welders exposed for more than 10 years urinary concentration did not change despite cessation of exposure. In these welders, the urine half-life was more than 6 months (Sjögren et al., 1988).

Elinder et al. (1991) analysed urinary, blood and bone aluminium content in two aluminium welders exposed to welding fumes for more than 20 years. The urinary values varied from 107 to 351 µg aluminium/litre. The daily urinary aluminium elimination was estimated to be 0.06% of the estimated body burden (on the basis of bone aluminium content), which corresponds to a half-life of about 3 years.

Ljunggren et al. (1991) studied workers occupationally exposed to aluminium flake powder after acute exposure and after periods of non-exposure of varying length. The calculated half-life during 4-5 weeks of exposure-free vacations was 6.8 weeks. In workers retired (for 6 months to 14 years) after exposure periods of 9 to 50 years, the calculated half-life varied between 0.7 and 7.9 years, depending on the length of the exposure-free period.

6.3.2.2 Biliary excretion

There is insufficient information to comment on biliary excretion of aluminium in humans.

6.4 Biological indices of exposure, body burden and organ concentration

Aluminium levels in blood and urine have been used to determine exposure levels. However, this relation is relatively weak. Blood aluminium levels are a poor indicator of tissue stores, rather indicating acute intake or rate of tissue store mobilization. In patients with impaired renal function, blood and urine levels are poor indicators of tissue levels.

High occupational exposure levels seem to be reflected better by urine levels than by blood levels, but the quantitative relation is not well established. Balance studies by current methodologies are not possible. Increased blood and urine concentrations have been observed in several groups of occupationally exposed workers and a quantitative relationship between the amount inhaled and the urinary aluminium concentration has been suggested (Sjögren et al., 1983).

A linear relationship has been observed between the air levels of aluminium exposure, the number of exposure years and the post-shift urine level in aluminium welders (Sjögren et al., 1988):

$$U_{Al} = 41.7 \times A_{Al} + 6.7 \times E - 4.6$$

where U_{Al} = urine aluminium level (µg/litre)
A_{Al} = air aluminium level (mg/m^3)
E = years of exposure

Owing to intra-individual variation, this equation can only be used for groups, not individuals. There have been no adequate investigations of the relation between air levels of exposure and urine or blood levels in workers apart from welders.

No information exists regarding the use of biological exposure indices in general populations.

7. EFFECTS ON LABORATORY MAMMALS AND *IN VITRO* TEST SYSTEMS

7.1 Single exposure

The acute toxicity is influenced by the solubility and bioavailability of the aluminium compounds administered. Aluminium compounds are only poorly absorbed after exposure by the gastro-intestinal, respiratory and dermal routes. The acute toxicity of aluminium metal and aluminium compounds is relatively low. No LC_{50} has been identified in inhalation studies.

Lethal doses of soluble aluminium compounds, such as $AlCl_3$, $Al(NO_3)_3$ and $Al_2(SO_4)_3$, have been determined by the oral or parenteral routes. Some LD_{50} values are given in Table 18.

Table 18. LD_{50} values for various aluminium compounds

Compound	Species	Route of administration	LD_{50} (mg Al/kg b.w.)	Reference
$AlCl_3$	mouse (male	oral (gavage)	770	Ondreicka
$Al_2(SO_4)_3$	Dobrá Voda)		980	et al. (1966)
$Al(NO_3)_3$	mouse (Swiss;	oral (gavage)	286	Llobet et al.
	20/sex)	i.p.	133	(1987)
$AlCl_3$		oral (gavage)	222	
		i.p.	105	
$Al_2(SO_4)_3$		oral (gavage)	> 730	
		i.p.	40	
$AlBr_3$		oral (gavage)	164	
		i.p.	108	
$Al(NO_3)_3$	rat (Sprague-	oral (gavage)	261	Llobet et al.
	Dawley, 20/sex)	i.p.	65	(1987)
$AlCl_3$		oral (gavage)	370	
		i.p.	81	
$Al_2(SO_4)_3$		oral (gavage)	> 730	
		i.p.	25	
$AlBr_3$		oral (gavage)	162	
		i.p.	82	

7.2 Short- and long-term exposure

7.2.1 *Oral administration*

Available data on the toxicity of aluminium compounds following repeated oral administration are presented in Table 19. Few of the studies reviewed are adequate to serve as a basis for the determination of effect levels, since many were designed to address principally aspects such as effect of citrate and decrements in kidney function on the body burden of aluminium; a very limited range of toxicological end-points was also examined in these studies (Ecelbarger & Greger, 1991; Greger & Powers, 1992).

There have been several repeated dose toxicity studies in which a wide range of end-points, including clinical signs, food and water consumption, growth, haematological and serum analyses, tissue and plasma concentrations of aluminium, histopathology, has been examined following oral exposure to various aluminium compounds. There were no treatment-related effects in rats fed up to 288 mg Al/kg body weight per day as sodium aluminium phosphate or 302 mg Al/kg body weight per day as aluminium hydroxide in the diet for 28 days (Hicks et al., 1987). In a subchronic study in which aluminium nitrate was administered in drinking-water to rats, the only effect observed was a significant decrease in body weight gain associated with a decrease in food consumption at 261 mg Al/kg body weight per day. (NOEL = 52 mg Al/kg body weight per day) (Domingo et al., 1987b).

When small groups of Beagle dogs were given sodium aluminium phosphate for 6 months in the diet, there were no treatment-related effects except for a decrease in food consumption not associated with a decrease in body weight (NOEL = approximately 70 mg Al/kg body weight) (Katz et al., 1984). Similarly, in small groups of Beagle dogs administered up to 80 mg Al/kg body weight per day as sodium aluminium phosphate for 26 weeks, the only treatment-related effect was a sharp, transient decrease in food consumption and concomitant decrease in body weight in males (LOEL = 75 to 80 mg Al/kg body weight per day; Pettersen et al., 1990).

In a study that was not well reported, mild histopathological effects on the kidney and liver of rats, which increased in severity with dose, were reported at doses as low as 17.2 mg Al/kg body weight (as aluminium sulfate) administered by gavage for 21 days (Roy et al.,

Table 19. Toxicity of aluminium compounds after repeated oral administration

Protocol description[a]	End-points examined	Results	Reference
5-10 male rats (Weizman strain) per group; $Al_2(SO_4)_3$ (200 or 350 mg Al/kg body weight per day in drinking-water), $AlCl_3$ (250 mg Al/kg body weight per day in drinking-water), $Al(OH_3)$ (150 mg Al/kg body weight per day by gavage) for an unspecified period; groups of animals that were 5/6 nephrectomized similarly exposed	clinical signs, histo-pathology (appears to have been limited to animals that died during study), tissue concentrations	periorbital bleeding in 3 of 5 animals at 350 mg/kg body weight per day $Al_2(SO_4)$; tissue and serum levels highest in nephrectomized animals; clinical signs of toxicity and death in all groups of nephrectomized animals; **comments:** protocol and results poorly documented; inadequate for establishment of effect levels	Berlyne et al. (1972)
Controls: 56 male Sprague-Dawley rats 10.5 mg Al/kg exposed groups 16 animals, ingesting: aluminium hydroxide, 1079 mg Al/kg diet (29 days) or 1012 mg Al/kg diet plus 4% citrate (29 days), 2688 mg/kg and 4% citrate (12 or 29 days); 24 h prior to sacrifice, all animals injected i.p. with desferrioxamine (DFO) or buffer	aluminium concentrations in tibia, liver, kidney and serum; serum aluminium concentrations after DFO; urinary aluminium excretion with and without DFO treatment; body and organ weight gain and haematological status	five of these measures (concentrations in tibia, liver, and serum and urinary excretion with and without DFO treatment); were highly correlated with oral exposure; changes induced by DFO were very small; ingestion of citrate had small but significant effects on aluminium retention; rats fed citrate weighed less (not associated with differences in intake of feed) and had significantly enlarged kidneys and livers and significantly smaller tibias; haematocrits were inversely correlated to tissue concentrations of aluminium - more evident with oral than parenteral exposure; hepatic iron was elevated with the citrate-containing diets but was only weakly correlated with hepatic aluminium concentrations;	Greger & Powers (1992)

Table 19 (contd).

		comments: comparisons of aluminium exposure in tibias and sera of rats exposed parenterally and orally indicated that 0.01 to 0.04% of dietary aluminium was absorbed; inadequate for establishment of effect levels owing to limited range of end-points examined; primarily an investigation to monitor aluminium body burdens	Greger & Powers (1992)
Administration to groups of 6 rats exposed in a 2x2x2x2 factorial design of diets containing 13 or 1112 mg Al/kg as aluminium hydroxide, citrate (0 or 5.2 mmol/kg diet) and calcium (2.7 or 10.0 g/kg diet) for 30 days; groups of 6 rats exposed in a 4x2 factorial design to 14 or 904 mg Al/kg diet and one of 4 levels of citrate (0, 10, 21 or 31 mmol/kg diet) for 28 days; groups of 7 rats exposed in 2x2x2 factorial design to 9 or 1044 mg Al/kg diet and citrate (0 or 21 mmole/kg diet) sham-operated or with one kidney removed for 28 days	tissue concentrations of aluminium; body and organ weight changes	ingestion of citrate increased retention of aluminium in bone of rats fed 1000 mg Al/kg diet and increased apparent absorption of zinc; when dietary calcium intake was increased from 67 to 250 mmol/kg diet, aluminium concentrations in bone were reduced without a change in growth of rats; reduction in kidney function (by removal of one kidney), which was insufficient to alter growth, increased aluminium retention in bone by 13% in rats fed aluminium; rats fed aluminium retained only 0.01 to 0.5% as much as those injected; **comments:** authors concluded that tissue concentrations and, presumably, toxicity can be altered by moderate changes in diet and kidney function even though overall retention of orally administered aluminium is low, inadequate for establishment of effect levels owing to limited range of end-points examined; designed primarily to investigate effect of dietary citrate, calcium and decreases in kidney function on absorption of aluminium	Ecelbarger & Greger (1991)

Table 19 (contd).

Protocol description[a]	End-points examined	Results	Reference
Groups of 10 female Sprague-Dawley receiving 1, 26, 52 or 104 mg Al/kg body weight per day as $Al(NO_3)_3$ in drinking-water for 28 days	clinical signs, food and water consumption, growth, haematological and serum analyses, tissue and plasma concentrations of aluminium, histopathology	no effects on any end-points examined except for mild histopathological changes in the spleen and liver of high dose group (hyperaemia in the red pulp of the spleen and liver; periportal lymphomonocytic infiltrate in the liver); dose-dependent accumulation of aluminium in spleen, heart and gastrointestinal tract; **comments:** well-conducted repeated dose toxicity in which a wide range of end-points was examined, though short term; NOEL = 52 mg Al/kg body weight per day; LOEL = 104 mg Al/kg body weight per day (aluminium nitrate)	Gómez et al. (1986)
Groups of female Sprague-Dawley rats receiving 0, 26, 52 or 261 mg Al/kg body weight per day as $Al(NO_3)_3$ in drinking-water for 100 days	clinical signs, food and water consumption, organ and body weights, haematological and serum analyses, tissue and plasma concentrations of aluminium, histopathology	significant decrease in body weight gain at highest dose associated with decrease in food consumption; no dose-dependent accumulation of aluminium in tissues; **comments:** well-conducted repeated dose toxicity in which a wide range of end-points; LOEL = 261 mg Al/kg body weight per day; NOEL = 52 mg Al/kg body weight per day for subchronic period of exposure	Domingo et al. (1987b)

Table 19 (contd).

Groups of Beagle dogs (4/sex) administered 0, 0.3, 1.0 or 3.0% sodium aluminium phosphate in the diet for 6 months (118, 317 and 1034 mg/kg body weight per day in males and 112, 361 and 1087 mg/kg body weight per day in females	clinical signs, food and water consumption, organ and body weights, haematological and serum analyses, urinalysis, ophthalmological examinations, tissue and plasma concentrations of aluminium, histopathology	statistically significant decreases in food consumption in females but no associated decrease in body weight; no other treatment-related effects; **comments:** wide range of end-points examined; subchronic period of exposure for dogs; small group sizes; NOEL = 1087 mg/kg body weight per day (approximately 70 mg Al/kg body weight per day)	Katz et al. (1984)
Groups of Beagle dogs (4/sex) administered 0, 10, 22 to 27 or 75 to 80 mg Al/kg body weight per day as sodium aluminium phosphate in the diet for 26 weeks	clinical signs, food and water consumption, organ and body weights, haematological and serum analyses, urinalysis, ophthalmological examinations, tissue and plasma concentrations of aluminium, histopathology	sharp, transient decrease in food consumption and concomitant decrease in body weight in high-dose males; in same group, decrease in testes weight and histopathological changes in the liver and kidney considered to be secondary to decreased food consumption; slight increase in concentration of aluminium in the brain in high-dose females but not males; **comments:** wide range of end-points examined; subchronic period of exposure for dogs; small group sizes; minimal toxicity at the highest dose; LOEL = 75 to 80 mg Al/kg body weight per day	Pettersen et al. (1990)
Groups of 25 male Sprague-Dawley rats fed control diets or 30 000 mg/kg KASAL I (6% aluminium-sodium aluminium phosphate), 7000 or 30 000 mg/kg KASAL II (13% aluminium-sodium aluminium phosphate) or 14 470 mg/kg aluminium hydroxide for 28 days (5, 141, 67, 288, 302 mg Al/kg body weight per day, respectively)	clinical signs, food and water consumption, organ and body weights, haematology and clinical chemistry urinalysis, ophthalmological examinations, concentrations of aluminium in the femur, histopathology	no treatment-related effects or significant deposition of aluminium in bone; **comments:** wide range of end-points examined; short-term exposure; no effects at 141 mg Al/kg body weight per day KASAL I; NOEL for KASAL II = 288 mg Al/kg body weight per day; no effects at 302 mg Al/kg body weight per day aluminium hydroxide	Hicks et al. (1987)

Table 19 (contd).

Protocol description[a]	End-points examined	Results	Reference
Groups of 15 albino male rats administered aluminium sulfate (0, 17, 22, 29, 43, 86 and 172 mg Al/kg body weight) and potassium aluminium sulfate (43 mg Al/kg body weight, 29 mg Al/kg body weight) in deionized water for 21 days; 5 rats killed weekly	histopathological examination of heart, liver, kidney, brain, testes, stomach and femur	dose-related cytotoxic effect in the liver - cytoplasmic degeneration at 17 to 29 mg Al/kg body weight with multifocal degeneration and fibrous tissue proliferation at higher doses. Dose-related effects in the kidney at 17 mg Al/kg body weight per day as aluminium sulfate, slight swelling of the tubules. With increased dose, increased swelling and degeneration of the cortical tubules. Degeneration of the nerve cell at 29 and 43 mg Al/kg body weight per day aluminium sulfate and potassium aluminium sulfate, respectively, which was more severe at higher doses. Some evidence of spermatological cell decrease at doses of 43 mg Al/kg body weight per day and above. Multifocal degeneration and decalcification at 43 mg Al/kg body weight per day and above for both salts, which increased with increasing dose; degeneration of calcified bone and irregularity of osteoblasts in animals exposed to 86 and 171 mg Al/kg body weight as aluminium sulfate. Hyperplasia and ulceration of stomach at highest doses. **Comments:** difficult to verify reported effect levels based on limited information presented in paper.	Roy et al. (1991b)

[a] Strain, number of animals/group and vehicle specified, where available; doses reported as mg/kg body weight, unless specified

1991b). Data presented in the report were inadequate to verify the reported effect levels.

7.2.2 Inhalation exposure

Many inhalation/intra-tracheal instillation studies have been conducted using aluminium compounds, including chloride, chloro-hydrate, oxyhydrate and oxides (Stacy et al., 1959; Corrin, 1963; Christie et al., 1963; Gross et al., 1973; Drew et al., 1974; Steinhagen et al., 1978; Stone et al., 1979; Finelli et al., 1981; Thompson et al., 1986). However, in the case of the inhalation studies, little data is available concerning exposure conditions and the size of the ambient aerosol, and some studies were of relatively short duration compared with the life-span of the animal employed. Consequently, although no toxic effects were reported in nearly all cases, it is not possible to assess how much, if any, of the compound was deposited in the lungs of the experimental animal, and the time-span of the experiment may have been too short to demonstrate delayed effects. The only inhalation study that demonstrated an effect was that of Finelli et al. (1981) who described increased lung size. Where aluminium oxide particles were administered by intra-tracheal instillation, fibrosis has been consistently reported (Stacy et al., 1959; Corrin, 1963). Dinman (1988) described this disease as "alumina-related pulmonary disease". However, such fibrosis is a common consequence of the inhalation of many particles, including silica and coal; it is unlikely to be related to aluminium *per se*, but rather to the physical properties of the particle inhaled.

7.2.3 Parenteral administration

Aluminium compounds were found to possess an increased toxicity when administered parenterally rather than orally. The effect depends on the dose, the aluminium compound used and the particular animal model. It can vary from death to behavioural alteration (loss of memory), loss of weight or minor changes in aluminium accumulation in bone. A LOAEL of approximately 1 mg/kg body weight per day can be obtained by this route for osteomalacia or for deterioration of renal function (Chan et al., 1983; Henry et al., 1984; Quarles et al., 1985; Bräunlich et al., 1986). Partially nephrectomized animals exhibited greater susceptibility to aluminium (Ittel et al., 1992).

7.3 Reproductive and developmental toxicity

7.3.1 Reproductive effects

The limited number of studies are not able to provide adequate information on reproductive toxicity (Domingo, 1995). Of these, few provide direct and complete evaluations of reproduction.

Domingo et al. (1987a) administered aluminium nitrate at 0, 13, 26 or 52 mg Al/kg body weight per day by intubation to male rats for 60 days prior to mating and to virgin females treated for 14 days prior to mating. The same doses were administered by gavage to pregnant animals from 14 days gestation to 21 days of lactation in a separate study (Domingo et al., 1987c). Domingo et al. (1987a) reported no reproductive effects on fertility (number of litters produced), litter size, or intrauterine or postnatal offspring mortality. Numbers of corpus lutea on day 13 of gestation were significantly lower at 52 mg Al/kg body weight per day. However a dose-dependant delay in the growth of the pups was observed in all treatment groups; female offspring were affected at 13 mg Al/kg body weight per day and males at 26 and 52 mg Al/kg body weight per day. Because of the design of the study by Domingo et al. (1987a) it is not clear whether the postnatal growth effects in offspring represented general toxicity to male or female parents, or represented specific effects on reproduction or development. However, the reported LOAEL for adverse effects in females in this study was 13 mg Al/kg body weight per day.

Dosing of pregnant animals from 14 days gestation to 21 days lactation with 13, 26 or 52 mg Al/kg body weight per day did not produce overt fetotoxicity (Domingo et al., 1987c), but growth of offspring was significantly delayed (body weight, body length and tail length) from birth to weaning.

7.3.2 Developmental effects

Details of the study designs of oral or gavage dosing studies of developmental toxicity are given in Table 20. Aluminium chloride administered i.p. to rats (Benett et al., 1975) or i.v. to mice (Wide, 1984) during embryogenesis produced a syndrome characterized by delayed and incomplete ossification of skull and vertebrae, skeletal variations and malformations, internal haemorrhage and reduced fetal

Table 20. Developmental toxicity after oral administration of aluminium salts[a]

Species	Route of application	Compound	Dose	Duration	Reference
Mouse (Swiss, 20/group)	oral (gavage)	$Al(OH)_3$	66.5, 133, 266 mg/kg b.w./day	gest. day 6-15	Domingo et al. (1989)
Mouse (BALB/c, 6-7 mice/group)	oral (gavage)	$AlCl_3$	oral: 200, 300 mg/kg b.w./day	gest. day 7-16	Cranmer et al. (1986)
Mouse (Swiss Webster, 15/group)	oral (feed)	Al lactate	500, 1000 mg Al/kg diet	gest. day 0 to day 21 p.p.	Golub et al. (1987)
Mouse (16 Swiss Webster)	oral (feed)	Al lactate	25, 500, 1000 mg Al/kg diet	gest. day 0, until weaning	Donald et al. (1989)
Mouse (Swiss albino CD-1, 10-13/group)	oral (gavage)	$Al(OH)_3$ Al lactate $Al(OH)_3$ + lactic acid	57.5 mg/kg b.w./day 166 mg/kg/day 627 mg/kg/day	gest. day 6-15	Colomina et al. (1992)
Mouse (Swiss Webster)	oral (feed)	Al lactate	25, 1000 mg/kg diet/day	gest. day 0 - day 20 p.p.	Golub et al. (1992)
Mouse (CBA)	oral (water)	$Al_2(SO_4)_3$	750 mg/litre	gest. day 10-17	Clayton et al. (1992)

Table 20 (contd).

Species	Route of application	Compound	Dose	Duration	Reference
Rat (Sprague-Dawley)	oral (feed)	$AlCl_3$	50 mg/kg b.w.	gest. day 6-19	McCormack et al. (1979)
Rat (Wistar, 14/group)	oral (feed)	Al lactate	100, 200, 300 mg Al/kg b.w.	gest. day 8 to parturition	Bernuzzi et al. (1986, 1989a,b)
Rat (Sprague-Dawley)	oral (gavage)	$Al(NO_3)_3$	180, 360, 720 mg/kg day	gest. day 14-21	Domingo et al. (1987a)
Rat (Sprague-Dawley, 10/group)	oral (gavage)	$Al(NO_3)_3$	180, 360, 720 mg/kg b.w.	gest. day 6-14	Paternain et al. (1988)
Rat (Sprague-Dawley, 15-19/group)	oral (gavage)	$Al(OH)_3$ Al citrate $Al(OH)_3$ + citric acid	384 mg/kg/day 1064 mg/kg/day	gest. day 6-15	Gómez et al. (1991)
Rat (Wistar, 18-19/group)	oral (gavage)	$Al(OH)_3$	192, 384, 768 mg/kg/day	gest. day 6-15	Gómez et al. (1990)
Rat (Wistar, 6-9/group)	oral (feed)	Al lactate	400 mg Al/kg diet	gest. day 1-7 gest. day 1-14 gest. day 1-20	Muller et al. (1990)

[a] b.w. = body weight; gest. = gestational; p.p. = postpartum

growth. Abnormal digits were also noted in rats. Administration of aluminium chloride in the diet with accompanying parathyroid hormone (PTH) injection (McCormack et al., 1979) also produced reduced skeletal ossification and increased incidence of skeletal variations. Maternal toxicity in the study of Benett et al. (1975) included reduced weight gain, hepatic granulomas and necrosis and maternal death at the highest dose levels (100 and 200 mg Al/kg per day). Resorption and embryolethality were seen primarily at highly maternally toxic doses (200 mg Al/kg per day). Maternal monitoring and reduced gestational weight gain were not seen at the LOAEL for developmental toxicity (75 mg Al/kg per day; day 9-13 of gestation). At this dose mean fetal weight and crown rump were reduced, and the number of resorptions increased. The use of i.p. administration makes it difficult to interpret these results with regards to human health effects.

The severity of developmental aluminium toxicity by the oral route is highly dependent on the form of aluminium and the presence of organic chelators that influence bioavailability, as demonstrated in a series of studies by Domingo (1995) using gavage administration during embryogenesis. Aluminium nitrate (nonahydrate) produced developmental effects in rats (Paternain et al., 1988) similar to the effects seen after i.p. injections (Benett et al., 1975), including skeletal variations, poor ossification, haemorrhage, oligodactyly and some soft tissue malformations. Aluminium hydroxide did not produce either maternal or developmental toxicity when it was administered by gavage during embryogenesis to rats (Gómez et al., 1990) or mice (Domingo et al., 1989). When aluminium hydroxide was administered with ascorbate (Colomina et al., 1994), no maternal or developmental toxicity was seen in mice in spite of elevated maternal tissue concentrations of aluminium, whereas aluminium hydroxide given with citrate produced maternal and fetal toxicity in rats (Gómez et al., 1991). Aluminium hydroxide given with lactate was not toxic, but aluminium lactate administration produced developmental toxicity, in mice including poor ossification, skeletal variations and cleft palate (Colomina et al., 1992).

In summary, developmental toxicology syndromes described above commonly included growth retardation, such as lower fetal weights and length (Bennet et al., 1975; Paternain et al., 1988; Gómez et al., 1990; Colomina et al., 1992). A study using s.c. administration of aluminium lactate did not demonstrate any developmental effects other than lower fetal length (Golub et al., 1987). Postnatal growth retardation has also been demonstrated in rats exposed in late gestation to aluminium nitrate (Domingo, 1987c) and in rabbits treated postnatally with aluminium lactate s.c. (Yokel, 1984). Reduced bone formation demonstrated when postnatal aluminium lactate was administered subcutaneously in rabbits (Yokel, 1987) supports the importance of bone as a target organ for developmental effects of aluminium.

Effects of aluminium exposures on brain development have also been studied in mice (Donald et al., 1989; Golub et al., 1992, 1994, 1995; Clayton et al., 1992) and rats (Bernuzzi et al., 1986, 1989a,b; Muller et al., 1990; Cherroret et al., 1992) by the oral route, and in rabbits (Yokel, 1984, 1985, 1987) using subcutaneous injections. Effects recorded in immature animals in more than one study in rats and mice included impaired performance of reflexes and simple behaviours (e.g., righting reflex, grasping, negative geotaxis, rod climbing). Other effects included footsplay and temperature sensitivity (tail withdrawal); (Donald et al., 1989; Golub et al., 1992) and auditory startle (Golub et al., 1994). Postnatal mortality and growth were also affected at the higher doses in only some of these studies. Studies of cognitive parameters in immature animals are limited to evaluation of classical conditioning of the nictating membrane response in rabbits. No effect of aluminium was seen after postnatal subcutaneous injection of aluminium lactate (Yokel, 1987); both enhancement and impairment of conditioning were seen after exposure during gestation to aluminium lactate, depending on the dose (Yokel, 1985).

Adult rats and mice have also been evaluated for brain function after developmental exposures. Reduced grip strength and startle responsiveness were found to persist up to 150 days of age in mice (Golub et al., 1995). No effect was found on a light avoidance task in rats after gestational (Bernuzzi et al., 1989b) or postnatal exposure (Cherroret et al., 1992). Radial maze learning/performance was also unaffected by postnatal exposure (Cherroret et al., 1992). No effects on delayed alternation or discrimination reversals were recorded in mice after dietary exposure during gestation and lactation (Golub et al., 1995).

The lowest-observed-adverse-effect level (LOAEL) for developmental effects after oral dosing was 13 mg Al/kg body weight per day by oral gavage of aluminium nitrate (Paternian et al., 1988). A dose-response relationship was noted with the highest dose of this extremely soluble aluminium salts (52 mg Al/kg body weight) representing 1/5 the LD_{50} (see Table 18). At 13 mg Al/kg per day, decreased ossification of skull bones, increased incidence of vertebral and sternebrae, and reduced fetal weight and tail length were reported with higher incidence of these effects at the higher doses (26 and 52 mg Al/kg body weight). Maternal toxicity (reduced weight gain during pregnancy) was reported to occur in a dose-dependent manner. No developmental toxicity was noted using much higher doses of aluminium hydroxide (266 mg Al/kg per day) in a similarly designed study (Gómez et al., 1990).

After administration of aluminium lactate in the diet of mice and rats a LOAEL of 100 mg Al/kg body weight per day was reported (Donald et al., 1989; Bernuzzi et al., 1989a,b).

The effect reported at 100 mg Al/kg per day by Bernuzzi et al. (1989a,b) in rats was impaired grip strength in the 6-day-old offspring of dams fed aluminium lactate in diet throughout gestation. Dose response was indicated in this study; at higher doses (200 and 400 mg Al/kg per day) impaired grip strength was reported along with impaired righting reflex and locomotor coordination. No effects on maternal or offspring weight were reported at 100 mg Al/kg although they occurred at the higher doses. Litters were not culled to a standard size at birth in this study. The litter was used as the unit of statistical analysis to avoid litter effect.

The effects reported at 100 mg Al/kg per day by Donald et al. (1989) in mice were increased landing foot splay, increased hindlimb grip strength and decreased temperature sensitivity in 21-day-old offspring of mice fed aluminium lactate in the diet throughout gestation and lactation. There was no effect on negative geotaxis or startle reflexes in the offspring. Dose response was not indicated in this study; similar effects were reported at a higher dose (200 mg Al/kg). No effects on maternal or offspring weights were found at either dose. It is not stated whether litters were culled to a standard number at birth. To address litter effects, litter was nested under treatment group in the statistical analysis. In this study, daily aluminium intake was estimated based on food intake at the beginning of pregnancy.

7.4 Mutagenicity and related end-points

7.4.1 Interactions with DNA

A number of observations indicate that aluminium is able to form complexes with DNA and can cross-link chromosomal proteins and DNA. In thermal denaturation, circular dichroism and fluorescence studies, Karlik et al. (1980) found that aluminium had a stabilizing effect upon the DNA double helix at a pH > 6, while at lower pH levels, binding of aluminium de-stabilized the DNA double helix. A recent investigation of NMR spectra and circular dichroism of DNA-aluminium complexes indicated that Al^{3+} binds to the phosphate oxygen while hydroxylated aluminium-species probably prefer other sites such as DNA bases (Rao & Divakar, 1993).

Cross-linking of various cytoplasmic proteins to DNA was investigated in live Novikoff ascites hepatoma cells exposed to aluminium *in vitro* (Wedrychowski et al., 1986). Cross-linking agents frequently produce clastogenic effects, owing to conformational distortions that prohibit proper replication of the DNA. More recently it was shown that AlF_4^- stimulates the glycation of the histone H1 in the proximity of its nucleotide-binding site, thus interfering with nucleoside triphosphate hydrolysis by H1 and with nucleotide modulation of H1 DNA binding (Tarkka et al., 1993).

In addition, it has been shown that micro-molar levels of aluminium reduce ^{3}H-thymidine incorporation in a transformed cell line (UMR 106-01) by impeding the cell cycle progression (Blair et al., 1989). More specifically, aluminium was shown to inhibit the ADP-ribosylation, a mechanism important for DNA repair, *in vivo* and *in vitro* (Crapper McLachlan et al., 1983).

7.4.2 Mutations

The rec-assay using *Bacillus subtilis* strains failed to show mutagenic activity for Al_2O_3, $AlCl_3$ or $Al_2(SO_4)_3$ at concentrations of 1-10 mM (Nishioka, 1975; Kada et al., 1980; Kanematsu et al., 1980; Léonard & Gerber, 1988; Bhamra & Costa, 1992). No reverse mutations were observed in the Ames test using *Salmonella typhimurium* strain TA102 with $AlCl_3$ (concentration range 10-100 nM per plate; Marzin & Phi, 1985). No morphological transformations were seen in Syrian hamster embryo cells after application of aluminium salts (no further specification) (Di Paolo & Casto, 1979). No induction of forward mutations were observed at the thymidine kinase locus in L5178Y mouse lymphoma assay with AlCl$_3$ when tested at concentrations up to 625 µg AlCl$_3$/ml (Oberly et al., 1982).

7.4.3 Chromosomal effects

A significant increase of chromatid-type aberrations (including gaps, breaks, translocation and ring formations), with non-random distribution over the chromosome complement, was found in bone marrow cells from mice that were dosed interperitoneally with AlCl$_3$ (Manna & Das, 1972). Prolonged treatment of rats with Al$_2$(SO$_4$)$_3$ or KAl(SO$_4$)$_2$ caused a dose-dependent inhibition of dividing cells (bone marrow) and an increase in chromosomal aberrations (Roy et al., 1991a). Chromosomal aberrations were also induced in peritoneal cells from rats, mice and Chinese hamsters (Bhamra & Costa, 1992) as well as in human leukocyte cultures (Roy et al., 1990). Aluminium caused a concentration-dependent bimodal change in the number of sister chromatid exchange in cultured human lymphocytes and increased the unscheduled DNA synthesis in cultured human astrocytes (De Boni et al., 1980).

7.5 Carcinogenicity

Based on limited early studies, there is little indication that aluminium is carcinogenic (Leonard & Gerber, 1988; Bhamra & Costa, 1992). Some studies indicated that inhalation of aluminium-containing fibres and particles may induce carcinomas in the lung. However, in these cases it is likely that the toxicity reflects the physical properties of the particles/fibres (3.5 µm median diameter). Similarly, aluminium implanted subcutaneously has induced soft tissue carcinomas at the site of implantation, but in these cases also the effects are probably related to a chronic foreign body reaction rather than to the aluminium ion itself (Stanton, 1974; Pigott & Ishmael, 1981; Pigott et al., 1981; Krueger et al., 1984).

7.6 Neurotoxicity

Considerable evidence indicates that aluminium is neurotoxic to experimental animals, but species variation exists. In susceptible animals, the toxicity is characterized by progressive neurological impairment resulting in death associated with status epilepticus. Morphologically, the progressive encephalopathy is associated with neurofibrillary pathology in large and medium size neurons predominantly in the spinal cord, brain stem, and selected areas of cortex (hippocampus and cingulate gyrus). However the nature of the accumulated fibrils at the light microscopic level and under the electron microscope differ from those found in AD. The tangles are not birefringent and are composed of 10 nm neurofilaments. The proteins involved in the aluminium-induced neurofibrillary tangles also differ from those found in the human diseases (see section 8.1.3.1). However, aluminium is the only known trace element capable of inducing this type of mylo-encephalopathy in susceptible animals (rabbit, cat, guinea-pig, ferret). The epileptogenic property of aluminium, in contrast to the progressive encephalopathy, occurs in all species studied (e.g., primates, rodents, fish). Routes of administration of aluminium sufficient to induce the encephalopathy include intrathecal intracerebral and subcutaneous injections. There have been no reports of progressive encephalopathy or epilepsy when aluminium compounds were given orally.

The brain aluminium concentration necessary to achieve LD_{50} in rabbits is about 6 µg aluminium/g dry weight (Crapper McLachlan et al., 1989; McLachlan & Massiah, 1992). The normal brain aluminium concentration in healthy rabbits is approximately 1.1 µg/dry weight.

7.6.1 *Impairments of cognitive and motor function*

Cats and adult or infant rabbits given intracerebral injections of soluble aluminium compounds revealed a progressive impairment in learning and memory performance after an asymptomatic period of 8 to 10 days (Crapper & Dalton, 1973a,b; Petit et al., 1980; Rabe et al., 1982; Solomon et al., 1990). Repeated subcutaneous injections of aluminium in rabbits affected classical conditioning (Yokel, 1983).

The intracisternal injection of a single or repeated low doses of metallic aluminium in rabbits resulted in altered motor function (Wisniewski et al., 1982; Bugiani & Ghetti, 1982; Strong et al., 1991; Strong & Garruto, 1991b). The animals developed progressive myelopathy and topographically specific motor neuron degeneration. They exhibited myoclonic jerks and muscular weakness. Histopathologically a neurofibrillary degeneration with swelling of the proximal axonal processes of anterior horn neurons was present. The authors proposed these preparations as possible models of human amyotrophic lateral sclerosis.

Behavioural impairment has been reported in laboratory animals exposed to aluminium in the diet or drinking-water in the absence of overt encephalopathy or neurohistopathology. Both rats (Commissaris et al., 1982; Thorne et al., 1987; Connor et al., 1988) and mice (Yen-Koo, 1992) have demonstrated such impairments at doses exceeding 200 mg Al/kg body weight. While significant alterations in acquisition and retention of learned behaviour were documented, the possible role of organ damage (kidney, liver, immunological) due to aluminium was incompletely evaluated.

7.6.2 *Alterations in electrophysiological properties*

The progressive encephalopathy and morphological alterations are also associated with electrophysiological changes. The epileptic seizures are associated with slowing of the EEG and epileptic activity. The mechanisms that evoke the neuronal hyperexcitability have not yet been completely elucidated but may involve altered membrane electrotonic properties, K^+ conductance, and synaptic processes (Franceschetti et al., 1990). Associative long-term potentiation (LTP), describes strengthening of a previously weak synaptic input by concomitant activation of a strong synaptic input. LTP can last up to several weeks and has been used as a model for the hippocampal contribution to memory. LTP was not sustained normally in hippocampal slices from rabbits exposed to intracranial injections of aluminium about 7 days prior to sacrifice. The occurrence of this electrophysiological alteration corresponds to the onset of behavioural changes but is not necessarily accompanied by neurofibrillary pathology in the hippocampal neurons exhibiting impaired LTP. The loss of LTP can be partially reversed by an increase in the calcium concentration in the bath (Farnell et al., 1985; Crapper McLachlan & Farnell, 1986).

In summary, aluminium exposure has been used as an animal model for the study of epilepsy, information processing, cognitive dysfunction and motor neuron disease.

7.6.3 *Metabolic effects in the nervous system*

Considerable experimental evidence implicates aluminium in alterations in the second messenger systems of cAMP and G proteins (Steinweis & Gilman, 1982; Johnson & Jope, 1987; Johnson et al., 1990, 1992). An increased cAMP concentration in brain tissue is a prerequisite for an increase in the phosphorylation of proteins. An elevation of protein kinase C activity and in the basal activity of cAMP-dependent protein kinase resulted in hyperphosphorylation of 12 proteins in rats chronically treated with aluminium (Johnson et al., 1990). In rats chronically treated with low oral doses of aluminium, hyperphosphorylation of MAP-2 was increased by 150% and the neurofilament H subunit by 150-200%, while the phosphorylation of several other proteins including tau was not different from that of control rats (Johnson et al., 1990; Jope & Johnson, 1992). It was suggested that abnormal phosphorylation may impair the axonal transport of cytoskeletal proteins.

Ohtawa et al. (1983) showed that Al^{3+} binding to ferritin reduced the binding of Fe^{2+} in rats fed aluminium. The free intracellular Fe^{2+} augmented the peroxidation of membrane lipids. Lipid peroxidation in kidney, lung, liver and spleen were not affected. The increased lipid peroxidation is at least, in part, due to inhibition of superoxide dismutase in the brain but not in other organ systems. An increase in lipid peroxidation was also shown in chickens fed with aluminium sulfate (Chainy et al., 1993). It is presumed that an increase in lipid peroxidation may be part of the mechanisms underlying aluminium neurotoxicity.

Aluminium is not equally distributed among chromatin fractions within the nucleus in control and aluminium-treated preparations. Concentrations of aluminium on highly condensed, non-transcribed chromatin are 15 to 20 times higher than those on active, decondensed chromatin (Crapper et al., 1980). Several experimental models have demonstrated that aluminium inhibits RNA synthesis and therefore may have an effect on gene expression.

Transient change in the blood-brain barrier to [^{14}C]sucrose have been observed following low-dose intraperitoneal injection of aluminium compounds (Kim et al., 1986). Intraperitoneal administration of aluminium compounds increased the permeability of the blood-brain barrier for a number of peptide and steroid hormones, such as prolactin, growth hormone, luteinizing hormone, thyroxine and cortisol. The greatest increase in penetration was observed for thyroxine, which is transported by a carrier-mediated mechanism (Banks & Kastin, 1985). From further studies on other transport systems, it was suggested that aluminium selectively alters the transport systems of the blood-brain barrier (Banks et al., 1988a; Vorbrodt et al., 1994).

7.7 Effects on bone

The skeleton is the principal site of aluminium deposition in the body. Aluminium deposited in this organ is important both because of its toxic effects on bone tissues and because the deposits act as a reservoir. Aluminium continues to be released from this reservoir to the blood stream for a long time after intake as a consequence of bone turnover, commonly referred to as bone remodelling.

Within the skeleton aluminium, in common with most other polyvalent metal ions, deposits on bone surfaces within a very thin layer (van de Vyver & Visser, 1990). How metal ions deposit in this way is unclear, but three modes of uptake have been suggested. Firstly, the metal may become trapped within the hydration shell of the bone mineral crystal, secondly, it may become incorporated into new bone crystals as they form at sites of bone accretion, and, finally, they may become bound by acidic organic components of the bone matrix, such as phosphoproteins (Priest, 1990). Subsequently, much of the aluminium may remain on surfaces until it back-exchanges into tissue fluids or may become locked into the bone matrix. "Locked in" ions may then become buried to form volume deposits below bone surfaces, as a result of bone accretion, or may be released by the bone resorption process. Resorbed aluminium first enters osteoclasts and macrophages and then returns to tissue fluids, including blood, for recycling or excretion. The burial and resorption processes take many years in man, where only a minority of surfaces show remodelling activity, but occur rapidly in most experimental animals. As the rate of bone turnover is largely under hormonal control, it follows that hormones also regulate the retention by and release from the skeleton of the more permanent deposits of aluminium. In this respect the most important hormones are calcitonin and parathyroid hormone (PTH), which act to increase either the rate of bone formation or the rate of bone resorption in response to serum levels of calcium.

7.7.1 *Toxic effects of aluminium in the skeleton*

Excess deposits of aluminium in the skeleton may result in a syndrome commonly referred to as "aluminium-induced bone disease" (AIBD). This has been reviewed by Goodman (1986, 1990), van de Vyver & Visser (1990) and Quarles (1991). A summary of some of the animal models used to study osteomalacia induced by aluminium is given in Table 21. It should be noted that all models utilize intraperitoneal or intravenous routes of administration, making it impossible to extrapolate to the risk in humans exposed to aluminium primarily by the oral route. AIBD presents as a moderate to severe low bone turnover osteomalacia, which is often insensitive to the vitamin D complexes that reverse the osteomalacia of rickets. It may also result in the de-coupling of the bone resorption and bone accretion processes producing an excess volume of structurally incompetent bone (neo-osteogenesis) and in disturbances in the normal processes of endochondral ossification in the long-bone metaphyses. In osteomalacic bones, osteoid (the unmineralized bone matrix) fails to mineralize or is increased (Goodman et al., 1984a,b; Sedman et al., 1987; Quarles et al., 1988), tetracycline markers of bone mineralization are not incorporated (Ellis et al., 1979) and bone resorption is reduced, resulting in an increase in the volume of unmineralized bone. Associated with these changes is a reduction in the number of osteoblasts (bone-forming cells) (Robertson et al., 1983) and a reduction in the level of circulatory osteocalcin produced by these cells. If osteomalacic bones are stained for aluminium then the metal may be demonstrated as being present at the mineralized bone/osteoid interface. Where present it would seem that the aluminium inhibits the mineralization of osteoid, this amounting to a complete block in severe cases. However, the mechanism for this block is unknown. Goodman (1990) has suggested that it results from an impairment of the movement of calcium and phosphate ions from the tissue fluids to the face of the forming hydroxyapatite bone-mineral crystals.

Aluminium, like some other metals, e.g., strontium, when present in bone crystals reduces the ability of the osteoclast (the bone resorbing cells) to resorb the mineral. As expected, reduced bone turnover may result in a reduced level of calcium in blood (hypocalcaemia), which, in turn, might be expected to produce changes in the levels of bone-active hormones in the circulation.

Table 21. Experimental animal models of aluminium-induced osteomalacia[a]

Species	Route of appli- cation	Compound	Dose	Duration of treatment	Al concentration in bone[b]	Histomorphometry	Reference
Rat (20 Wistar)	i.p.	AlCl₃	0.27-2.7 mg Al/day	once daily; 5 days/ week; 48-85 days	(15.4 µg/g), 109.3-176 µg/g	n.d.	Ellis et al. (1979)
Rat	i.p.	AlCl₃	N (control), LD: 0.1 mg Al/day; HD: 1.0 mg Al/day	once daily; 5 days/ week; 90-120 days	n.d.	% osteoid: N: 6.6; LD: 7.8; HD: 1.8; osteoid width (µm): N: 3.3; LD: 3.7; HD: 14.9; tetracycline uptake: irregular, attenuated in HD	Robertson et al. (1983)
Rat (74 male SD)	i.p.	AlCl₃	1.5 mg Al/kg b.w. per day	5 days/week; 35-79 days	55 mg/kg d.w.		Alfrey et al. (1985)
Rat (weanling, male H, 10/group)	i.p.	Al, elemental	2 mg/day	5 days/week, 4 weeks	not specified	decreased bone formation and osteoid maturation in Al-treated animals	Goodman et al. (1984b)
Rat (weanling male H, 10/group)	i.p.	Al, elemental	2 mg/day	5 days/week, 44 days	not specified	formation of periosteal bone and matrix reduced	Goodman (1984)

Table 21 (contd).

Species	Route of appli-cation	Compound	Dose	Duration of treatment	Al concentration in bone[b]	Histomorphometry	Reference
Rat (male W, 23)	i.p.	$AlCl_3$	1.5 mg Al/kg day;	5 days/week, 9 weeks	control: 1.8 mg/kg d.w.; Al-treated: 47.0 mg/kg d.w.	osteoid width (µm): normal: 3.5; Al-treated: 3.0	Chan et al. (1983)
Rat (male H, 18/group) weanling, adult	i.p.	$AlCl_3$	10 mg/kg per day	5 days/week	3, 6, 9 weeks, 3 weeks recovery	9 w: trabecular and endo-steal bone formation decreased; periosteal bone formation normal, recovery to normal level	Ott et al. (1987)
Dog (Beagle, 6/group)	i.v.	$AlCl_3$	1 mg/kg b.w.	3 times weekly 3 weeks	control: 10.5 mg/kg d.w. Al-treated: 73.6 mg/kg d.w.	% osteoid surface: control: 35.6% Al-treated: 35.8%	Quarles et al. (1985)
Dog (6 female mongrel)	i.v.	$AlCl_3$	1 mg Al/kg b.w. per day	3-5 weeks	(1.3 mg/kg), 94 mg/kg d.w.	% osteoid: (2.8)[b] 7.0 osteoid width: (5.7)[b] 8.0 poor tetracycline uptake	Goodman et al. (1984a)

Table 21 (contd).

Species	Route	Compound	Dose	Schedule	Concentration in bone	Effects	Reference
Dog (female mongrel, 7/group)	i.v.	AlCl₃	0.75 mg Al/kg b.w.	5 days/week, 3 months	(7.4 mg/kg d.w.) 202.6 mg/kg d.w.	number of osteoblasts 8-fold decreased	Galceran et al. (1987)
Dog (18 male Beagles)	i.v.	AlCl₃	0.75 mg Al/kg b.w. / 1.2 mg Al/kg b.w.	3 days/week, 16 weeks	(2.2 µg/g) low dose, 8 weeks: 65.8 mg/kg low dose, 16 weeks: 161.7 mg/kg / high dose, 8 weeks: 125.2 mg/kg high dose, 16 weeks: 152.2 mg/kg	low dose, 8 weeks; reduced bone resorption and osteoblastic surfaces; low turnover: low dose, 16 weeks; increased trabecular number; uncoupled bone formation / high dose, 8 and 16 weeks: uncoupled bone formation	Quarles et al. (1988)
Dog (8 male Beagles), normal	i.v.	AlCl₃	1.25 mg/kg b.w. per day	3 days/week: 8 weeks	(4.2 ng/litre) sham op. + Al: 147 ng/litre	sham op. + Al bone volume, tabecular number increased	Quarles et al. (1989)
Piglets (8 Yorkshire)	i.v.	AlCl₃	1.5 mg/kg per day	8 weeks	(1.6 mg/kg d.w.) 241 mg/kg d.w.	osteoid seam width, osteoid volume, mineralization lag time: increased; reduction of active bone forming surface	Sedman et al. (1987)

[a] b.w = body weight; d.w. = dry weight; H = Holtzman; i.p. = intraperitoneally; i.v. = intravenous; n.d. = no data; SD = Sprague-Dawley; W = Wistar; N = control; LD = low dose; HD = high dose; op = operation

[b] Control values are given in parentheses

In particular aluminium-induced hypocalcaemia would be expected to result in increased production of parathyroid hormone (PTH), in an attempt to stimulate bone resorption and restore normal blood calcium levels. However, the available evidence suggests that this does not occur and that the levels of circulating PTH are normal or even reduced (Goodman et al., 1984a). Rodriguez et al. (1990) found that PTH is able to stimulate osteoblasts in the presence of aluminium, but that it cannot improve mineralization. Similarly, there is also much evidence to suggest that fluoride (a potent stimulator of osteoblast numbers) interacts with aluminium in the skeleton by antagonizing the aluminium-induced reduction in osteoblast numbers, but does not ameliorate the aluminium-induced decrease in mineralization (Ittel et al., 1992).

Of the available animal models, only the larger species, e.g., dogs and pigs, consistently show osteomalacia as it presents in man (Goodman, 1990). In rodents bone remodelling is an unimportant feature of normal bone turnover (bone growth continues throughout life), and in these animals aluminium does not produce classical osteomalacia, although the changes in bone accretion, mineralization and resorption seen in the larger species are also seen in rats and mice. In these species, the disturbances seen in the ossification and resorption of bone under the growth cartilages may indicate a risk of similar occurrences in aluminium-contaminated children. Animal studies have shown that osteomalacia in trabecular bone is induced faster than in cortical bone, a result of the lower bone turnover in the latter (Goodman et al., 1984a,b).

Neo-osteogenesis, resulting in large increases in the volume of trabecular bone, following aluminium administration has been observed in a number of animal studies (Galceran et al., 1987; Quarles et al., 1988, 1990) and has even been suggested as a possible treatment for post-menopausal osteoporosis in women. In these studies a dose and time-dependent effect was seen, lower levels of aluminium suppressing bone formation but higher doses for long periods of time resulting in an increased bone volume. Under such conditions it is likely that bone apposition has become uncoupled from bone resorption processes - a pathological change.

7.7.2 *Dose response*

As indicated above, the extent of pathological changes in bone produced by aluminium after parenteral administration is dose-dependent (Goodman, 1986), being barely perceptible at low doses, but marked or severe at high doses. However, dose response will be much affected by the period of aluminium accumulation, so that a single high intake of aluminium may produce transient changes that are more marked than in the case of higher accumulations over a long period. In general, the available evidence suggests that, as in humans, bone aluminium levels in the order of 100-200 µg/kg bone ash are required to produce these changes. The study of Ellis et al. (1979) showed that levels of aluminium in bone in the order of 100 µg/g bone ash produced few bone changes in rats, but that higher levels produced marked changes in the rat metaphysis and osteomalacic changes, these being most marked in rats with excess aluminium levels of about 200 µg/g bone ash. The authors found that osteotoxic doses of aluminium were similar in humans and rats. Longer term studies in dogs (see Table 21) show that low exposures to aluminium for short times produced few morphological changes in bone, but that similar or higher dose levels for a longer period did result in observable changes. Uncoupled bone formation (neo-osteogenesis) was produced after 16 weeks at a final bone aluminium level of 170 µg/g dry weight (Quarles et al., 1988). An earlier study by the same authors showed no observable bone changes after 9 weeks at a final bone aluminium content of 70 µg/g dry weight (Quarles et al., 1985). Similarly, human aluminium levels of this order are unlikely to result in osteomalacia.

7.8 Effects on mineral metabolism

Oral application of $AlCl_3$ (300 to 1200 mg/kg diet) to cattle for 84 days did not change plasma or tissue levels of calcium, phosphorus, magnesium or iron, although increased levels of zinc were seen in liver and kidney (Valdivia et al., 1978). In sheep (20 lambs) fed a diet supplemented with $AlCl_3$ (2000 mg/kg for 56 days), Valdivia et al. (1982) observed a reduction of the apparent calcium absorption and lower plasma/serum phosphate levels. The ingestion of moderate concentrations of aluminium (aluminium lactate, aluminium palmitate, aluminium phosphate, aluminium hydroxide; 5-272 µg Al/g diet) also had no effect on tissue calcium, magnesium or iron levels in male Sprague-Dawley rats (Greger et al., 1985a). Small effects were seen on tissue levels of phosphorus, zinc and copper. In rats receiving high intraperitoneal doses of aluminium (AlCl$_3$, 2.7 mg Al/day) repeatedly for 10 days, the calcium concentration was increased in brain, liver and spleen, but not in the heart, and serum calcium levels were not significantly affected (Burnatowska-Hledin & Mayor, 1984). No changes in plasma magnesium levels were seen in this study.

Reduced plasma magnesium concentrations were observed in cows (Kappel et al., 1983; Allen et al., 1986) and sheep (Valdivia et al., 1982) after feeding a diet supplemented with various amounts of aluminium chloride, sulfate or citrate. In sheep (24 lambs) fed an aluminium-rich diet (1450 µg/g), the magnesium content of kidney and bone was reduced (Rosa et al., 1982).

From their experiments in dogs (female mongrel) receiving i.v. injections of AlCl$_3$ (1 mg Al/kg body weight, 5 days/week, for 3-5 weeks), Henry et al. (1984) concluded that the increased serum calcium concentration was due to an increased liberation from bone.

In cows fed a diet supplemented with aluminium citrate (1730 mg Al/kg dry weight for 56 days), serum and urinary calcium concentrations were increased (Allen et al., 1986).

The effect of vitamin D and its metabolites on calcium metabolism following aluminium intoxication was studied by Hodsman et al. (1984) and by Henry & Norman (1985). In vitamin-D-deficient rats receiving repeated intraperitoneal injections of AlCl$_3$ (9.25 mg aluminium for 33 days), serum calcium levels were increased regardless of the vitamin D status of the animals (Hodsman et al., 1984). Treatment of chickens with AlCl$_3$ (5 mg Al/kg body weight intraperitoneally for 5 days) partially blocked the intestinal calcium absorption response to vitamin D in vitamin-D-deficient animals, although serum calcium levels were elevated (Henry & Norman, 1985). No consistent effects of aluminium on the bone calcium mobilization response to vitamin D or 1,25(OH)$_2$D$_3$ were noted. The authors concluded that the ability of the intestine to respond normally to 1,25(OH)$_2$D$_3$ may be compromised by the aluminium application.

A depression of the serum phosphate level was also observed in vitamin-D-deficient rats receiving repeated intraperitoneal injections of AlCl$_3$ (9.25 mg aluminium for 33 days; Hodsman et al., 1984).

Aluminium forms complexes with fluoride, which are considerably more stable than the respective Fe^{3+} complexes. Ingestion of relatively small amounts of aluminium decreases the fluoride concentration available in the intestinal lumen by complexation and thus fluoride absorption from the intestine. Fluoride and AlF_4^- stimulate the enzyme adenylate cyclase (Sternweis & Gilman, 1982). This effect presumably proceeds by complexation of Al^{3+} that is present as a contaminant of the substrate ATP, thus raising the effective ATP concentration (Martin, 1986).

Aluminium exerts its protective effect from fluorine toxicosis, which has been reported in hens (Hahn & Guenter, 1986), turkeys (Cakir et al., 1977) and sheep (Saia et al., 1977), also by formation of a stable complex between Al^{3+} and F^-, thus increasing the fecal fluoride excretion.

8. EFFECTS ON HUMANS

8.1 General population exposure

Aluminium is a potential neurotoxic agent in humans (Steinegger et al., 1990). Humans have highly efficient natural barriers to limit aluminium concentration within the central nervous system except under specific conditions such as renal failure. Encephalopathy attributed to aluminium intoxication in patients receiving treatment for chronic renal failure is discussed in section 8.3.1.

8.1.1 Acute toxicity

There is little indication that aluminium is acutely toxic by oral exposure despite its widespread occurrence in foods, drinking-water and many antacid preparations.

8.1.2 Effects of short-term exposure

In 1988 a population of perhaps 20 000 local residents and numerous tourists were exposed for 5 days or more to unknown levels of aluminium sulfate, subsequent to 20 tonnes of concentrated aluminium sulfate being accidentally placed in the Lowermoor water treatment plants in Camelford, England. The drinking-water also contained elevated concentrations of lead and copper, which leached from the plumbing systems due to increased water acidity. In view of the anecdotal reports of nausea, mouth ulcers, skin rashes and increased arthritic pain, some lasting for months after the exposure, the Cornwall District Health Authority convened a Health Advisory Group which prepared an official report on the incident (Clayton, 1989). The report described the exposure scenario and made conclusions based on expert knowledge of aluminium toxicity and interviews with local residences and tourists claiming long-lasting adverse health effects. No one was exposed to levels of aluminium over 100 mg/litre since such water is unpalatable. Levels between 10 and 50 mg/litre were found for only 1-3 days and water levels for the next month were above 0.2 mg /litre but below 1 mg/litre. The report concluded that such exposures should not pose a hazard to human health. Furthermore, the report concluded that there is no evidence to support the causation by the levels of aluminium, zinc, lead and sulfate of joint and muscle pain, memory loss, hypersensitivity or gastrointestinal disorders reported by residents and tourists some months after the incident. The report stated: "In our view it is not possible to attribute the very real current health complaints to the toxic effects of the incident, except insofar as they are the consequence of the sustained anxiety naturally felt by many people". Other reports, such as that of McMillan et al. (1993), despite containing major scientific deficiencies, do not provide evidence contrary to this conclusion.

8.1.3 Neurotoxic effects

8.1.3.1 Aluminium and Alzheimer's disease (AD)

It has been suggested that aluminium exposure is a risk factor for the development or acceleration of onset of Alzheimer's disease (AD) in humans (Crapper McLachlan, 1986; Crapper McLachlan et al., 1989). The precise pathogenic role of aluminium in AD is judged controversial and remains to be defined (Wisniewski & Wen, 1992; Wischik et al., 1992; Edwardson, 1992).

The purported association is based on six points:

1. The experimental induction of neurofibrillary changes in the neurons of certain species of animals, which suffer a unique progressive neurological impairment after parenteral administration of aluminium salts (see chapter 7). However, these neurofibrillary changes differ from those seen in AD in staining properties and ultra-structural and biochemical composition (Wisniewski & Wen, 1992).

2. The presence of elevated aluminium levels in bulk grey matter of AD-affected brains, which have been found by most investigators using various techniques, including graphite furnace atomic absorption spectroscopy (Crapper et al., 1973, 1976), neutron activation techniques, and inductively coupled mass spectroscopy. However, some investigators using the same techniques have failed to find elevated aluminium levels in the brains of patients with AD (McDermott et al., 1979; Jacobs et al., 1989).

3. The reported detection of aluminium in the amyloid core of classical plaques, neurofibrillary tangles and neuronal nuclei affected by neurofibrillary pathology in AD. Increased aluminium levels have been found within the neurofibrillary tangles of AD using laser

microprobe mass spectrometry (LMMS) (Good et al., 1992). However, using the same technology, others have been unable to replicate these results (Lovell et al., 1993). These techniques are difficult. There may be technical reasons for the disparity in the results, or some of the differences may relate to aluminium contamination of fixatives and stains (Landsberg et al., 1992). AD patients may have an altered blood-brain barrier that allows excess aluminium to accumulate in the brain (Wisniewski & Kozlowski, 1982; Liss & Thornton, 1986; Banks et al., 1988b), although this may in turn be secondary to deposition of amyloid fibrils in the walls of large and small cerebral vessels (amyloid angiopathy) (Wisniewski et al., 1992). If it is accepted that aluminium levels are raised in classical plaques and neurofibrillary tangles in AD, it has been proposed that this may be a secondary phenomenon rather than the primary etiological agent.

4.   Epidemiological studies showing an association between aluminium intake in drinking-water and an increase in the prevalence of AD. The methodology and interpretation of these studies is still under debate, and is considered further in section 8.1.3.2.

5.   The reported decrease in the rate of disease progression in clinically diagnosed AD patients in one, single-blind, oral-versus-placebo controlled trial of desferrioxamine, a trivalent ion chelator administered by intramuscular injection (McLachlan et al., 1992). However, this study has been criticized on three grounds: a) desferrioxamine also chelates iron, which has been linked to free radical damage in AD (Andorn et al., 1990; Crapper McLachlan et al., 1991); b) desferrioxamine may have acted through an anti-inflammatory effect in this (at least partly) inflammatory disease (Crapper McLachlan et al., 1991); c) the absence of a double-blind placebo controlled design may have resulted in differential treatment of patients in the active arm (Wisniewski & Rabe, 1992).

6.   The reported interactions of aluminium with β-amyloid protein (the major component of AD plaques) and with purified paired helical filament tau protein (the major component of neurofibrillary tangles, NFTs). The neurotoxicity of β-amyloid and the formation of plaque deposits is dependent on its aggregation, which has been found to be promoted by low millimolar concentrations of aluminium, iron and zinc (Mantyh et al., 1993). However, this pattern of results has been attributed to iodination-induced alteration of the β-protein structure by Bush et al. (1994), who reported that zinc is a much more potent

metallic ion aggregator of native β-protein than aluminium, being active at low micromolar concentrations. *In vitro* studies have failed to induce Alzheimer-type paired helical filaments (PHFs) in any cellular system. However, human neuroblastoma cells in tissue culture, exposed to aluminium, exhibit epitopes found in AD tangles. Mesco et al. (1991) reported aluminium induction of the well-known Alz50 epitope-recognizing NFT, and Guy et al. (1991) reported the development of an epitope, recognized by an antibody staining for NFT and neuropil threads. Alz50 expression is also observed in experimental aluminium encephalopathy. Shin et al. (1994) have found that aluminium binds to and stabilizes paired helical filament tau, both *in vitro* and *in vivo*. Although aluminium-stabilized PHF tau induced co-deposition of β-protein *in vivo*, the relevance of these recent unconfirmed findings to AD is as yet unclear.

It seems likely that the causation and pathogenesis of AD is multi-factorial (i.e. it may be regarded as a syndrome rather than a disease) and that genetic factors and environmental factors each contribute to a greater or lesser extent in the individual case. Recent genetic studies show that in a small proportion of dominant familial cases, a single point mutation near or in the β-protein segment of the amyloid precursor protein is necessary to cause the disease - a situation of great theoretical importance despite its rarity (Goate et al., 1991).

Other familial AD pedigrees have been linked to a locus on chromosome 14 (St. George-Hyslop et al., 1992; van Broeckhoven et al., 1992). Apo-E allele status is also a major risk factor, the presence of one E4 allele conveying a relative risk of about 3 (Saunders et al., 1993). Other environmental risk factors include low educational and socio-economic status, and head injury (van Duijin et al., 1991). It is against this knowledge base that the possible contribution of aluminium to AD must be evaluated.

8.1.3.2 *Epidemiological studies on AD and environmental aluminium levels*

Many studies have examined risk factors for AD. Among the many case control studies that have been carried out, head trauma, family history, thyroid status, maternal age, child with Down syndrome all stand out as important risk factors (van Duijin et al., 1991). Aluminium exposure as a single risk factor began to be examined in the early 1980s, when reports of the increased level of aluminium in brains of AD patients suggested that this might also be a factor. The availability of water-borne aluminium measurements in many public water supplies and of readily available vital statistics made the study of this exposure relatively accessible.

Studies that examine the relationship between aluminium in drinking-water and AD have been carried out in five separate populations: Norway (Flaten, 1990), Ontario, Canada (Neri & Hewitt, 1991; McLachlan, 1996), France (Michel et al., 1991; Jaqmin et al., 1994), Switzerland (Wettstein et al., 1991) and England (Martyn et al., 1989). These are summarized in Table 22. Several studies examined the water aluminium-AD relationship in the course of investigating other associations (Wood et al., 1988; Frecker, 1991). In addition, exposure from aluminium-containing antiperspirants (Graves et al., 1990) and aluminium-containing antacids (Flaten et al., 1991) have also been explored as risk factors for dementia and/or AD.

Each of the studies that relate aluminium in drinking-water to AD can be assessed systematically for comparability of exposed and control groups, precision of exposure assessment and outcome definition. Ideally, exposed and control groups should be controlled for age, sex, socio-economic status and other variables that can confound results (e.g., education, family history, etc.). Exposure should include concentration and duration for each member of the study group and include a dose range which can be used to assess dose-response relationships. The outcome should be measured preferably by standard criteria, not by surrogates (e.g., dementia for AD), and latency should be incorporated into the analysis (Smith, 1995).

In addition, a variety of study designs from least powerful to most powerful will allow a progressive assessment of the relationship under study (e.g., ecological, cross-sectional, case control, cohort). Nearly 20 studies that examine the relationship between AD and drinking-water aluminium levels have been published.

Studies in five populations using different design are of sufficient quality and meet the general criteria for exposure and outcome assessment and for the adjustment of at least some confounding factors (e.g., age and sex) in order to be used here to evaluate the relationship between water-borne aluminium and AD.

Table 22. Summary of epidemiological studies of aluminium in drinking-water and dementia or Alzheimer's disease (AD)[a]

Type of study	Exposure measure of aluminum intake	Outcome measure/ data source	Results RR			Reference
Ecological	aluminum in drinking-water (concurrent) 4 seasonal samples	mention of dementia ICD9 290, 290.1 (dementia) 342.0 (Parkinson's disease) 348.0 (ALS); sex-adjusted death certificate	AD only Al	Males	Females	Flaten (1990)
			< 0.05	1.00	1.00	
			0.05-0.2	1.15	1.19	
			> 0.2	1.32	1.42	
			PD and ALS - no gradient			
Morbidity prevalence	aluminum in finished drinking-water; historical	dementia by diagnostic category (not standard) CT scan center records age-sex-adjusted	all males and females RR 1.3-1.5, no dose-response < 65 males and females 1.4-1.7[b], dose response			Martyn et al. (1989)
Morbidity prevalence case control	finished drinking-water aluminum; historical	"cases" were hospital discharges with Dx of AD (ICD9 331.0), presenile dementia (ICD9 290). age/sex/residence-matched controls with other Dx HMRI data base - Ontario	RR from OR, gradient for AD Al	RR from OR		Neri & Hewitt (1991)
			< 0.01	1.00		
			0.01-0.099	1.13		
			0.10-0.199	1.26		
			> 0.2	1.46		
Morbidity prevalence	aluminum in finished drinking-water; residence >15 years	mnemic skills in octogenerarians urinary and serum Al	no difference in mean scores of tests for cognitive function			Wettstein et al. (1991)

Table 22 (contd).

Type of study	Exposure measure of aluminum intake	Outcome measure/ data source	Results RR	Reference
Morbidity	urinary aluminum and serum aluminum; historical and concurrent	sample of 800 residents in high & low aluminum areas 10 AD patients & controls in each area age, sex, education population based	slightly higher serum aluminium in AD in low aluminium areas; similar urinary excretion in AD and controls hypothesis of association not supported	Wettstein et al. (1991)
Morbidity prevalence	aluminum in drinking-water; historical	cognitive function in sample of > 65 years by test battery (DSM III) population-based (2792); age, sex, education, ses, Al in water - many sources for the data	probable AD - gradient-adjusted for age, education, residence RR 4.53/100 µg/litre aluminium (NSS); RR corrected to NS with current aluminium measurement	Michel et al. (1991)
Case control	aluminium in drinking-water; residence-weighted historical	pathological; confirmation of diagnosis in all cases and controls no age-sex-education adjustment	RR 1.7 aluminium $\geq$ 100 µg/litre RR 2.5 aluminium $\geq$ 100 µg/litre based adjustment for 10-year weighted exposure history	McLachlan et al. (1996)
Morbidity prevalence case control	aluminum in water, pH, calcium	cognitive function	calcium protective RR = 1.2 with pH < 7.3 NS /all other pH values	Jacqmin et al. (1994)

[a] AD = Alzheimer's disease; PD = Parkinson's disease; RR = relative; OR = odds ratio; NS = not significant; ses = socioeconomic status
[b] Significant (P < 0.05) of highest exposure only

144

Results of four studies are consistent for a positive relationship between water-borne aluminium and AD (Martyn et al., 1989; Neri & Hewitt, 1990; Flaten et al., 1991; McLachlan et al., 1996). Three found a "dose-response" relationship (McLachlan, 1989; Flaten, 1990; Neri & Hewitt, 1991) and one found a significant relationship between high and low aluminium exposure (Martyn et al., 1989). Adjustment for sex was performed in two of these studies (Martyn et al., 1989; Flaten, 1990). One study (McLachlan et al., 1996) did not adjust for age, sex or any other confounding factor but did correct for "during life" exposure.

With regard to exposure assessment, all of the positive studies used ecological assessment of exposure but from only one source, the public water supply. Total exposure to aluminium was not determined. It is therefore impossible to determine if the relationship observed is due to water aluminium alone without explicit adjustment for, and information about, other sources of aluminium intake.

Studies that showed no association between water aluminium and AD (Wettstein et al., 1991; Michel et al., 1991) were more precise in their outcome measure. However, the water aluminium levels were very low and corresponded to the water aluminium levels found as the lowest concentrations of the studies that showed a positive association.

Initial results reported by Michel et al. (1991) in the Bordeaux cohort study showed a high, though not significant, risk (4.5) for exposure to water aluminium levels greater than 0.10 mg/litre when 10- to 15-year historical analyses of water were used. When current analyses of water were used, the relationship disappeared (Jacqmin et al., 1994). However, other relationships appeared, such as the increase in risk of cognitive impairment when the pH was below 7.3, a decrease in risk with a pH greater than 7.3, and no elevated risk when pH was not considered. An inverse relationship was found between cognitive impairment and calcium concentration (Jacqmin et al., 1994).

The initial observation of elevated risk for cognitive impairment with a set of numbers that were possibly random (Flaten, 1990) and the changes in risk level with other water quality parameters such as calcium and pH are difficult to interpret and require further evaluation.

Studies with more precise outcome and exposure measures would be expected to show the highest relative risks or odds ratios.

McLachlan et al. (1996) examined the relationship between autopsy-confirmed AD and aluminium in drinking-water. The odds ratio of exposure to water above 100 µg/litre was calculated for confirmed cases of AD and a combination of AD and other neuropathology, compared to controls. Cases and controls were obtained from brains donated to a tissue bank supported by lay organizations. Control neuropathology included normal brains and brains with non-AD neuropathology. The aluminium level in water was obtained from a data bank of water measurements for public water supplies. A next-of-kin interview was used to refine exposure by weighing for length of residence by assigning exposure to residence not to place of death.

The odds ratio of exposure to water with an aluminium concentration of ≥ 100 µg/litre for AD alone compared to controls was 1.7 (1.2-2.5). The use of weighted exposure measures (residential group levels of aluminium in water) increased the odds ratios for the same comparison groups to 2.5 or more.

The use of pathologically confirmed outcome measures and of accurate exposure measures brings added strength to the studies examining the relationship between aluminium and AD. Notwithstanding, this study is subject to selection bias of the sample (voluntary donation to a tissue bank), the possibility of misclassification of the ecological measure of exposure and a failure to account for confounding factors.

The study of McLachlan et al. (1996) does show the highest relative risks of any of these studies. However, this study suffers from lack of adjustment for very important known risk factors, such as age, sex, education and socioeconomic status.

8.1.3.3 *Epidemiological studies relating aluminium concentrations in water to cognitive dysfunction*

Wettstein et al. (1991) looked for a relationship between water aluminium levels up to 98 µg/litre and cognitive function in a male population (800 men) of octogenarians but found none (OR = 0.92) (CI = 0.66-1.29).

Forbes et al. (1994) examined a cohort of 2000 men followed since 1959 in a longitudinal study of ageing. The outcome measure examined was "any evidence of mental impairment" as measured by skills of daily living assessment. In the survivors of the cohort for whom information was available (290 individuals), exposure was linked to the level of aluminium in their drinking-water obtained from the Ontario Canada Drinking Water Surveillance database. In an analysis that considered fluoride and aluminium in drinking-water, the odds ratio after exposure to water with high aluminium and low fluoride levels was 3.98 [CI = 1.72-9.19]. In a multi-variate analysis, which adjusted for a variety of confounding factors, the adjusted odds ratio for high aluminium level (> 85 µg/litre) was 1.72 (1.08-2.75).

8.1.3.4 *Other neurological conditions in the general population*

Other severe neurological diseases, such as amyotrophic lateral sclerosis, Parkinsonism and the dementia complex of Guam, have been related to aluminium accumulation in the brain (Gajdusek & Salazar, 1982; Perl et al., 1982; Garruto et al., 1984). However, the role of aluminium in these conditions is still under considerable scientific debate.

8.1.3.5 *Conclusions regarding neurological effects of aluminium*

The positive relationship between aluminium in drinking-water and AD, which has been demonstrated in several epidemiological studies, cannot be totally dismissed. However, strong reservations about inferring a causal relationship are warranted in view of the failure of studies to account for demonstrated confounding factors and for aluminium intake from all sources.

Taken together, the relative risks for AD from exposure to aluminium in drinking-water at levels above 100 µg/litre as determined in these studies are low. But, because the risk estimates are imprecise for a variety of methodological reasons, a population-attributable risk cannot be calculated with precision. Such predictions may, however, be useful in making decisions about the need to control the exposure to aluminium in the general population.

In light of the above studies, which consider water-borne aluminium as the sole risk factor, and the recent findings that water accounts for less than 5% of daily uptake of aluminium, it is difficult to reconcile a presumable impact on cognition. Several lines of investigation should be pursued to elucidate further the nature of the relationship found in these studies (see Chapter 12).

8.1.4 Allergic effects

Although human exposure to aluminium is widespread, hypersensitivity has been reported following exposure to some aluminium compounds in only a few cases, either after dermal application or parenteral administration.

A case of contact sensitivity to aluminium was reported in Sweden. The patient had regularly been using an aluminium chloride roll-on antiperspirant and developed an itchy dermatitis in the axillae. Patch-tests with aluminium chloride were positive (Fischer & Rystedt, 1982). Contact allergy to aluminium also occurred in a patient hyposensitized with aluminium-precipitated grass pollen (Clemmensen & Knudsen, 1980). Two cases of contact allergy to aluminium after use of topical medications containing aluminium acetotartrate have been reported (Meding et al., 1984).

Childhood immunization with an aluminium-bound vaccine can lead to delayed hypersensitivity to aluminium. Children who had had previous injections with these vaccines showed positive patch-tests to aluminium chloride (Böhler-Sommeregger & Lindemayr, 1986; Veien et al., 1986).

In Denmark a follow-up study was made of 202 children (age 6-15 years) who had received hyposensitization therapy with various aluminium-containing extracts (subcutaneous application) for an average of 3 years. One to three years after cessation of hyposensitization, 4% (13 children) still had severely pruriginous treatment-resistant subcutaneous nodules in their forearm (application site). Six of these 13 children were patch-tested and four reacted positively on aluminium chloride administration (Frost et al., 1985).

8.2 Occupational exposure

This section deals with the effects observed in occupations where workers are exposed to aluminium metal and aluminium compounds. Where exposures are to mixed dusts and/or chemical mixtures, one cannot infer causality between aluminium exposure and effects from studies on such workers.

8.2.1 Respiratory tract effects

Respiratory disorders among workers in the aluminium industry have been reviewed in detail (Dinman, 1988b; Abramson et al., 1989).

8.2.1.1 Restrictive pulmonary disease

Historically, pulmonary fibrosis has been associated with various jobs within the aluminium industry. Shaver's disease (described in the 1940s) was a form of silicosis associated with the production of corundum abrasives (Shaver & Riddell, 1947). Another historically important occupational exposure associated with pulmonary fibrosis was experienced by "pyro powder" workers, who were exposed to very fine stamped aluminium powder (generally < 1 μm), including that used in the manufacture of explosives and fireworks (Doese, 1938; Meyer & Kasper, 1942; Mitchell et al., 1961; Jordan, 1961; McLaughlin et al., 1962; Gross et al., 1970). In that process, oils and solvents were used to coat particles to prevent naturally occurring oxidation, and nearly all cases of fibrosis were reported in workers exposed to mineral-oil-coated particles. That process is no longer used (Dinman, 1988a) and only one case has been reported since 1960 (McLaughlin et al., 1962). This syndrome indicates the potential pulmonary effect of non-oxidized aluminium metal, but such exposures do not occur in nature.

In a report of nine cases of workers exposed to aluminium oxide (mean duration of exposure 25 years), abnormal chest roentgenograms were described, as well as pathological lung functions in three of the cases (Jederlinic et al., 1990). Biopsies were taken from these three patients and analysed by electron microscopy and microprobe analysis. Interstitial fibrosis was the main histological finding. Metals occurred in amounts several orders of magnitude above background levels and the majority was aluminium oxide. The authors stated that aluminium oxide was the most likely cause for the development of interstitial fibrosis in these workers and that asbestos could be ruled out. Exposure to a "mixed dust", including free silica, also seemed to be a possible explanation.

With the exception of this exposure, pathological findings associated with aluminium exposure listed in Table 23 refers to mixed exposures, and cannot be solely attributed to aluminium. Other exposures, such as to silica or other metals, must be considered.

Table 23. Clinical and pathological pulmonary findings in aluminium-exposed workers[a]

Exposure	Clinical effects	Pathological changes	Confounding exposures	Reference
Aluminium powder grinder for 6 years	cough, DOE, abnormal X-ray, restrictive PFTs	pulmonary alveolar proteinosis	iron, kaolinite, mica, rutile, calcium at biopsy	Miller et al. (1984)
Polisher for 24 years	cough, DOE	bronchogenic cancer; diffuse interstitial fibrosis	stainless steel, chromium, nickel, cigarettes (45 packet-years), silica (biopsy)	de Vuyst et al. (1986)
Catalyst fabrication	cough, DOE, mild restriction, no clinical evidence of sarcoid	non-caseating granuloma; T-lymphocyte alveolitis	iron, copper, zinc, nickel, chromium, manganese, cobalt, molybdenum, vanadium, palladium, silica, nobellium on biopsy; cigarettes	de Vuyst et al. (1987)

Table 23 (contd).

Exposure	Clinical effects	Pathological changes	Confounding exposures	Reference
Welding fumes	mild ventilatory restriction	diffuse and focal fibrosis; pig-mented content of macrophages	iron, cigarettes	Vallyathan et al. (1982)
Welding fumes, intermittent welder (1965-1970)	X-ray interstitial pattern; dyspnoea	interstitial granuloma, macro-phages, foreign body giant cells, crystals, EDA indicated aluminium crystals	smoker, no TB	Chen et al. (1978)
Welder for 16 years	dyspnoea, X-ray bilateral, hazy basal infiltrates, reduced TLC (3.5/6.8)	lung biopsy, diffuse chronic interstitial pneumonia, predominantly desquamative	ex-smoker	Herbert et al. (1982)

DOE = dyspnoea on exertion; TLC = total lung capacity (measured/predicted (6.8 litres)); EDA = energy dispersive analysis; PFT = pulmonary function test; TB = tuberculosis

8.2.1.2 *Obstructive pulmonary disease*

a) *Asthma*

A potentially persistent form of occupational asthma related to primary aluminium smelting (pot room asthma) has been reported over the past 35 years; reversible symptoms, airflow limitation and increased bronchial responsiveness have been described (O'Donnell et al., 1989). The likely causes are irritant airborne particulate and fumes contributed by cryolite (sodium aluminium fluoride), gaseous hydrogen fluoride and other agents that may be adsorbed onto aluminium. A close relationship in aluminium potroom workers between levels of exposure to fluoride, which may be one of a number of general inhalant irritants, and the work-related asthmatic symptoms has been shown (Kongerud et al., 1990; Kongerud, 1991). A positive association between plasma levels of fluoride and increased bronchial responsiveness has also been reported (Söyseth et al., 1994).

A similar occupational asthma ascribed to irritant particulate has also been described among workers following technical failure in plants producing aluminium fluoride and aluminium sulfate (Simonsson et al., 1985) and in solderers working with potassium aluminium tetrafluoride flux (Hjortsbert et al., 1994).

b) *Chronic bronchitis*

Aluminium production and processing may lead to high levels of workplace exposure to dusts and particulate.

In Italy the possible association of aluminium exposure and pneumoconiosis was investigated (Saia et al., 1981). Chronic bronchitis symptoms were found in 39% of the 119 exposed workers and in 13% of the 119 control subjects. The X-ray findings showed one kind of pneumoconiosis with small irregular opacities or accentuation of broncopulmonary markings in 29% of the exposed workers and in 15% of the controls.

A case study of 2086 employees at the Arkansas operations of a large aluminium production company was performed (Townsend et al., 1985). The study indicated that long-term high accumulative dust exposure was associated with decreased levels of pulmonary function in active workers at a bauxite refinery and aluminium-based chemical products plant. A follow-up study of this cohort (Townsend et al., 1985) supported the conclusion regarding respiratory effects of dust in the workplace related to lung function.

In a cross-sectional study (Sjögren & Ulfvarson, 1985) on 64 aluminium welders and 64 age-matched controls (non-welding industrial workers), an increased prevalence of chronic bronchitis was observed but there were no effects on pulmonary function. The prevalence of chronic bronchitis among aluminium welders was similar to that of welders working with stainless steel or iron.

8.2.2 *Central nervous system effects*

A number of neurological effects have been associated with occupational exposure to aluminium, including impairment of cognitive function, motor dysfunction and peripheral neuropathy.

Welders exposed to aluminium fumes for about 13 years had significantly more neuropsychiatric symptoms (ascertained from positive answers in a questionnaire) than railway track welders not exposed to aluminium (Sjögren et al., 1990). Despite the potential bias associated with the questionnaire methodology used in this study, a dose-response effect was seen.

In a further study (Sjögren et al., 1994b) 38 aluminium-exposed welders (median urinary aluminium level, 22 µg/litre; median exposure time, 4.5 years) were compared with a group of 39 iron-exposed welders. Small decrements in the speed of repetitive motor functions were found, but there were no differences in other neurophysiological or neuropsychological parameters.

A mixture of finely ground aluminium (85%) and aluminium oxide (15%) powder was used between 1944 and 1979 as a prophylactic against silicosis. Underground gold and uranium miners were exposed to an aluminium dust concentration of 20 000-34 000 particles/ml air (approximately 30 mg/m^3) in their changing room before each shift for 10 min (Rifat et al., 1990). Exposure to aluminium powder in the cohort ranged from 6 months to 36 years. A yearly deposition in each miner of about 375 mg of aluminium powder has been calculated.

From the 29 000 underground miners examined in provincial chest clinics between 1955 and 1979, a sampling frame was constructed containing a cohort of 6604. Two samples were drawn from this cohort. One sample consisted of 369 exposed and 369 unexposed matched miners adjusted for age and year of their first mining experience in Ontario, Canada, and total mining time. The second sample consisted of 678 randomly drawn miners in equal numbers from the exposed and unexposed populations. Between 1988 and 1989, miners who could be traced were interviewed and psychometric testing was performed. Cognitive test scores and proportions impaired in at least one test indicated a disadvantage for exposed miners. A positive exposure-related trend in increased risk was described.

A group of 87 workers (average age 40.7 years) from an aluminium foundry exposed to workplace aluminium concentrations ranging between 4.6 and 11.5 mg/m^3 air, with an exposure time of at least 6 years, was studied by Hosovski et al. (1990). Sixty non-exposed workers matched for age, job, seniority and social status served as control. Psychomotor and psychometric tests were performed, except on workers who consumed alcohol or who had taken psychotropic drugs within a month prior to the test. A significant difference in complex reaction time, oculomotor coordination and the sum of manipulative tests was noted in exposed workers compared to controls. In the Weschler Adult Intelligence Scale (WAIS), the most significant differences were found in the memory subtest.

In contrast, Bast-Petersen et al. (1994) did not find any impairments in small groups of foundry workers (8) or potroom workers (14) in a broad battery of psychometric tests. A cluster of aluminium potroom workers exposed to unhooded pots for 4 or more years displayed an increased incidence of impairment of cognitive function and/or defects in motor control. However, insufficient biochemical investigations were undertaken to determine whether aluminium or other potential neurotoxins were the causative agent (Longstreth et al., 1985; White et al., 1992).

In a case where a man was exposed to ultrafine aluminium powder for 13.5 years in the ballmill area of an aluminium factory, the individual died following a rapidly progressive encephalopathy, and his brain was found to contain elevated aluminium levels (McLaughlin et al., 1962).

8.3 Cancer

There is insufficient information to allow for the classification of the cancer risk from human exposures to aluminium and its compounds.

8.4 Genotoxicity

In an abstract, Haugen et al. (1983) reported no increase in the number of sister chromatid exchanges in peripheral blood lymphocytes of workers employed in an aluminium factory. There have been no reports concerning genetic effects of aluminium in humans following oral exposure to aluminium.

8.5 Reproductive toxicity

There is no information regarding reproductive toxicity in humans following exposure to aluminium.

8.6 Subpopulations at special risk

Aluminium intoxication developed over weeks or months in patients with chronic renal failure when dialysis fluids or parenteral solutions contained aluminium (Alfrey et al., 1972; Klein, 1991), or when the main source was aluminium-containing oral phosphate binders. In patients suffering from renal failure, increases in serum and tissue aluminium concentration were observed. The increased aluminium content in brains of patients with renal failure seems to be the major etiological factor in the development of the neurological syndrome termed either dialysis encephalopathy or dialysis dementia. The development of a specific form of osteomalacia and of microcytic, hypochromic anaemia is also attributed to aluminium (Ward, 1991).

Aluminium intoxication is caused by using haemodialysis fluids made from tap water without removal of the aluminium (Elliot et al., 1978). After the introduction of water treatment with a combination of filtration, softening, carbon absorption, reverse osmosis and de-ionization, these clinical syndromes were prevented. Nephrologists limit the exposure to aluminium from dialysis fluids and drugs. This follows the introduction of guidelines in the USA, Canada, Japan and the EEC. As a consequence, in most dialysis centres the dialysis fluids are monitored and the aluminium level is kept below 0.4 µmol/litre (10 µg/litre). Aluminium-free phosphate-binding agents such as calcium carbonate are preferably used for oral medication. The same clinical syndromes have been described in patients with renal impairments, including premature infants who have not been dialyzed, and are a consequence of aluminium accumulation from aluminium-containing pharmaceutical products and parenteral solutions (Finberg et al., 1986).

8.6.1 Encephalopathy

Dialysis encephalopathy is a complication of prolonged haemodialysis first described in 1972 (Alfrey et al., 1972). The main symptoms are speech disorder followed by the development of dementia, convulsions and myoclonus. The mean duration of dialysis was 48 months and the dialysis fluids were made with untreated tap water. Elevated aluminium contents were found in the brain, muscle and bone tissues of the affected patients. The same findings were reported from other dialysis centres in Europe and the USA. Many outbreaks of encephalopathy have been described in association with the use of dialysis fluids containing a high concentration of aluminium, usually above 200 µg/litre (Flendrig et al., 1976; McDermott et al., 1978; Alfrey, 1978).

In a study with 55 patients suffering from dialysis encephalopathy in six dialysis centres using a uniform clinical classification, the incidence of dialysis encephalopathy rose significantly with increasing cumulative exposure to aluminium via the dialysate (Schreeder et al., 1983).

Epidemiological studies of dialysis centres in England showed that encephalopathy was almost non-existent in those centres using water with aluminium concentrations less than 50 µg/litre to prepare dialysis fluids. The incidence of encephalopathy rose progressively with higher water concentrations of aluminium. The Registration Committee of the European Dialysis and Transplant Association made a European survey, which showed clusters of encephalopathy in certain areas of Britain, Spain, Greece and Scandinavia. In Britain, 92% of the patients in these areas had been treated with dialysis fluids made from softened tap water (Kerr & Ward, 1988). No signs of overt aluminium toxicity were observed in 27 long-term haemodialysis patients on dialysis fluids containing low aluminium concentrations

(Altmann et al., 1989) and these subjects had only mildly elevated serum aluminium levels. However, defects in several tests of psychomotor function, including digit coding, were found.

8.6.2 *Osteomalacia*

Osteomalacia has also been observed in patients with chronic renal failure, exposed to aluminium in dialysis fluids, or in infants with renal failure treated with aluminium hydroxide to control hyper-phosphataemia (Ward et al., 1978; Andreoli et al., 1984). Bone pain, myopathy, pathological fractures and poor response to vitamin D therapy are the characteristic symptoms of osteomalacia, accompanied by radiological changes, including partial and complete non-healing fractures, osteopenia, and reduction in calcified bone area (Simpson et al., 1973). When aluminium was removed from fluids used for dialysis, the incidence of osteomalacia diminished. The level without undue risk was estimated to be 30 µg/litre or less (Platts et al., 1984). The aluminium content of the bone is increased in patients with renal disease, treated by haemodialysis, and this aluminium may remain in the bone even after successful renal transplantation (Ellis et al., 1979). The aluminium in patients with osteomalacia was found to be mainly localized at the interface between the osteoid and the calcified matrix (Cournot-Witmer et al., 1981). Vitamin-D-resistant osteomalacia due to aluminium is a progressive metabolic bone disease. The mechanism for the disordered bone formation remains to be clarified.

8.6.3 *Microcytic anaemia*

In a study of ten aluminium-intoxicated dialysis patients, microcytic anaemia was observed. The disease was reversible after deionization of the dialysis water (Touam et al., 1983). The mechanism by which an excess of aluminium induces microcytic anaemia remains to be clarified (Wills & Savory, 1983, 1989).

9. EFFECTS ON OTHER ORGANISMS IN THE LABORATORY AND FIELD

9.1 Laboratory experiments

9.1.1 *Microorganisms*

Den Dooren de Jong (1971) inoculated a medium containing aluminium chloride (10^{-4} mol/litre) with three *Azobacter* strains. After incubation for 1 to 2 days, the aluminium had produced an inhibition zone of 14 mm with increased pigmentation at the edges. The inhibition zone, when compared with that produced by other metals, was found to indicate intermediate toxicity.

9.1.1.1 *Water*

Sheets (1957) studied the effect of shock loadings of aluminium sulfate on the biochemical oxygen demand of sewage sludge and found that a concentration of 18 mg/litre caused a 50% reduction.

Panasenkov (1987) found that aluminium sulfate at concentrations of 0.1 and 1 mg/litre had no effect on the heterotrophic fixation of $^{14}CO_2$ or the number of saprophytes of a natural bacterial coenosis. However, at 10 mg/litre aluminium sulfate reduced these two parameters by 50% and 60%, respectively.

Dobbs et al. (1989) studied the effect of complexation on the toxicity of aluminium using the Microtox system based on measurement of the light output of a luminescent bacterium. Aluminium citrate complexes were essentially non-toxic up to levels of at least 25 mg Al/litre. The one-hour EC_{50}, defined as a 50% reduction in light output, was 300 µg/litre in the absence of citrate. Complexation by fluoride was complicated by a toxic response to fluoride itself. Correction for this effect still revealed an appreciable toxicity of aluminium fluoride complexes. The toxic response in the presence of 9 and 36 mg/litre fulvic acid was reduced by 24% and 61%, respectively. Hoke et al. (1992) reported 15-min EC_{50} values (Microtox tests) for aluminium chloride (as aluminium) of 5.57 and 3.31 mg/litre for solutions osmotically adjusted with 22% sodium chloride and 20.4% sucrose, respectively.

9.1.1.2 *Soil*

Zwarun et al. (1971) found the soil bacterium *Bacillus* sp. to be resistant to aluminium. Increasing acidity from pH 6.6 to pH 4.5 reduced the number of surviving cells suspended for 3 h in an acetate buffer. Addition of 80 mg Al/litre produced no further reduction, even though the cell walls were saturated with aluminium. Zwarun & Thomas (1973) exposed the soil bacterium *Pseudomonas stutzeri* to acidic conditions at aluminium concentrations of 1, 10 and 80 mg/litre for 3 h. Increasing the acidity reduced the number of surviving cells. The addition of aluminium (10 mg/litre) at pH 4.5 significantly reduced the survival rate of cells, and 80 mg/litre was lethal.

Thompson & Medve (1984) studied the effects of aluminium (0-500 µg/ml) on the growth of the ectomycorrhizal fungi *Cenococcum graniforme*, *Suillus luteus*, *Thelephora terrestris*, and three isolates of *Pisolithus tinctorius* (all four species are commonly found on spoil tips). *T. terrestris* was the most sensitive species showing no growth at aluminium concentrations $\geq$ 150 µg/ml, whereas *S. luteus* was the most tolerant, being unaffected at aluminium concentrations < 350 µg/ml. The other species showed reduced growth at all aluminium concentrations. However, the results obtained were not consistent with field observations.

The severity of the incidence of the fungal disease potato scab was reduced by the addition of aluminium (Mizuno & Yoshida, 1993).

9.1.2 Aquatic organisms

9.1.2.1 *Plants*

Algal assays are often carried out in culture media containing high concentrations of nutrients, including phosphate. These nutrients ameliorate the toxicity of aluminium, and limit the application of the results to natural waters. For example, in culture medium the green alga *Chlorella pyrenoidosa* successfully grew at concentrations of up to 12 mg total aluminium/litre at pH 4.6, but an aluminium concentration of 24 mg/litre was toxic. By selecting those algae which tolerated high levels of aluminium, the authors were able to develop algal cultures that grew at up to 48 mg/litre (Foy & Gerloff, 1972). However, Helliwell et al. (1983) found that maximum toxicity of aluminium to algal growth was achieved at pH 5.8 to 6.2, 5 µg labile

Al/litre significantly inhibiting the growth of the alga *Chlorella pyrenoidosa* in a synthetic hard water. The assay showed that toxicity is a function of the labile, rather than the total, aluminium. It was found that Al $(OH)_2^+$ was the aluminium species most toxic to the alga. Similar results were reported by Parent & Campbell (1994), although they found that polymerized aluminium species were also toxic.

Bringmann & Kühn (1959) found a toxic threshold of 1.5 to 2 mg/litre aluminium chloride for the green alga *Scenedesmus quadricauda*. Rueter et al. (1987) found that a concentration of 60 µmol aluminium/litre at pH 5.7 is required to produce any inhibitory effect on the growth rate of the *S. quadricauda*. In an experiment studying the effect of both copper and aluminium on the growth of *Scenedesmus* it was found that the majority of the toxic action was due to indirect chemical interactions that result in higher cupric ion activities.

Hörnström et al. (1984) studied the effects of aluminium on 19 freshwater algal species in lake water at pH 5.5. The biotests showed that 13 of the species, including all of the desmoids and diatoms, experienced complete growth inhibition at 200 µg/litre. In fact, two of the four diatom species (*Nitschia actinastroides* and *Synedra nana*) showed 47% inhibition at 100 µg/litre. The most insensitive group was the Chrysophyceae, where three out of five species were unaffected at 400 µg/litre.

Lindemann et al. (1990) studied the impact of aluminium (4-220 µmol/litre) on green algae (*Scenedesmus* sp. and *Chlorella* sp.) isolated from acidic and alkaline headwater streams in a semi-continuous culture media at pH 5. The threshold for inhibition was found to be less than 4 µmol aluminium/litre when the aluminium was added to the medium abruptly. When the aluminium was added gradually there was a lag period, which can be explained by the formation of polymeric aluminium hydroxy compounds and the precipitation of aluminium hydroxides and phosphates; this reduces the amount of aluminium bioavailable to the algae. Folsom et al. (1986) studied the toxicity of aluminium (0, 10, 25 and 50 mg/litre) to the acid-tolerant green alga *Chlorella saccarophila* at pH 3.0 and found a concentration-dependent growth inhibition. Addition of the fast-exchange ions Ca^{2+}, Mg^{2+}, Na^+ and K^+ (150 mg/litre) caused some reversal of the toxic effects of aluminium.

Exley et al. (1993) studied the effect of aluminium on the freshwater diatom *Navicula pelliculosa* and the amelioration of this toxicity with silicon. An aluminium concentration of 10 μmol/litre significantly inhibited diatom growth at all but the highest silicic acid concentration (100 μmol/litre). The mechanism of action was found to be independent of a direct effect on cell biomass, chlorophyll *a* content per cell or the protein content of each cell. The toxicity of aluminium was mitigated by increasing the nominal phosphorus concentration from 1 to 10 μmol/litre. Further growth experiments were carried out on the non-silicon-requiring green alga *Chlorella vulgaris*. The rate of growth was significantly inhibited at 48 μmol/litre. The inhibitory effects were again removed at the highest silicic acid concentration. The authors concluded that the mechanism of aluminium toxicity was a reduction in the bioavailability of phosphorus.

Genter & Amyot (1994) exposed freshwater benthic algal populations to aluminium concentrations of 50, 100 and 500 μg Al/litre (as aluminium sulfate) at pH 4.8 in artificial streams. During the 28-day test, aluminium in acidified water inhibited the abundance of diatoms and cyanobacteria (blue-green algae) more than the acidity alone. Aluminium decreased chlorophyll abundance beyond the effects of acidity alone at 500 μg/litre.

Nalewajko & Paul (1985) studied the effect of aluminium on phytoplankton collected from a circumneutral and an acid-stressed lake. Addition of aluminium (50 μg/litre) caused significant decreases in microbial phosphate uptake and photosynthesis. The effects were more pronounced at pH 5.2-6.9 (lake water pH range) than at pH 4.5, there being larger decreases in phytoplankton from the acid-stressed lake. The authors reported that the toxicity was due to both the precipitation of phosphate as particles after addition of aluminium and the direct effect of aluminium.

Stanley (1974) grew the aquatic angiosperm Eurasian milfoil (*Myriophyllum spicatum*) in solutions of aluminium for 32 days. There was a 50% inhibition of root dry weight, shoot dry weight, root length and shoot length at aluminium concentrations of 2.5, 7.6, 5.1 and 12.7 mg/litre, respectively.

9.1.2.2 Invertebrates

a) *Acute toxicity*

The acute toxicity of aluminium to aquatic invertebrates is summarized in Table 24; 48-h and 96-h LC_{50} values range from 0.48 mg/litre (polychaete) to 59.6 mg/litre (daphnid). However, care must be taken when interpreting the results because of the significant effects of pH on the availability of aluminium.

Bringmann & Kühn (1959) found no effect on *Daphnia magna* immobilization at aluminium chloride concentrations of up to 1000 mg/litre over a 48 h exposure period at pH 7.5.

Havens (1990) exposed two acid-sensitive cladocerans (*Daphnia galeata* and *D. retrocurva*) and one acid-tolerant cladoceran (*Bosmina longirostris*) to aluminium concentrations of 200 µg/litre at pH 5.0 for 24 h. The exposure consistently resulted in nearly 100% mortality for *D. galeata* and *D. retrocurva*, but mortality rates for *B. longirostris* were not significantly different from those of controls (2-6%). Haematoxylin staining procedures revealed that the daphnids showed marked aluminium binding at the maxillary glands (the site of ion exchange), whereas *B. longirostris* showed no noticeable aluminium binding.

Havas & Hutchinson (1982) studied the tolerance of crustaceans, collected from acid (pH 2.8) and alkaline (pH 8.2) tundra ponds, to low pH and elevated levels of aluminium. When adjusted to pH 4.5, water from acid ponds was more toxic than water from alkaline ponds, probably due to elevated concentrations of aluminium (up to 20 mg Al/litre). Removal of heavy metals and aluminium by co-precipitation significantly reduced the toxicity of adjusted pond water to crustaceans. The subsequent addition of 20 mg/litre aluminium resulted in 100% mortality of *Daphnia* within 20 h, whereas the addition of other metals (iron, nickel and zinc) did not restore the toxicity.

Havas (1985) studied the effect of aluminium chloride (0.02, 0.32 and 1.02 mg Al/litre), pH (6.5, 5.0 and 4.5) and calcium (2.5 and 12.5 mg/litre) on the survival of *Daphnia magna* during a 48-h exposure period. Maximum aluminium toxicity was observed at pH 6.5 and a calcium concentration of 2.5 mg/litre. A pH of 5.0 was

Table 24. Toxicity of aluminium (LC_{50}) to aquatic invertebrates

Organism	Size/age	Stat/flow[a]	Temper- ature (°C)	Hardness[b] (mg/litre)	pH	Salt	Duration (h)	LC_{50}[c] (mg/litre)	Reference
Bivalve *Pisidium* *casertanum*		stat stat	20-25 20-25		3.5 4.5		96 96	> 1.0 m > 0.4 m	Mackie (1989)
Bivalve *Pisidium* *compressum*		stat stat	20-25 20-25		3.5 4.5		96 96	> 1.0 m > 0.4 m	Mackie (1989)
Gastropod *Amnicola* *limosa*		stat stat	20-25 20-25		3.5 4.5		96 96	> 1.0 m > 0.4 m	Mackie (1989)
Hyallela *azteca*		stat stat	20-25 20-25		3.5 4.5		96 96	> 1.0 m > 0.4 m	Mackie (1989)
Enallagma sp.		stat stat	20-25 20-25		3.5 4.5		96 96	> 1.0 m > 0.4 m	Mackie (1989)
Polychaete *Neanthes* *arenaceodentata*		stat	20-25		7.6-8.0	chloride	96	> 2.0 n	Petrich & Reish (1979)

Table 24 (contd).

Organism	Size/age	Stat/flow[a]	Temperature (°C)	Hardness[b] (mg/litre)	pH	Salt	Duration (h)	LC_{50}[c] (mg/litre)	Reference
Polychaete		stat			7.6-8.0	chloride	96	2.0 n	Petrich &
Polychaete *Ctenodrilus serratus*		stat			7.6-8.0	chloride	96	0.48 n	Reish (1979)
Copepod *Nitocra spinipes*	adult	stat	20	7[d]	8.0	chloride	96	10 (7.5-13.4)	Bengtsson (1978)
Water flea *Daphnia magna*	< 24 h	stat	17-19	44-53	7.4-8.2	chloride	48	3.9 n	Biesinger & Christensen (1972)
		stat	12-15	240	7.2-7.8	ammonium sulfate	48	59.6 (45.8-73.3) n[e]	Khangarot & Ray (1989)

[a] Stat = static conditions (water unchanged for duration of test)
[b] Hardness expressed as mg $CaCO_3$/litre
[c] n = based on nominal concentrations; m = based on measured concentrations
[d] Salinity (%)
[e] EC_{50} based on immobilization

164

toxic to *D. magna* in soft water, 50% of the daphnids being immobilized within 24 h. Aluminium marginally increased the toxicity of water at pH 5.0. At pH 4.5, high concentrations of aluminium significantly reduced the hydrogen ion toxicity. However, this amelioration was short lived and all of the *Daphnia* had died within 24 h. Havas & Likens (1985) exposed the crustaceans *Daphnia catawba* and *Holopedium gibberum*, and the insect larvae *Chaoborus punctipennis* and *Chironomus anthrocinus* to the same aluminium concentrations (0.02, 0.32 and 1.02 mg Al/litre) at pH levels of 3.5, 4.0, 4.5, 5.0 and 6.5. The crustaceans were exposed for 72 h and the insect larvae for 168 h. *D. catawba* was the most acid-sensitive species, mortality being significantly increased at and below pH 5.0; high concentrations of aluminium significantly increased mortality only at pH 6.5. *H. gibberum* was less sensitive to both hydrogen ions and aluminium than *D. catawba*. The highest aluminium concentration was moderately toxic at pH 6.5; however, as with *D. catawba*, the effect of aluminium at lower pH was completely masked by hydrogen ion toxicity. Neither aluminium nor hydrogen ions affected the mortality of *C. punctipennis* or *C. anthrocinus*.

Lamb & Bailey (1981) studied the effects of aluminium sulfate on larvae of the midge *Tanytarsus dissimilis* at pH 7.8. There was no apparent effect of aluminium on either second or third instar larvae at aluminium sulfate doses of between 80 and 960 mg/litre after 96 h. Owing to the polymeric, coagulant nature of aluminium sulfate, a white grey precipitate (up to 3-4 mm) formed in all solutions.

Six common macro-invertebrates were exposed to 200 µg/litre aluminium sulfate at pH 4.5 and a calcium concentration of 2.45 mg/litre. The order of acid sensitivity (mean 48-h survival is given in parentheses) for the species tested was: *Caenis* sp. (2%) > *Hyalella azteca* (12%) > *Enallagma* sp. (20%) > *Gyraulus* sp. (55%) > Chironomidae (94%) > Hydracarina (99%). Aluminium significantly reduced survival still further in *H. azteca*, *Gyraulus* sp. and Chironomidae. However, the addition of aluminium significantly increased survival for *Enallagma* sp. and *Caenis* sp. when compared with the acid-only group (Havens, 1993).

b) *Long-term toxicity*

France & Stokes (1987) studied the effect of nominal aluminium concentrations of 0.05 to 0.70 mg/litre on the hydrogen ion toxicity to the amphipod *Hyalella azteca* over an 8-day period. Aluminium concentrations of 0.25 and 0.40 mg/litre at pH 4.8 and 0.40 mg/litre at pH 4.3 significantly increased the mortality of *H. azteca* compared with that in reference aluminium concentrations of 0.05 mg/litre. Mortality rates remained unchanged with the addition of 0.25 mg Al/litre at pH 4.3 or 5.3 and with either 0.40 mg Al/litre or 0.70 mg Al/litre at pH 4.0. The authors predicted from these results that mortality of this amphipod from springmelt pulses will be determined primarily by hydrogen ions and only secondarily by aluminium in the pH range 4.3 to 5.3. Berrill et al. (1985) found no effect of aluminium (up to 200 µEq/litre) on the accumulated 10-day mortality caused by hydrogen ions in the crayfish *Orconectes rusticus*, *O. propinquus* and *Cambarus robustus*.

Biesinger & Christensen (1972) exposed water fleas (*Daphnia magna*) to aluminium chloride for a period of three weeks in Lake Superior water (pH 7.4-8.2). An LC_{50} of 1.4 mg total aluminium/litre was calculated and the EC_{50}, based on reproductive impairment, was found to be 0.68 mg/litre.

Burton & Allan (1986) exposed three species of stream invertebrates (*Nemoura*, *Asellus* and *Physella*) to aluminium concentrations of 250 or 500 µg/litre at pH 4, 5 and 7 for 28 days in experimental streams. Survival of all species was significantly decreased at pH 4; the addition of aluminium at 15 °C did not cause additional mortality. However, at 2 °C or with low organic matter the addition of 500 µg/litre caused a significant additional mortality for both *Nemoura* and *Asellus*. Addition of citrate reduced the effect of aluminium in low-organic treatments.

Petrich & Reish (1979) studied the effect of aluminium chloride (pH 7.6-8.0) on the polychaetes *Neanthes arenaceodenata*, *Capitella capitata* and *Ctenodrilus serratus*. Neither *Capitella* nor *Neanthes* were affected by a 7-day exposure to 2 mg/litre aluminium chloride (the maximum concentration that could be used without precipitation in seawater). *Ctenodrilus* showed significant reproductive suppression during a 28-day exposure to aluminium chloride concentrations of 0.5 mg/litre or more.

c)   *Physiological and biochemical effects*

Herrmann & Andersson (1986) exposed the nymphs of three mayfly species *Heptagenia fuscogrisea*, *H. sulphurea* and *Ephemera danica* to total inorganic monomeric aluminium levels of 500 and 2000 µg/litre at pH 4.0 and 4.8 for 10 days. The oxygen consumption rate of nymphs was monitored. The rate showed a tendency to increase at 500 µg/litre for *H. sulphurea* and *E. danica*. At 2000 µg/litre there were significant increases in the oxygen consumption rate for all three species at both pH levels. *E. danica*, which is restricted to less heavily acidified regions, was the most severely affected by the aluminium treatments. Exposure of *E. danica* and *H. sulphurea* to the same aluminium and pH regimes for 14 days caused significant aluminium-related decreases in sodium levels (Herrmann, 1987).

Malley & Chang (1985) studied calcium-45 uptake by postmoult crayfish (*Orconectes virilis*) exposed to aluminium chloride concentrations of 200, 500 and 1000 µg Al/litre for 2 to 3 h at pH 5.3 to 7.2. An aluminium concentration of 200 µg/litre had no effect on calcium uptake at neutral pH. However, reducing the pH to 5.5 caused an inhibition of calcium uptake. Exposure of crayfish to 500 µg/litre, under acidic conditions, also caused a significant reduction in calcium uptake. However, exposure to acidic conditions alone revealed that most of the reduction was due to acidic conditions rather than aluminium. In fact, transferring the crayfish from 500 µg Al/litre to 1000 µg Al/litre, under acidic conditions, had no significant effect. Witters et al. (1984) maintained the air-breathing water bugs (*Corixa punctata*) at aluminium chloride concentrations of 0.15, 0.3 (the natural level), 2.5, 5, 10 and 50 mg Al/litre at pH 3 and 4. A dose-related decrease in sodium-influx was observed and there was a significant 50% decrease when comparing the lowest concentration with 10 mg/litre.

d) *Population studies*

Havens (1991) studied the effect of aluminium on the survival of littoral zooplankton species collected from alkaline lakes. Toxicity tests were performed at pH 4.5 with or without aluminium (500 µg/litre) for 24 h. The four cladocerans *Simocephalus serrulatus*, *Diaphanosoma birgii*, *Acantholeberis curvirostris* and *Chydorus sphaericus* were unaffected by either the acidic conditions or aluminium. The cladoceran *Eurycercus lamellatus* and the copepod *Acanthocyclops vernalis* suffered 100% mortality at pH 4.5 with or without aluminium. The cladocerans *Camptocercus rectirostris*, *Alona costata* and *Pleuroxus denticulatus* and the copepod *Mesocyclops edax* showed decreased survival at pH 4.5 and a significantly greater decrease in survival under acid conditions and aluminium exposure.

Havens & Heath (1989) carried out an *in situ* mesocosm study of zooplankton responses to acidification and aluminium. Large plastic enclosures were acidified (pH 4.5) with or without the addition of aluminium, giving an inorganic monomeric aluminium concentration of 180 µg/litre. The populations of acid-sensitive species declined more rapidly in the acid-plus-aluminium treatment than in the acid-alone treatment. Two cladocerans (*Bosmina longirostris* and *Chydorus sphaericus*) were tolerant to acidity and aluminium. Havens & Decosta (1987) performed bioassays using *in situ* enclosures to expose zooplankton to acidified waters (pH 4.7) with and without the addition of aluminium (300 µg/litre) for up to 49 days. Acidification did not affect abundance of zooplankton or succession because all species were acid-tolerant. However, addition of aluminium resulted in a reduction in zooplankton abundance.

9.1.2.3 Fish

The bioavailability and toxicity of aluminium varies with its chemical speciation. In the case of fish, higher polymers are less toxic than monomers and polymers of low relative molecular mass. Polymerization is a slow process, hence the biological activity of aluminium in water depends not only on aluminium concentration and conditions such as pH, temperature and the presence of complexing ions, but can also depend on the pre-history of the water. The various aluminium species differ in their effects on fish gills, either disturbing the ion balance or interfering with respiration. The toxicity diminishes if the aluminium is inactivated by complexation with organic ligands, fluoride or silicate, or by extensive polymerization to large molecules in the water (Rosseland & Staurnes, 1994).

a)   *Acute toxicity*

The acute toxicity of aluminium to fish is summarized in Table 25. The 96-h LC_{50} values range from 0.095 mg/litre (American flagfish) to 235 mg/litre (mosquito fish). However, care must be taken when interpreting these results because of the significant effects of pH on the availability of aluminium. The wide range of LC_{50} values probably reflects this variable availability. LT_{50} values for salmonids

Table 25. Toxicity of aluminium to fish (laboratory studies)

Organism	Size/age	Stat/flow[a]	Temperature (°C)	Hardness[b] (mg/litre)	Calcium concentration (mg/litre)	pH	Salt	LT_{50} (mg inorganic monomeric (Al/litre)	96-h LC_{50}[c] (mg Al/litre)	Reference
Atlantic salmon (*Salmo salar*)	1 +	flow	5.2	5	2.0	4.95	sulfate	59	0.245 m	Rosseland & Skogheim (1984)
	2 +					4.95		33	0.245 m	
	1 +	flow	5.2	5	2.0	4.94	sulfate	57	0.313 m	
	2 +					4.94	sulfate	22	0.313 m	
	1 +					4.90		27	0.463 m	
	2 +					4.90		15	0.463 m	
Brown trout (*Salmo trutta*)	2 +	flow	5.2	5	2.0	4.94	sulfate	40	0.313 m	
	1 +					4.90		57	0.463	
	2 +					4.80		30	0.463	
Atlantic salmon (*Salmo salar*)	2 + (38 g)	stat	3.7		1.3	5.06	chloride	108	0.075	Skogheim & Rosseland (1986)
					1.3	4.92		38	0.137 m	
					1.3	4.90		32	0.177 m	
Mummichog (*Fundulus heteroclitus*)	2.7 g	stat	20	6.6[d]			ammonium sulfate		3.6 n	Dorfman (1977)
	2.7 g	stat	20	17[d]			ammonium sulfate		27.5 n	

Table 25 (contd).

Organism	Size/age	Stat/flow[a]	Temper-ature (°C)	Hardness[b] (mg/litre)	Calcium concen-tration (mg/litre)	pH	Salt	LT_{50} (mg inorganic monomeric (Al/litre)	96-h LC_{50}[c] (mg Al/litre)	Reference
Mummichog (*contd*).	2.7 g 2.7 g	stat stat	20 20	7.9[d] 18.8[d]			chloride chloride		3.6 n 31.5 n	Dorfman (1977)
Mosquito fish (*Gambusia affinis*)		stat stat	20-21 19-22			4.3-7.2 4.4-7.7	chloride sulfate		133 n 235 n	Wallen et al. (1957)
Fathead minnow (*Pimephales promelas*)	0.45 g 0.45 g	stat stat	22 22	38 38		7.4 7.4	nitrate[e] sulfate[f]		4.25 (3.3-5.5) 4.4 (3.4-5.6)	Mayer & Ellersieck (1986)
American flagfish (*Jordanella floridae*)	2-3 days	stat	25	6.0		5.8			0.095 m	Hutchinson & Sprague (1986)

[a] Stat = static conditions (water unchanged for duration of test)
[b] Hardness expressed as mg $CaCO_3$/litre
[c] n = based on nominal concentrations; m = based on measured concentrations
[d] Salinity (%)
[e] 7.2% technical material
[f] 8.1% technical material

are also summarized in Table 25. Muramoto (1981) found that addition of the complexans NTA and EDTA reduced the acute (48-h) toxicity of aluminium to carp (*Cyprinus carpio*).

Rosseland & Skogheim (1984) exposed three salmonid species, Atlantic salmon (*Salmo salar*), brown trout (*Salmo trutta*) and brook trout (*Salvelinus fontinalis*), to inorganic monomeric aluminium concentrations of 120, 225 and 415 µg/litre (as aluminium sulfate) under flow-through conditions. Owing to the acidity of the aluminium sulfate the pH decreased from 6.6 to 4.9. Pre-smolt salmon were the most sensitive, showing 100% mortality within 48 h at 245 µg/litre. Brook trout were the least sensitive, mortalities only occurring at 463 µg/litre (less than 25% over the 64-h exposure). The authors reported that whenever aluminium sulfate was added excessive mucus was observed between the gill lamellae; or all species mucus clogging increased with an increased addition of aluminium. However, there was no excessive mucus on gills of fish that died in acid brook water with naturally occurring aluminium concentrations.

Schofield & Trojnar (1980) exposed brook trout (*Salvelinus fontinalis*) fry to aluminium (0.1-0.5 mg/litre) at various pH levels (4.0-5.2). At pH 4.0 survival of fish was not related to aluminium concentration, the LT_{50} values ranging from 2.8 to 5.2 days. However, at pH levels of $\geq$ 4.4, mortality increased with increasing aluminium concentration. At pH 4.9 and 5.2 neither acidity nor 0.1 mg Al/litre affected fish mortality; 0.5 mg Al/litre produced LT_{50} values ranging from 1.6 to 3.3 days. Symptoms of stress were darkening of skin coloration and cessation of feeding. All fish at pH 4.0 and 4.4 showed these symptoms, although they took longer to develop at pH 4.4 with 0 or 0.1 mg/litre aluminium. No symptoms were observed at pH 4.9 and 5.2 for aluminium concentrations of 0.1 mg/litre; however, stress symptoms were seen in all groups exposed to $\geq$ 0.25 mg/litre aluminium at any pH level. Heavy accumulations of mucous and cellular debris on the gills were found in trout exposed to $\geq$ 0.25 mg/litre aluminium at pH levels of $\geq$ 4.4. Histopathological changes observed in sections of gills from fish exposed to aluminium levels $\geq$ 0.5 mg/litre included cell proliferation at the distal ends of gill filaments, lamellar oedema and fusion, epithelial desquamation, filament collapse, and general loss of gill structure.

Gundersen et al. (1994) exposed rainbow trout (*Oncorhynchus mykiss*) to aluminium at pH values ranging from 7.97 to 8.56 in 96-h tests. No significant mortality was observed at pH 8.33 or less and filterable aluminium concentrations of 0.52 mg/litre or less. However, 100% mortality was found at pH 8.58 and a filterable aluminium concentration of 1 mg/litre. The 96-h LC_{50} values ranged from 0.36 to 0.79 mg filterable aluminium/litre at weakly alkaline pH levels.

Young brown trout (*Salmo trutta*) exposed for 5 days to pH 5 in high calcium water at temperatures of 4 and 12 °C showed no alterations in growth or in mucous cell concentration and volume. However, exposure to aluminium (230 µg/litre) under the same testing regime resulted in significant growth depression but no changes to mucous cell morphometrics (Segner et al., 1988).

Freeman & Everhart (1971) found that the toxicity of aluminium hydroxide complexes (5.2 mg/litre) to rainbow trout (*Oncorhynchus mykiss*) increased with the amount of aluminium dissolved. At pH 6.8, 8.0, 8.5 and 9.0 the amounts of aluminium dissolved were 1%, 10%, 31% and 97%, respectively, and the respective LT_{50} values were 38.90, 31.96, 7.46 and 2.98 days. Surviving fish recovered rapidly in all groups, except those exposed at pH 8.0, with normal growth being resumed within 2 weeks (Freeman, 1973).

b) *Long-term toxicity*

Hickie et al. (1993) exposed rainbow trout (*Oncorhynchus mykiss*) to aluminium for 23-26 days after hatching at pH 5.8 and 4.9. The 144-h LC_{50} for total aluminium was found to be > 1050 and 91 µg/litre at the two pH levels, respectively. An LC_{50} of 1.17 µg/litre was calculated for fish exposed from 16 to 19 days after hatching at pH 4.9.

Neville & Campbell (1988) exposed juvenile rainbow trout (*Oncorhynchus mykiss*) to aluminium (2.8 µmol/litre nominal concentration) in a flow-through system over a pH range of 4.0 to 6.5 for up to 11 days. The response of trout to aluminium was most severe at pH 4.5 (electrolyte loss) and 6.1 (asphyxia). At pH 4.0 there was competition between hydrogen ions and aluminium for binding at the gill surface which reduced toxicity. However, the toxic response at pH 6.1 appeared to be more complex being either a bimodal response to two different aluminium species or a physical response to precipitation on the gill surface.

Driscoll et al. (1980) studied the toxic effect of aluminium on brook trout (*Salvelinus fontinalis*) fry. At pH values of 4.4 and 5.2 there was no effect on survival during the 14-day exposure period. The addition of inorganic monomeric aluminium (0.42-0.48 mg/litre) produced an LT_{50} of 115 h at pH 5.2 and 256 h at pH 4.4. Treatment with excess fluoride or citrate reduced the toxicity of aluminium. Skogheim & Rosseland (1986) exposed Atlantic salmon (*Salmo salar*) to aluminium at varying pH levels. No mortality occurred during a 20-day exposure to pH 5.07 alone. At pH 5.06 and 75 µg Al/litre the LT_{50} was 108 h, at pH 4.92 and 137 µg Al/litre the LT_{50} was 38 h, and at pH 4.9 and 177 µg Al/litre the LT_{50} was 32 h. Brown (1983) exposed brown trout (*Salmo trutta*) to aluminium (0, 0.25 and 0.5 mg/litre) at pH values ranging from 4.5 to 5.4 and calcium concentrations ranging from 0.5 to 2.0 mg/litre for 16 days. Survival was relatively unaffected by pH except at a calcium level of 0.25 mg/litre and a pH of 4.5. High mortality was observed at both aluminium exposure levels at calcium levels of 0.25 and 0.5 mg/litre. At calcium levels of 1.0 and 2.0 mg/litre there was increased mortality at the highest aluminium concentration.

Gundersen et al. (1994) studied the effects of aluminium on rainbow trout (*Oncorhynchus mykiss*) in 16-day tests. Growth rates were higher at weakly alkaline pH (7.97-8.10) than at near-neutral pH (7.30-7.35). The authors concluded that polymeric and colloidal forms of aluminium are more potent than soluble forms in restricting growth. Trout exposed to aluminium at 0.53 to 2.56 mg/litre and humic acid at 4.31 to 5.23 mg/litre had higher specific growth rates and lower mortality than those exposed to aluminium and no humic acid at all the pH values tested. When exposed to sub-lethal concentrations of aluminium (38 µg/litre nominal concentration) in a synthetic soft water of pH 5.2, rainbow trout became acclimated to aluminium and showed increased resistance when exposed to lethal levels of aluminium (162 µg/litre nominal concentration) in the same soft water. Acclimation was associated with reduced disturbances of ionoregulation and respiration (Wilson et al., 1994a). Acclimation to 38 µg/litre (nominal concentration) also caused a 4-fold increase in gill mucous density and a reduction in apparent lamellar surface area (Wilson et al., 1994b). Acclimation to sub-lethal levels of aluminium could explain the continued presence of fish populations in acidified lakes and rivers containing more than 100 µg Al/litre. Wicklund Glynn et al. (1992) exposed minnows (*Phoxinus phoxinus*) to acidic water (pH 5.0) with and without aluminium (150 µg/litre) at various calcium

(0, 0.07 and 2 mmol/litre) and humus (5 and 25 Pt) concentrations for 15 days. Mortality among fish exposed to aluminium was higher than among unexposed fish but was less at the highest calcium level. At 0.07 mmol calcium/litre, the aluminium-induced mortality was reduced by the presence of humus. Gill morphology was altered after exposure to aluminium at pH 5.0, but was not affected by different concentrations of calcium or humus.

Juvenile brook trout (*Salvelinus fontinalis*) were intermittently or continuously exposed to aluminium (0.2 to 1.2 mg/litre) at pH 4.4 or 4.9 for 24 days. There was 100% survival of fish at both pH levels in the absence of aluminium, regardless of exposure regime. Aluminium significantly reduced survival at 0.2 mg/litre or more for all exposure regimes except the intermittent exposure at pH 4.4 where significant mortality was observed at 0.4 mg/litre or more. When aluminium concentration was expressed as the 24-day mean, it was shown that intermittent exposure was more toxic than continuous exposure (Siddens et al., 1986). Ingersoll et al. (1990) exposed 1-year-old brook trout (*Salvelinus fontinalis*) to combinations of aluminium, pH and calcium during a 28-day experiment. Survival was reduced at inorganic monomeric aluminium concentrations of 29 µg/litre at pH 5.2 and $\geq$ 228 µg/litre at pH 4.4 or 4.8. Fish weight was reduced at an aluminium concentration of $\geq$ 34 µg/litre and pH < 4.8. The gills sampled from low pH groups showed lifting of the outer epithelium and hypertrophy of chloride and epithelial cells. These effects were more pronounced at low pH with elevated aluminium concentrations. Effects such as vacuolation and degeneration of epithelial and chloride cells and the presence of dense cells were also observed at low pH and elevated aluminium concentration.

No mortality of lake trout (*Salvelinus namaycush*) embryos occurred during 5-day exposures to aluminium sulfate (0, 100 and 200 µg Al/litre) at pH 5.0 or during 21- and 32-day recovery periods. None of the embryos or later alevins displayed erratic swimming behaviour or mucus accumulation around the mouth or gills. After 21-day (late embryos) and 32-day (early embryos) recovery periods, fish at the highest aluminium concentrations were significantly smaller in length, had reduced whole body concentrations of calcium and potassium, and were significantly less successful as predators on *Daphnia magna* (Gunn & Noakes, 1987).

Cleveland et al. (1991) exposed brook trout (*Salvelinus fontinalis*) to a nominal aluminium concentration of 200 µg/litre for 56 days under flow-through conditions at pH 5.3, 6.1 and 7.2. The weights of trout exposed to pH 5.3 and 6.1 did not differ significantly throughout the study. After day 3 fish exposed to pH 7.2 weighed significantly more than those at pH 5.3 and 6.1. Mortality was significantly higher in brook trout exposed to pH 5.3 than in those exposed to pH 6.1 (except on day 56) or 7.2.

c)   *Lifestage effects*

Not only do species differences in response to a given pH and aluminium concentration exist but great differences in sensitivity also exist between strains of the same species as well as between different life-history stages (Rosseland et al., 1990; Rosseland & Staurnes, 1994).

Fivelstad & Leivestad (1984) studied the toxicity of aluminium to different life-stages of Atlantic salmon (*Salmo salar*) and brown trout (*Salmo trutta*). To study the effect of acidity citrate was added. Only 1 of 200 swim-up salmon larvae died during a 108-h exposure at pH 4.9; no behavioural responses were observed. However, when exposed to aluminium concentrations ranging from 110 to 300 µg/litre, salmon swim-up larvae were more sensitive than the postlarval stage. Toxicity was found to be most significantly correlated with inorganic monomeric aluminium concentration, survival time decreasing with increasing aluminium concentration. The LT_{50} at an inorganic monomeric aluminium concentration of 148 µg/litre was 26 h for swim-up larvae. Exposure of salmon parr to natural aluminium variations (50-180 µg/litre) at pH 5.3 induced hyperventilatory responses together with increases in haematocrit and small decreases in chloride. The authors concluded that coughing, hyperventilation and excessive mucous clogging on the gill surface was due to an irritant effect of aluminium. Brown trout exposed at pH 5 to the same aluminium regime showed no sublethal stress symptoms.

Rosseland & Skogheim (1984) demonstrated the increased sensitivity of Atlantic salmon undergoing smoltification compared to younger year classes. In a laboratory study at pH 4.9-5.0 and inorganic monomeric Al concentrations of 130-463 µg/litre, pre-smolt (age 2 years) were more sensitive than parr (age 1 year) in all combinations of pH and aluminium. For instance, at pH 4.95 and 245 µg Al/litre, the LT_{50} for pre-smolt was 35 h whereas the LT_{50} for parr was 60 h.

Early life-stage (fertilized eggs, alevins and swim-up fry) golden trout (*Oncorhynchus aguabonita aguabonita*) were exposed to low pH (4.5-6.5) and aluminium (50-300 µg Al/litre, nominal concentration) for 7 days. Significant mortality occurred at pH 4.5 in the absence of aluminium, at pH 5.5 in the presence of 100 µg aluminium/litre for larvae and at pH 5.0 with 300 µg aluminium/litre for alevins. The duration of swimming and feeding activity was unaffected by treatment in golden trout exposed as eggs. Locomotory behaviour of alevins was severely inhibited at both pH 5.0 and 5.5 irrespective of treatment and at pH 4.5 and 6.0 in aluminium-exposed fish. Feeding activity was reduced at pH 4.5, at pH 5.0 with ≥ 50 µg aluminium/litre and at pH 5.5 with 100 µg/litre. Swimming activity was not greatly affected among fish exposed as swim-up larvae. Feeding activity was greatly inhibited at all aluminium concentrations and at pH 4.5 (DeLonay et al., 1993).

Farag et al. (1993) studied the effect of aluminium (50-300 µg Al/litre, nominal concentration) on eggs, eyed embryos, alevins and swim-up larvae of cutthroat trout (*Oncorhynchus clarki bouvieri*) at pH values ranging from 4.5 to 6.5 for either 7 days or during continuous exposure until 40 days after hatching. Fish survival decreased when pH was lowered to 5.0 or 4.5 for 7 days during the egg stage. Alevin and swim-up larval stages were less sensitive to low pH and more sensitive to aluminium, with 100 µg/litre at pH 5.0 significantly decreasing survival. The eyed embryo stage was the most resistant; there was > 90% survival in all groups except in the presence of > 100 µg/litre at both pH 5.0 and 5.5. During continuous exposure, survival decreased with time and individuals died earlier in each life-stage when exposed to combinations of pH and aluminium than did those exposed to pH alone. Swim-up larvae were the most sensitive group with regard to growth and all larvae exposed to 50 µg/litre showed significantly reduced growth.

Buckler et al. (1987) exposed striped bass (*Morone saxatilis*) of different ages to total aluminium (up to 400 µg/litre) at various pH levels (pH 5.0-7.2) in a flow-through diluter system for 7 days. Eleven-day-old fish showed significant mortality at pH 6.0 irrespective of aluminium exposure; significant mortality was observed at 25 µg/litre for pH 6.5 and at 400 µg/litre for pH 7.2. Older fish

(160 days) were less sensitive, showing significant mortality at 50 µg Al/litre for pH 6.0, 200 µg/litre for pH 6.5, and 400 µg/litre for pH 7.2. In a similar test, 300 µg/litre was lethal to 100% of both 159- and 195-day-old bass at pH 5.5, but produced no observable adverse effects at pH 6.5 or 7.2. Mortality among 159-day-old fish held in water at pH 5.5 without aluminium was 22% after 7 days, there being no deaths among control fish. No mortality was observed among 195-day-old fish exposed to pH 5.5 alone.

Eggs, larvae and post-larvae of white suckers (*Catostomus commersoni*) and brook trout (*Salvelinus fontinalis*) were exposed to pH levels of 4.2 to 5.6 and inorganic monomeric aluminium concentrations ranging from 0 to 0.5 mg/litre. White sucker embryos were very sensitive to low pH levels, with none surviving to the eyed stage at pH levels of 5.0 or less. The addition of aluminium increased embryo survival through the eyed stage but did not increase hatching. At pH levels of 5.4 and 5.6 survival to eyed stage increased to 38% to 69% and was 74% to 81% in controls. At pH levels above 5.2 the presence of aluminium resulted in embryo deformities. Survival of trout eggs through the eyed stage was unaffected at pH 4.6 or more irrespective of aluminium treatment. However, in the absence of aluminium at pH levels of 4.4 survival decreased and at pH 4.2 no embryos survived. The addition of aluminium to low pH groups significantly increased survival through the eyed stage to hatching. All white sucker larvae died within 146 h at pH levels below 5.0 with or without aluminium. In the absence of aluminium at pH levels greater than 5.0, more than 80% survived the 13-day experiment; however, the addition of aluminium further decreased the survival of larvae. At pH levels of 4.4 or more > 97% of trout larvae survived without aluminium. The addition of more than 0.1 mg Al/litre at all pH levels decreased the survival of larvae. White sucker post-larvae were sensitive to low pH levels, only 16 to 68% surviving at pH 4.6. The addition of aluminium to acidic solutions further decreased survival. In the presence of high levels of aluminium (0.3 or 0.5 mg/litre) at all pH levels, all post-larvae died within 75 h. At aluminium levels of 0.1 and 0.2 mg/litre at low pH levels all post-larvae died within 145 h. Brook trout post-larvae were tolerant of low pH levels. All post-larvae survived at pH levels ranging from 6.99 to 4.22 without aluminium. At aluminium levels of 0.2 mg/litre or more survival was decreased at all pH levels (Baker & Schofield, 1982).

Cleveland et al. (1986) carried out a partial life-cycle toxicity study on brook trout (*Salvelinus fontinalis*) for 60 days in a flow-through proportional diluter. Eyed brook trout eggs and the resultant larvae were exposed in water containing 3 mg calcium/litre at nominal pH values of 7.2, 5.5 and 4.5 with and without aluminium (300 µg Al/litre, nominal concentration) until 30 days after hatching. Mortality of trout eggs was not influenced by aluminium but was significantly increased by low pH. Larval growth and mortality was unaffected by aluminium at pH 7.2 and 4.5, but mortality was significantly increased and growth decreased by aluminium at pH 5.5. DNA and RNA content was significantly reduced by aluminium at pH 5.5. In general swimming and feeding behaviour were unaffected by aluminium at pH 7.2 and significantly reduced by aluminium at pH 5.5. At pH 4.5 behaviour was inhibited to such an extent that possible effects of aluminium were masked. In a second experiment 37-day-old trout were exposed to similar conditions. Mortality was significantly increased by aluminium at pH 5.5 and 4.5. Aluminium significantly reduced growth at pH 7.2 and 5.5. DNA and RNA content was significantly increased by aluminium at pH 5.5. Juvenile trout behaviour was less affected by acid conditions than in the case of larvae; there were significant decreases in behaviour in the presence of aluminium at pH 5.5 and 4.5. Hunn et al. (1987) utilizing a similar experimental set-up found that embryo mortality exceeded 80% at pH 4.5, averaged 15% to 18% at pH 5.5 and was less than 2% at pH 7.5. Aluminium significantly increased mortality at pH 4.5 but did not affect mortality at pH 5.5 or 7.5. Hatching success was pH-dependent and was not influenced by aluminium exposure. Brook trout larvae suffered 100% mortality at pH 4.5, 20% mortality at pH 7.5 with or without aluminium, 69% mortality at pH 5.5 without aluminium and 100% mortality within 15 days with aluminium. Cleveland et al. (1989) reported that 60-day no-observed-effect nominal concentrations for aluminium at pH 5.6 to 5.7 were 29 µg/litre for swimming capacity, 68 µg/litre for weight and 142 µg/litre for frequency of movement (2 min period), strike frequency (directed at prey), fry mortality and length. At pH 6.5 to 6.6 no-observed-effect concentration (NOEC) values were 88 µg/litre for length and weight, 169 µg/litre for fry mortality and > 350 µg/litre for movement, strike frequency and swimming capacity.

d)   *Physiological and biochemical effects*

Physiological and biochemical effects have recently been reviewed by Rosseland & Staurnes (1994).

Witters (1986) studied the effect of total aluminium (350 µg/litre), pH (4.1 and 6.1) and calcium concentration (38 and 190 µEq/litre) on ion balance and haematology in rainbow trout (*Oncorhynchus mykiss*) exposed for 3.5 h. None of the treatment combinations affected the number of erythrocytes or the haemoglobin content. However, exposure to aluminium under acidic conditions significantly reduced plasma osmolarity and increased plasma potassium levels. Plasma sodium and chloride levels were significantly reduced under acidic conditions with or without aluminium. The haematocrit value was significantly increased and plasma ammonium decreased by aluminium only under acidic conditions and at low calcium concentration.

Muniz & Leivestad (1980) reported that brown trout (*Salmo trutta*) exposed to acidic conditions (pH 4.3 to 5.5) showed plasma losses of both chloride and sodium. These losses were enhanced by the addition of total aluminium at 900 µg/litre. Fish showing signs of stress exhibited hyperventilation, coughing and excessive mucus clogging of the gills. The authors reported that the changes in blood electrolytes indicate that aluminium toxicity is similar to that seen with hydrogen ion stress. However, aluminium can cause such effects at pH levels that are not physiologically harmful.

Wood & McDonald (1987) studied the physiology of brook trout and rainbow trout exposed to inorganic monomeric aluminium concentrations ranging from 111 to 1000 µg/litre (as aluminium chloride) at pHs ranging from 4.4 to 6.5. Acid stress alone for 10 days was not lethal to adult brook trout, but there was a net loss of sodium and chloride ions. The addition of aluminium resulted in an increased loss of ions and severe mortality. At pH 4.8, low calcium level (25 µEq/litre) and an aluminium concentration of 333 µg/litre, the LT_{50} was found to be 39 h. At a lower pH (4.4) the average survival time was twice as long. The cause of death was ionoregulatory failure. However, increasing the calcium levels (400 µEq/litre) still killed fish almost as quickly but the cause of death was respiratory disturbance. Rainbow trout were more sensitive to both acid and acid/aluminium than brook trout. Respiratory disturbances were found to be the cause of death in both high and low calcium groups exposed to acid/aluminium conditions. For both species there was a correlation between toxic effects and aluminium accumulation in gills.

Dalziel et al. (1986) exposed brown trout to nominal aluminium concentrations of 8 µmol/litre at pH levels ranging from 7.0 to 4.0 and calcium levels of 10 or 50 µmol/litre. Low pH had little effect on the influx of sodium, but the addition of aluminium significantly reduced influx at pH 4.5 and 4.0. Efflux of sodium tended to be increased by low pH, but no further effect was caused by aluminium. Aluminium at higher pH values appeared to have no effect on sodium fluxes. Dalziel et al. (1987) found that reduced pH levels had no effect on the sodium influx in brown trout (*Salmo trutta*). However, the presence of aluminium at concentrations of 2 µmol/litre at pH 4.5 and 4.0 significantly decreased sodium influx. At pH 5.4 there was no effect of aluminium on influx. Sodium efflux was significantly increased at low pH. Increasing the aluminium concentration at pH 5.4, and to a smaller extent at pH 4.5, tended to increase efflux. There was no effect of aluminium on sodium efflux at pH 4.0.

Booth et al. (1988) studied the effects of total aluminium at concentrations of 333 and 1000 µg/litre and at low pH (5.2-4.4) on net ion fluxes and ion balance in the brook trout (*Salvelinus fontinalis*) over a period of 11 days. Low pH caused a pH-dependent net loss of sodium and chloride ions and the addition of aluminium increased this loss. The authors reported that any fish losing more than 4% of total sodium ions during the initial 24 h of aluminium exposure was 90% more likely to die. All fish exposed to aluminium accumulated it on gill surfaces; fish that died accumulated more aluminium than survivors.

Leivestad et al. (1987) studied the effect of inorganic monomeric aluminium on Atlantic salmon (*Salmo salar*) exposed for 28 weeks at pH levels of 4.8-6.5 and aluminium concentrations of 50-350 µg/litre. The authors found that failure in ionic regulation was the primary cause for mortality and that Na-K-ATPase activity was reduced at toxic aluminium levels. The symptoms were correlated with ion-exchangeable aluminium, precipitating aluminium hydroxide having low toxicity. Staurnes et al. (1993) maintained smolting Atlantic salmon in soft water at pH 5 both with and without 50 µg/litre total aluminium. Exposure to acid water resulted in osmoregulatory failure and high mortality, and aluminium greatly enhanced the toxicity.

Sensitivity to acid and acid-aluminium increased when fish had developed to seawater-tolerant smolts. Gill carbonic anhydrase activity was reduced by aluminium exposure. Fish in both treatment groups had low seawater tolerance and this was related to a decline in Na^+/K^+-ATPase activity.

Hutchinson et al. (1987) studied the effects of total aluminium (0-1000 μg/litre) at pH levels ranging from 3.8 to 6.0 on the early lifestages of lake trout (*Salvelinus namaycush*), brook trout (*Salvelinus fontinalis*) and pumpkin seed sunfish (*Lepomis gibbosus*). Three different responses were observed: a) aluminium toxicity at pH ≤ 5.0 represented joint action with hydrogen ions producing ionoregulatory failure; b) at pH 5.0-6.0 aluminium toxicity required concentrations of inorganic forms that greatly exceeded theoretical gibbsite solubility; c) at acutely lethal levels of pH and ionic strength, aluminium increased the resistance time of eggs, fry and adults.

Ogilvie & Stechey (1983) studied the respiratory responses of rainbow trout (*Oncorhynchus mykiss*) to aluminium exposure (50 to 500 μg/litre) at a pH of 6.0 and an exposure period of 26 h. Mean opercular rate was significantly increased at 500 μg aluminium/litre and mean cough rate was significantly increased at both 200 and 500 μg/litre. Spontaneous locomotion and mean activity levels were variable in all groups.

Neurotoxic effects on the olfactory organ of rainbow trout were demonstrated by Klaprat et al. (1988), who exposed the fish to pH 7.7 and pH 4.7 both with (5.0, 9.5 and 20.0 μmol total Al/litre) and without aluminium. At pH 4.7 alone, increased mucous was observed over parts of the olfactory epithelium. After Al additions, however, loss of receptor cell cilia, irregular shaped olfactory knobs, changed microvilli and swellings of microridge cells were observed. Electrical response from the olfactory nerve to L-serin was not changed by pH alone, but was depressed by aluminium additives. Since sensory organs play a very important role in the behavioural ecology of fish populations (feeding, alarm signals, pheromones, imprinting, spawning, etc), neurotoxic effects on the olfactory organ can have great adverse effects in nature (Rosseland & Staurnes, 1994).

e)   *Pathological effects*

Hunter et al. (1980) noted that rainbow trout (*Oncorhynchus mykiss*) which survived exposure to 50 mg/litre aluminium at pH 8.0 to 9.0 showed several pathological signs of toxicity. These included proliferative changes in the gills and congestion of the secondary lamellae, slight demyelination of the brain, extensive necrosis of the liver, severe inflammatory glomerular necrosis of the kidney and some evidence of skin hyperplasia. Karlsson-Norrgren et al. (1986b) exposed brown trout (*Salmo trutta*) to aluminium sulfate (50, 200 and 500 µg total aluminium/litre) at pH 5.5 and 7.0 for up to 6 weeks. Advanced gill lesions (enlargement of secondary lamellae due to the increased number of chloride cells in the epithelia) were observed in fish exposed to aluminium at pH 5.5 and a temperature of 2.5 °C. The lesions contained cytoplasmic aluminium precipitates. The addition of humus or increasing the pH to 7.0 reduced or inhibited the effects of aluminium. A water temperature of 15 °C reduced the gill lesions observed at 2.5 °C. However, prolonged exposure to higher water temperatures produced gill alterations even in controls. Eggs and the resulting fry of Atlantic salmon (*Salmo salar*) exposed to aluminium (38-300 µg/litre) at pH 5.5 were investigated. Scanning electron microscopy revealed gill abnormalities, which included poorly developed or absent secondary lamellae, fused primary lamellae, proliferation of epithelial cells and increased numbers of surface pits. These effects were not noted when fish were raised in aluminium-free water at pH values ranging from 4.5 to 7.2 (Jagoe et al., 1987).

9.1.2.4   Amphibians

Clark & LaZerte (1985) exposed eggs and tadpoles of the American toad (*Bufo americanus*) and the wood frog (*Rana sylvatica*) to total aluminium concentrations of 10, 20, 50, 100 and 200 µg/litre at pH ranging from 4.14 to 5.75. A nominal pH of 4.14 significantly reduced hatching in the absence of aluminium. Aluminium had no effect on hatching at pH 4.75 or pH 5.75. However, at pH 4.14 there was a significant reduction in hatching for eggs exposed to any aluminium concentration compared with eggs without aluminium at the same pH level. Tadpoles that hatched out were not affected by any aluminium concentration or pH level.

Clark & Hall (1985) studied the effects of total aluminium (7-210 µg/litre), pH (pH 4.41-6.29) and dissolved organic content

(2.2-9.9 mg/litre) at calcium concentrations of 2 mg/litre on *B. americanus*, *R. sylvatica* and the spotted salamander (*Ambystoma maculatum*). High aluminium, low pH and high dissolved organic content (DOC) significantly reduced hatching success of *B. americanus*. For *R. sylvatica* neither aluminium nor pH correlated significantly with hatching success over the range of pH tested. Hatching success for *A. maculatum* ranged from 41% at pH 4.4 to 68% at pH 6.1. Although pH was not significantly correlated with hatching success, a greater number of eggs hatched above pH 5.0 than below, the difference being significant. Decreased hatching success was correlated with high aluminium and high DOC. In a second experiment the authors studied the effects of aluminium (total aluminium 54-75 µg/litre) and pH (pH 4.23-5.8) at calcium concentrations of 2 mg/litre. Hatching success of *B. americanus* and *R. sylvatica* was unaffected at pH 4.8 and 5.8 with total aluminium concentrations of 54 to 63 µg/litre. However, there were significant reductions in hatching at a pH of 4.3 and total aluminium concentration of 75 µg/litre. Hatching success of *A. maculatum* was not correlated significantly with pH. However, hatching success was only 57% at the highest pH value and lowest aluminium concentration.

Gascon et al. (1987) studied the affects of total dissolved aluminium (7.4 µmol/litre), pH (4.5 and 6.2) and calcium (25 and 500 µEq/litre) on the eggs and tadpoles of *Rana sylvatica*. There was no egg mortality in any group. Hatching was significantly delayed in groups exposed to aluminium under acidic conditions. Tadpoles exposed to aluminium at pH 4.5 and calcium at 25 µEq/litre suffered 100% mortality. In a similar group where the pH was allowed to drift up to 5.3, mortality was not significant. Metamorphosis in surviving tadpoles was significantly delayed by acidic conditions and aluminium exposure. Growth, as measured by dry weight, was significantly depressed in the group suffering 100% mortality. In the groups exposed to aluminium with either pH rising to 5.3 or calcium at 500 µEq/litre, growth was significantly increased over controls.

Freda & McDonald (1990) exposed embryos (4 to 5 days) and tadpoles (96 h) of the leopard frog (*Rana pipiens*) to a range of total aluminium concentrations (250-1000 µg/litre) and pHs (4.2-6.5). The pH and the aluminium concentration had a significant effect on the survival of embryos. All control embryos hatched whereas 94% of embryos at pH 4.2 failed to hatch. At pH 4.2 and 4.4 the addition of aluminium ameliorated the effects of low pH, increasing hatchability to 78-99%. At pH 4.6 and 4.8 aluminium was found to be toxic. The LC_{50} values for aluminium at pH 4.6 and 4.8 were 811 and 403 µg/litre, respectively. Tadpoles (pre-stage 25) were less sensitive to low pH than embryos, showing 20% mortality at pH 4.2. However, they were much more sensitive to aluminium, all the tadpoles dying at aluminium concentrations ≥ 500 µg/litre and pH 4.4 or 4.6, and at ≥ 250 µg/litre and pH 4.8. Three-week-old tadpoles were less sensitive to lowered pH and elevated aluminium than embryos or newly hatched tadpoles. Low pH (4.2) had no effect on the survival of tadpoles, and aluminium was only toxic at pH 4.8 with 40% mortality at 1000 µg/litre.

Common frog (*Rana temporaria*) tadpoles were raised to metamorphosis at total aluminium concentrations of 800 and 1600 µg/litre and at pH 4.4. Decreasing pH reduced maximum body size and delayed metamorphosis. Growth was depressed and metamorphosis delayed at 800 µg Al/litre; at 1600 µg/litre small tadpoles had arrested growth and development and subsequently died, whereas large tadpoles metamorphosed at a very small size (Cummins, 1986).

9.1.3 Terrestrial organisms

9.1.3.1 Plants

Numerous studies exist of plants exposed to aluminium in nutrient solution or sand culture. They show that exposure causes diminished root growth and development, reduced uptake of plant nutrients (notably phosphorus, calcium and magnesium) and stunted plant growth (Bartlett & Riego, 1972a,b; Göransson & Eldhuset, 1987; Boxman et al., 1991; Keltjens & Tan (1993). The effect of aluminium on plants is complex. It can act directly on plant cell processes (Taylor, 1991) or indirectly by interfering with plant nutrition (Roy et al., 1988; Taylor, 1991).

Plant species vary in their response to aluminium (Roy et al., 1988; Taylor, 1995). Even within species (e.g., wheat, *Triticum aestivum*), aluminium sensitive and tolerant varieties exist (Taylor & Foy, 1985; Kinraide et al., 1992; Huang et al., 1992a; Wheeler et al., 1993). There are reports that aluminium can benefit plants (Hackett, 1962, 1964, 1967). Various proposed mechanisms are listed in the review by Roy et al. (1988). However, it seems that exposure to excessive concentrations of aluminium is detrimental to plants, but the level that is excessive is highly variable.

9.1.3.2 *Invertebrates*

No data have been reported on the effects of aluminium on terrestrial invertebrates.

9.1.3.3 *Birds*

Hussein et al. (1988) fed Japanese quail (*Coturnix coturnix japonica*) on diets containing 0.05, 0.1, 0.15 and 0.3% aluminium (as aluminium sulfate) for 4 weeks. Egg production was significantly decreased at 0.1% and body weight gain at 0.15%. Feed intake was significantly depressed temporarily at 0.1 and 0.15% and permanently at 0.3%. Eggshell breaking strength was temporarily reduced (after 1 week only) at 0.1, 0.15 and 0.3%.

Hussein et al. (1989a) fed white leghorn laying hens on a diet containing 0.05, 0.1 or 0.15% aluminium (as aluminium sulfate) for 28 days. Feed intake, body weight, tibia breaking strength and plasma inorganic phosphorus were significantly reduced at 0.15%. Egg production was only significantly depressed after 21 days at 0.15%. Eggshell breaking strength was unaffected by the treatment. In a second experiment hens were exposed to diets containing up to 0.3% aluminium for 42 days. Feeding 0.3% aluminium significantly decreased plasma inorganic phosphorus in samples collected immediately following oviposition (10 to 42 days). Plasma calcium, tibia weight and tibia breaking strength were unaffected. Egg production and feed intake were significantly reduced during days 1 to 21 but not during days 22 to 42. The effects of 0.3% aluminium on the egg production and shell quality of laying hens are similar to those obtained with conventional force-moulting procedures using feed restriction (Hussein et al., 1989b). White leghorn laying hens were maintained on a diet containing 0, 0.15 or 0.3% aluminium for 17 weeks. Hatchability of eggs was unaffected while fertility and body weight of chicks were significantly depressed at both aluminium treatments. Total egg production and feed consumption both were significantly reduced at the highest aluminium dose (Wisser et al., 1990).

Carrière et al. (1986) fed ring doves (*Streptopelia risoria*) on a diet containing 0.1% aluminium sulfate with reduced calcium and phosphorus levels (0.9% Ca; 0.5% P) for a period of 4 months. There were no significant effects on egg production, fertility, hatchability, growth or final weight of chicks. Egg permeability was initially decreased but subsequently recovered to normal levels. The diet had no effect on plasma calcium, phosphorus or magnesium. There was no effect on weight or growth rate in juvenile doves fed diets containing 500, 1000 or 1500 mg/kg aluminium sulfate from day 21 to day 63.

9.2 Field observations

9.2.1 Microorganisms

No data have been reported regarding effects in the field of aluminium on microorganisms.

9.2.2 Aquatic organisms

9.2.2.1 Plants

Hörnström et al. (1984) studied the effects of pH and different levels of aluminium on lake phytoplankton from the Swedish west coast area. They concluded that the absence of several phytoplankton species in acid lakes was not caused by the low pH but rather a raised aluminium supply from the surrounding land, which produced oligotrophic waters through precipitation of phosphorus. Comparing phytoplankton communities in strongly acid lakes with low and high levels of aluminium revealed that aluminium toxicity alone contributed significantly to the reduced numbers of phytoplankton species.

9.2.2.2 Invertebrates

Aston et al. (1987) found that for streams in Wales and the Peak district, United Kingdom, the population density and biomass of freshwater invertebrates were generally lowest in streams with low pH and high aluminium content. Hörnström et al. (1984) reported that most zooplankton species found in acidic lakes of the Swedish west coast were relatively resistant to acidity but were more susceptible to the oligotrophication process caused by the precipitation of phosphorus by aluminium. There was also an inverse correlation between the number of invertebrates and the aluminium concentration.

Hall et al. (1985) added aluminium chloride (0.28-3.8 mg total Al/litre) to a stream to simulate episodic release during acidic snowmelt. Significant decreases in pH and dissolved oxygen content accompanied increases in aluminium. There was an increased drift of invertebrates with increasing aluminium concentration. The gradually increasing drift rate of benthic macro-invertebrates appeared to be a stress response to the aluminium/hydrogen ion concentrations. Drift of terrestrial insects feeding at the water surface appeared to be due to the reduction in surface tension of the aluminium-treated portion of the stream. Hall et al. (1987) found that during second-order stream experiments, overall more aquatic invertebrates drifted at pH 5.0 during aluminium chloride addition (> 0.28 mg total Al/litre) than at pH 5.0 during hydrochloric acid addition (0.012 mg total Al/litre). McCahon et al. (1987) subdivided a stream into sections of low pH (4.3) and low aluminium concentration (0.052 mg total Al/litre) by adding sulfuric acid and high aluminium concentration (0.35 mg total Al/litre; pH 5.0) by adding aluminium sulfate. In the acid zone, mayfly mortalities of 20% and 5.3% after 24 h were observed for *Baetis rhodani* and *Ecdyonurus venosus*, respectively. Mortality rose to 52.6% after 48 h for *E. venosus*. Mayflies killed during the exposure did not stain for aluminium or mucus. Similar mortalities were observed for both species in the acid/aluminium zone. However, both species gave an aluminium-positive reaction for all parts of the body examined, aluminium being concentrated in the gut, within and surrounding the gill plates, and on the outer surface of the abdomen.

Ormerod et al. (1987a) created simultaneous episodes of low pH (4.28), and low pH (5.02) with increased aluminium content (347 µg Al/litre) in a soft-water stream in upland Wales. *In situ* toxicity tests were performed, and *Chironomus riparius*, *Hydropsyche angustipennis* and *Dinocras cephalotes* were found to have suffered no mortality. *Ecdyonurus venosus*, *Baetis rhodani* and *Gammarus pulex* showed up to 25% mortality in both treatment zones. Drift densities increased, especially in the aluminium-treated zone, *Baetis rhodani* showing an increase of 8 times. *Baetis rhodani* was the only invertebrate to show a significant decline in benthic density (in the aluminium zone), which was due mostly to drift. Weatherley et al. (1988) created 24-h experimental episodes by adding acid, aluminium and citric acid to different treatment zones of an upland stream. Drift density was only observed for the ephemeropteran *Baetis rhodani*, and was found to be unaffected by flow at pH 7 or organically-bound aluminium. Both acidity (pH 4.9) and labile aluminium (0.11 mg/litre) increased drift density. Benthic density was significantly decreased by both labile and organically bound aluminium.

9.2.2.3 Vertebrates

Grahn (1980) reported two fish kills in lakes Ransjön and Ämten, two pristine acid lakes in Sweden, during 1978 and 1979. In 1978 the main part of the ciscoe (*Coregonus albula*) population was wiped out. One week later the pH was found to be 5.4 at the surface and 4.9 at the bottom, with maximum aluminium levels of 0.91 mg/litre in groundwater and 0.31 mg/litre in stream water. One year later a similar incident occurred when the pH was 6.0 in surface water and 5.4 in bottom water. Total aluminium concentrations ranged from 0.36 to 0.52 mg/litre. Analysis of fish gills revealed that aluminium concentrations were at least 6 to 7 times higher than those found in fish gills from reference lakes in the area. The authors conclude that weather patterns caused an increase in phytoplankton, which in turn increased pH levels near the surface. Aluminium hydroxide was precipitated out in the epilimnion water. Ciscoes migrate to the surface to feed where the flocculated aluminium hydroxide caused fish gills to clog and fish to die of suffocation.

Hunter et al. (1980) investigated Black Cart water, a tributary of the River Clyde, Scotland, following sporadic occurrences of fish kills (brown trout *Salmo trutta*) during 1974 and 1975. Aluminium levels were 475 mg/kg (dry weight) in the lateral muscle of dead fish and 358 mg/kg in live fish. Effluent waters from an anodizing factory (pH 6.3-7.3; total aluminium 12-530 µg/litre and soluble aluminium 20-360 µg/litre) were mixed with waters of pH 8.35-8.70 and total and soluble aluminium concentrations of 190-220 µg/litre and < 20 µg/litre, respectively. Downstream of the confluent, which was the area of fish kills, the waters varied in pH between 8.1 and 8.5, and in total (200-1300 µg/litre) and soluble (20-33 µg/litre) aluminium. The authors suggested that when a high pH river receives high loadings of aluminium from water-treatment works soluble aluminium concentrations lethal to fish can occur.

Schofield & Trojnar (1980) reported that lakes in the Adirondack mountains, USA, in which stocked brook trout (*Salvelinus fontinalis*) were not recovered in netting surveys during 1975, were those with significantly lower mean pH (4.79 versus 5.25), calcium level (1.62 versus 1.87 mg/litre) and magnesium level (0.30 versus 0.39 mg/litre), and higher mean aluminium concentrations (0.29 versus 0.11 mg/litre). The covariance analysis of water quality suggested that aluminium intoxication may have been a primary factor in determining the success or failure of fish stocking, whereas both pH and calcium level showed a lack of significance.

Henriksen et al. (1984) showed the acid-aluminium-rich (pH 5.1; inorganic monomeric aluminium 30 µg/litre) waters of the river Vikedal, in southwestern Norway, during a period of increased water flow, to be toxic to pre-smolt Atlantic salmon (*Salmo salar*). Skogheim et al. (1984) reported massive deaths of adult Atlantic salmon in the River Ogna in south-west Norway in 1982. Newly run migrating spawners were killed when acid tributary water (pH 4.7; inorganic monomeric Al 340-360 µg/litre) was mixed into the falling main stream flow of better water quality (pH 5.96-6.18; inorganic monomeric Al 12-13 µg/litre). A near total mortality of salmon occurred for several km downstream of the confluent (pH 4.76-5.41; inorganic monomeric Al 110-307 µg/litre). Blood samples from highly stressed fish (plasma chloride 103-113 mEq/litre) demonstrated osmoregulative failure (normal values 120-135 mEq/litre), and gill aluminium accumulation (70-341 µg Al/g fresh weight) was around 10 times higher than normal values.

Harriman et al. (1987) studied the long-term fish population changes in streams and lochs of south-west Scotland during 1978, 1979 and 1984. Trout were not caught in areas known to have contained them in the past. Fish-less lochs and streams contained the levels of acidity (pH 4-5) and aluminium (up to 300 µg labile monoesic Al/litre) known to be toxic to fish. The authors concluded that acidic deposition was probably the major cause of the change in the fish population in this area.

Eaton et al. (1992) compared laboratory exposure of four embryo-larval fish species to aluminium (< 6.0-70 µg/litre) and pH levels of 4.5 to 7.0 with field observations. Laboratory results showed that monomeric aluminium concentrations of approximately 50 µg/litre, which were comparable to aluminium concentrations in the acidified half of a lake, increased low pH toxicity. However, the laboratory tests for largemouth bass (*Micropterus salmoides*) and rock bass (*Ambloplites rupestris*) underestimated field toxicity, those for black crappie (*Pomoxis nigromaculatus*) overestimated field toxicity and those for yellow perch (*Perca flavescens*) were similar to those observed in the field.

Karlsson-Norrgren et al. (1986a) collected and examined brown trout (*Salmo trutta*) from two fish farms within acid-susceptible areas in Sweden. The total aluminium concentrations in the water were 200 to 300 µg/litre. Trout from a third non-acidified location (aluminium levels in water 35 µg/litre) were also examined. Light and electron microscopic examination of fish from the acid-susceptible areas revealed two major types of gill lesion characterized by chloride cell hyperplasia, and enlargement of the intercellular spaces, in the secondary lamellar epithelium. The gills from the control area appeared normal, exhibiting features characteristic of salmonids.

Norrgren & Degerman (1993) transferred eyed eggs of Atlantic salmon (*Salmo salar*) and brown trout (*Salmo trutta*) in plastic boxes to various locations on the Morrum river, Sweden. The pH levels ranged from 5.1 to 6.7 and total mean aluminium levels ranged from 933 to 569 µg/litre (mean reactive aluminium concentrations ranged from 8 to 203 µg/litre). No significant effects were observed on hatching (13 days) or fry survival (77 days) at pH ≥ 5.7 and reactive aluminium concentrations of up to 49 µg/litre. At pH 5.1 and a total aluminium concentration of 569 µg/litre (reactive aluminium = 203 µg/litre), there was a significant reduction in the salmon hatch but not the trout hatch; total fry mortality after 77 days was 100% for salmon and 94% for trout. Histochemical studies revealed aluminium precipitates in the gills of dead fish; precipitates were associated with the apical plasma membrane.

Stoner et al. (1984) carried out 17-day survival studies of caged brown trout (*Salmo trutta*) in streams of the river Tywi catchment, Wales. All streams where fish died had concurrent mean total aluminium concentrations exceeding 21 µEq/litre and mean pH levels of less than 6. There was a high positive correlation between fish mortality (expressed as the inverse of LT_{50}) and mean filterable aluminium concentration. Differences in LT_{50} values reflected differences in aluminium at similar pH levels. There were considerable differences in gill aluminium concentrations between "control" fish (61 µg/g) and those that died most rapidly (3505 µg/g). There was also a positive correlation between mortality rate and gill aluminium concentration. Weatherley et al. (1990) studied the survival of eggs, alevins and parr of brown trout (*Salmo trutta*) in streams of different acidity (pH 4.7-6.9). Egg survival from fertilization to hatching was independent of the mean total monomeric aluminium concentration, which ranged from 3 to 397 µg/litre. However, the survival of alevins was strongly related to both aluminium and pH; LC_{50} values for 28- and 42-day exposures were approximately 19 and 15 µg total monomeric aluminium/litre, respectively (equivalent to 79 and 72 µg/litre of 0.45 µm filterable aluminium). The 21-day LC_{50} for parr (3 months) was between 84 and 105 µg/litre filterable aluminium.

Ormerod et al. (1987a) created an acidic episode in a softwater stream in upland Wales. Three stretches were identified: (a) upper reach with natural waters of pH 7.0 (40 µg total Al/litre), (b) addition of sulfuric acid to pH 4.2-4.5 (52 µg total Al/litre), and (c) pH 5.2 (347 µg total Al/litre). Caged salmon (*Salmo salar*) and brown trout (*Salmo trutta*) showed 7-10% mortality in the acid zone (b) and 50-87% in the aluminium zone (c). Salmon (14.7 h) had a significantly shorter LT_{50} than trout (23.5 h) in the aluminium zone (c). Ormerod et al. (1987b) reported that brown trout (*Salmo trutta*) exposed to similar episodes showed reduced plasma sodium at low pH (4.2), which appeared to be decreased by the addition of aluminium; however, at pH 4.8 to 5.1 aluminium increased the effect. At pH 4.8-5.1 with the addition of aluminium, fish showed an increased frequency of ventilation. At lower pH effects on ventilation were less consistent.

McCahon et al. (1987) reported that trout and salmon exposed to acid conditions (pH 4.3) alone and low aluminium concentration (0.052 mg/litre) did not stain for aluminium, although increased mucus production was demonstrated in the gills. Fish exposed to aluminium (0.35 mg/litre) at low pH (5.0) exhibited extensive aluminium and mucus coating of the secondary gill lamellae. Fish that died in the acid/aluminium zone showed large significant increases in gill aluminium content compared with controls or with fish from the acid-only zone. Mean aluminium concentrations in fish gills from the acid/aluminium zone were 2950 and 3050 µg/g (dry weight) for trout and salmon, respectively.

Rosseland et al. (1992) exposed *in situ* caged smolts of Atlantic salmon (*Salmo salar*) and sea trout (*Salmo trutta*) to waters in an acid tributary (pH 4.8; inorganic monomeric aluminium 236 µg/litre) and the mixing zone with the limed river Audna (Norway) (pH 7.0; inorganic monomeric aluminium 17 µg/litre). In the acid tributary LT_{50} values were 22 h and 40 h for the two species, respectively. However, in the mixing zone, between 1 and 3 min after mixing (pH 5.8-5.9; inorganic monomeric Al 78-111 µg/litre), both species gave an LT_{50} of 7 h. Fish showed osmoregulatory failure (loss of plasma ions and reduced gill Na/K-ATPase) and gill lesions. No mortality occurred 5 min after mixing or in the limed water. The authors concluded that the increased toxicity in the mixing zone was due to the transformation of aluminium from a low to a high molecular weight precipitating species. The ecological importance of these mixing zones was pointed out (especially being related to seasonal changes) as low temperatures (longer polymerization period) and high flows both would increase the river stretch being affected by these processes.

Poléo et al. (1994) used the same water sources to a channel experiment with control mixing of the waters. Caged Atlantic salmon were exposed to acid stream water (pH 4.89; inorganic monomeric Al 139 µg/litre), limed stream water (pH 6.41; inorganic monomeric Al 14 µg/litre) and the mixture of the two (pH 5.64; inorganic monomeric Al 70 µg/litre). No mortality occurred in the limed water, but there was a 27% mortality in the acid stream water after 72 h exposure. In the mixed water, mortality of up to 90% (mean of 75%) occurred in the first two metres and up to 1 min after mixing, the LT_{50} being 60 h. Within the next 3 min of reaction a total mortality of 16% was found. Fish in the most toxic zone lost plasma ions at a slower rate than in the acid, less toxic zone, apparently demonstrating a different mechanism of toxicity. Although no mortality occurred towards the end of the channel (4-7 min after mixing), loss of plasma ions and increased haematocrit were found, indicating suboptimal conditions.

Lydersen et al. (1994) exposed caged one-year-old parr of brown trout to mixing zone conditions in a channel, using as input water from an acid lake (pH 5.3; total Al 379 µg/litre and inorganic monomeric Al 350 µg/litre) and a neutral lake of pH 7.0, total Al 38 µg/litre. After mixing, a constant pH of 6.1-6.2 was achieved all along the channel. Total mortality in the lake water was 15% after 24 h. Downstream of the confluent (9 seconds of mixing) mortality started after 5 h, reaching 100% after 17 h. The LT_{50} values after 9, 18, 45, 136, 180 and 225 seconds of mixing were 7.5, 9, 12, 17, 23 and 26 h, respectively. Through the use of improved *in situ* aluminium-separation techniques, the authors could for the first time demonstrate the increase in high molecular Al forms (polymerization) at stations along the channel and relate this directly to toxicity.

Freda & McDonald (1993) transplanted embryos and tadpoles of the wood frog (*Rana sylvatica*), the American toad (*Bufo americanus*) and the spotted salamander (*Ambystoma maculatum*) to acidified ponds. Statistical analysis revealed that pH was the only significant parameter in determining mortality; the concentrations of total and labile aluminium were not correlated with the survival of any of these species.

9.2.3 Terrestrial organisms

9.2.3.1 Plants

Aluminium toxicity to plants is well known in agriculture and forestry (Wild, 1988). Direct and indirect effects of enhanced aluminium availability in soil due to soil acidification may be a cause of current problems in some European forests (Abrahamsen et al., 1994).

Reich et al. (1994) monitored the light-saturated net photosynthesis, dark respiration and foliar nutrient content of Scots pine (*Pinus sylvestris*) growing in polluted and non-polluted sites. At the polluted site soil pH and calcium and magnesium contents were 10 times lower and aluminium content 10 times higher than at the control site. The rate of photosynthesis was lower and that of dark respiration was higher at the polluted site. Photosynthesis was found to be negatively correlated to the aluminium:calcium ratio across both sites. Dark respiration rate increased with nitrogen and aluminium contents. Based on the data, the authors concluded that at the polluted site there were excessive soil aluminium levels and deficient levels of magnesium. Low needle magnesium level and high aluminium concentrations and aluminium:calcium ratios resulted in reduced photosynthetic capacity and increased respiration.

Cronan et al. (1987) reported that observed field total monomeric aluminium concentrations and aluminium ion activities were considerably lower than laboratory-based toxic thresholds for several tree species. However, analysis suggests that calcium/aluminium ratios for fine roots were near to critical levels. Aluminium toxicity could possibly have been acting as a stress factor either directly or indirectly by nutritional interference.

Joslin et al. (1988) sampled roots and foliage of spruce trees from five sites in North America and Europe. Aluminium concentrations in fine roots from B horizons were highly correlated with soil solution monomeric aluminium. Sites with higher levels of plant-available aluminium had spruce trees with lower foliage levels of calcium and magnesium. The authors concluded that this may be evidence of aluminium interference in calcium and magnesium uptake and transport. There was no obvious interference of aluminium in the uptake and translocation of phosphorus.

Godbold et al. (1988b) studied the effects of aluminium on nutrient fluxes in *Picea abies*. The authors reported that, using X-ray microanalysis, the distribution of aluminium, magnesium, calcium and potassium was found to be similar in roots to those collected from declining spruce stands in Solling, Germany.

Cuenca & Herrera (1987) reported that trees analysed from a tropical cloud forest growing in acid/aluminium-rich soil were found to have two distinct strategies for survival: accumulator plants, with aluminium levels of > 1000 mg/kg, and non-accumulators. Both types contained large amounts of aluminium in the roots, but in accumulators the plasmalemma in endodermic cells was permeable to aluminium. The authors found that both groups were able to accumulate aluminium in cell walls, alkalinize the surrounding rhizosphere and produce chelating agents, but all at a high ecological cost and with low growth rates as a result.

Most cultivated plants are non-accumulators and efficiently exclude aluminium from the harvested parts. A notable exception is tea (*Camellia sinensis*) where aluminium concentration in mature leaves can reach 1.7% Al/dry weight (Chenery, 1955; Coriat & Gillard, 1986).

Clarkson (1967) studied the aluminium tolerance of four species of *Agrostris* from different sites in the United Kingdom. The most sensitive species was *A. stolanifera* from a site with no detectable soil aluminium (as exchangeable ions) and the most tolerant was *A. setacea* from a site with soil levels of 3.6 mEq Al/kg. Growing the species in soils from each of the different sites revealed that peak growth was achieved in soil from the site where the plant was collected.

9.2.3.2 Invertebrates

No information has been reported regarding the field effects of aluminium on terrestrial invertebrates.

9.2.3.3 Vertebrates

Nyholm (1981) found aluminium in the bone marrow tissue of the humeri of pied flycatchers (*Ficedula hypoleuca*) with impaired breeding from the shores of Lake Tjulträsk, Sweden. The impairments included production of small clutches, defective eggshell formation and intrauterine bleeding. The authors stated that these impairments compare with the symptoms of aluminium intoxication in mammals. However, the effects may be indirect, the result of phosphate binding in the intestinal tract rather than direct toxicity of aluminium.

Ormerod et al. (1986) reported that sites without breeding dippers (*Cinclus cinclus*) had significantly higher mean concentrations of filterable aluminium, lower mean pH, fewer trichopteran larvae and ephemeropteran nymphs, and were on rivers with more conifer afforestation on their catchments than sites where dippers were present. Ormerod et al. (1988) found no evidence that aluminium (0.47-2.13 mg/g; dry weight) in the invertebrate prey of dippers (*Cinclus cinclus*) collected from streams of different pH from Wales and Scotland adversely affected shell thickness or mass of eggs.

10. EVALUATION OF HUMAN HEALTH RISKS AND EFFECTS ON THE ENVIRONMENT

10.1 Health effects

The overall assessment of the risks of aluminium exposure to healthy, non-occupationally exposed humans is rendered uncertain by several deficiencies in the database, namely:

i) the questionable relevance to humans of animal experiments designed for hazard identification, in which massive doses were administered by parenteral routes, and the lack of data based on oral dosing at relevant exposure levels;

ii) the dubious relevance to humans of the many biochemical findings from cell culture experiments and other *in vitro* models;

iii) the uncertainty in the analytical and estimated cumulative exposure data in epidemiological studies of the relationship of aluminium in drinking-water to Alzheimer's disease (AD), and the less than robust dose-response data obtained from such studies;

iv) the complete lack of epidemiological studies relating to total aluminium exposure, when it is considered that aluminium derived from drinking-water is responsible for only a small fraction of such exposure.

It should be noted, however, that animal models employing oral aluminium administration provide some limited support for cognitive and motor impairment in the absence of neuropathological changes.

Adverse health effects from aluminium exposure have been definitely established in one special group, i.e. patients with severely impaired renal function. These patients are at risk from severe neurological dysfunction and are also at risk of vitamin-D-resistant osteomalacia and microcytic anaemia from iatrogenic exposure to aluminium-containing preparations. The toxicity of oral aluminium-containing preparations is exacerbated by concurrent use of oral citrate-containing preparations under these circumstances.

An increased tissue loading of aluminium, especially in bone, has been shown in premature infants without azotaemia. Current paediatric practice is to warn about the potential risk that may be associated with increased tissue levels of aluminium following parenteral administration or oral intake of products with elevated aluminium content.

10.1.1 Exposure assessment

Human exposure to aluminium can vary greatly depending on diet, use of specific medications, sources of drinking-water and exposure to other ambient and occupational sources of aluminium. In many countries non-occupationally exposed adults are exposed to between 2.5 and 13 mg aluminium/day from air, water and food (0.08-0.18 mg/kg body weight per day for a 60-kg individual). However, large variations in daily intake can occur as a consequence of differing intakes of foods containing commonly encountered food additives. Infants consuming formulae based on cow's milk have very low aluminium intakes (0.1-0.8 mg/litre), whereas those fed soya-based formulae have much greater aluminium intakes (3.1-4.3 mg/litre). Moreover, use of aluminium containing antacids and/or buffered analgesics can increase daily intake between 10 and 1000 times. Actual exposures will vary from country to country, but the above figures can be used as a first approximation for assessing human health risks from aluminium exposure.

Occupationally exposed populations have background exposure levels similar to those of non-occupationally exposed populations, but their work can lead to significantly increased exposure. Actual levels of exposure depends on the specific work tasks performed, the type and form of aluminium compound encountered, and the adequacy of workplace hygiene practices. Inhalation is the most important route of occupational exposure, but the extent of pulmonary uptake and retention has not been determined in most occupational settings. Based on limited data, daily occupational aluminium exposure can range from <1 mg to 40 mg per 8-h shift.

10.1.2 Evaluation of animal data

Information from toxicokinetic studies in animals is consistent with and complementary to that obtained in humans. Available studies indicate that oral bioavailability is low (< 1%) and they provide valuable information on dose-related concentrations and effects in target tissues.

In general, the animal studies evaluated were not designed for risk assessment purposes. However, these studies provide information relevant to hazard identification and some data on dose-response.

The target tissues in animals are similar to those in humans and include the bone and nervous system.

In developmental studies in rodents, reduced intrauterine weight gains were noted in the female offspring of dams gavaged with aluminium nitrate at doses as low as 13 mg Al/kg body weight per day, whereas male offspring were not affected at this dose level. Neurobehavioural and motor development were affected at 100 and 200 mg Al/kg body weight per day when aluminium lactate was administered to mice in the feed.

There is no indication that aluminium is carcinogenic.

10.1.3 Evaluation of human data

There is no indication that aluminium is acutely toxic after oral intake. A causal relationship between short-term exposure to high levels of aluminium in drinking-water and adverse health effects is not supported by available data.

The information available is insufficient to classify the carcinogenic risk to humans from exposure to aluminium and aluminium compounds.

No information is available associating aluminium exposures with adverse reproductive effects.

Although human exposure to aluminium is widespread, only a few reports of hypersensitivity exist. In all cases the hypersensitivity followed dermal or parenteral administration.

In the healthy general population the major health concern relates to the purported association between the intake of aluminium and the development and/or acceleration of the onset of AD and other neurotoxic effects. After an in-depth analysis of the available epidemiological data (section 8.1.3 - Table 22), considering study design, exposure measurements and relative risks reported, it was concluded that:

- On the whole, the positive relationship between aluminium in drinking-water and AD, which was demonstrated in several epidemiological studies, cannot be totally dismissed. However, strong reservations about inferring a causal relationship are warranted in view of the failure of these studies to account for demonstrated confounding factors and for total aluminium intake from all sources.

- Taken together, the relative risks for AD from exposure to aluminium in drinking-water above 100 µg/litre, as determined in these studies, are low (less than 2.0). But, because the risk estimates are imprecise for a variety of methodological reasons, a population-attributable risk cannot be calculated with precision. Such imprecise predictions may, however, be useful in making decisions about the need to control exposures to aluminium in the general population.

- In light of the above studies, which consider water-borne aluminium as the sole risk factor, and the recent findings that water accounts for less than 5% of daily intake of aluminium, it is difficult to reconcile this with the presumed impact on cognition. Several lines of investigation should be pursued to further elucidate the nature of the relationship found in these studies.

Data from many clinical studies have firmly established the causal relationship between aluminium exposure in patients with chronic renal failure (including premature infants with kidney failure) and the development of encephalopathy (dementia), vitamin-D-resistant osteomalacia, and microcytic anaemia. The major sources of aluminium exposure have been indicated as the level of aluminium in the water used to prepare the dialysis fluids and treatment with aluminium-containing phosphate binders. Dialysis encephalopathy was found to be rare when the aluminium level in the dialysis fluid was maintained below 50 µg/litre. The use of aluminium-free phosphate-binding agents will also decrease the risk of developing encephalopathy in patients treated for kidney failure.

In many occupational settings workers are exposed not simply to aluminium fumes and dust, but rather to a complex mixture of chemicals and dusts, of which only some contain aluminium. Therefore, it is essential that urinary aluminium levels be determined as a measure of exposure (dose), in addition to workplace levels of particulates, if a causal association between aluminium and effects on the respiratory and nervous systems is to be developed with any degree of certainty. Only a few of the published surveys contain such information.

In the past, exposure to stamped pyrotechnic aluminium powder, usually coated with mineral oil lubricants, has caused pulmonary fibrosis. However, exposure to other forms of aluminium has not proved to be a cause of pulmonary fibrosis.

There is no evidence of specific toxicity of any immunological reaction to the element aluminium as a cause of occupational asthma. This disorder is considered to be irritant-induced following exposure during the production of compounds such as aluminium sulfate, aluminium fluoride and potassium aluminium tetrafluoride, or in production areas of primary aluminium smelting. Exposure to dust and particulate in workers fabricating (welding) aluminium have been associated with an increased level of chronic bronchitis or decreased lung function. A causative role of non-aluminium fume or dusts, e.g., fluorides, cannot be ruled out. It was reported that the chronic bronchitis noted in aluminium welders was similar to that in welders working with stainless steel or iron.

There is some evidence that aluminium exposure in welders, miners and foundry workers can lead to an impairment of cognitive and motor functions. However, owing to the small cohorts used in some studies, methodological deficiencies in most studies, and conflicting results from different studies, there is considerable uncertainty in ascribing a causative role for aluminium in the neurological effects reported. In one large study of miners exposed to aluminium powder, the difficulties in adequately controlling for confounding factors also lead to much uncertainty in accepting the positive effects observed on cognition. There is a need for additional studies to clarify the uncertainties in these data.

10.2 Evaluation of effects on the environment

10.2.1 Exposure

Aluminium is among the least mobile of the major elements of the geological sedimentary cycle. In air it is present mainly as wind-blown soil particles. Aluminium-bearing solid phases are relatively insoluble, particularly in the circumneutral pH range, and so most natural waters contain low concentrations of dissolved aluminium. However, the solubility of aluminium is highly dependent on pH, increasing at both low and high pH values, which reflects the amphoteric nature of the element. This fact, coupled with the large reservoir of aluminium in soils and sediments, means that aluminium concentrations can be substantially enhanced in acidic or poorly buffered environments subjected to sustained or periodic exposure to strong acidifying inputs. Under such conditions aluminium can be transported from soil to surface waters. Afforestation, the cessation of liming, and sulfide oxidation all contribute to acidification and thus to the release of previously bound aluminium. However, a major cause of acidification is acidifying deposition from the atmosphere.

10.2.2 Effects

Laboratory and field studies have revealed that the inorganic mononuclear aluminium complexes are more toxic to both aquatic organisms and terrestrial plant species than the organically complexed forms. Aluminium has been shown to affect adversely both aquatic organisms and terrestrial plants at concentrations found in acidic or poorly buffered environments. However, there exist large species, strain and life-history stage differences in sensitivity. Elevated concentrations of inorganic monomeric aluminium have detrimental biological effects that are mitigated in the presence of organic acids, fluoride, silicate, and high concentrations of calcium and magnesium. There is a substantial reduction in species richness associated with the mobilization of the more toxic forms of aluminium in acid-stressed waters; this loss of species diversity is reflected at all trophic levels. In waters with non-steady-state aluminium chemistry (ongoing polymerization), toxicity can become extreme in pH ranges not normally associated with toxicity.

11. CONCLUSIONS AND RECOMMENDATIONS FOR PROTECTION OF HUMAN HEALTH AND THE ENVIRONMENT

In reaching the following conclusions with regards to the risks from aluminium exposure the Task Group felt it was appropriate to consider separately the human populations at risk as well as the environment. The conclusions are, therefore, grouped as to the risk to the healthy general population, healthy workers and individuals with impaired kidney function. This is followed by conclusions regarding the risk to the environment from aluminium.

11.1 Conclusions

11.1.1 Healthy general population

Hazards posed by aluminium to intrauterine and neurological development and brain function have been identified through animal studies. However, aluminium has not been shown to pose a health risk to healthy, non-occupationally exposed humans.

There is no evidence to support a primary causative role of aluminium in Alzheimer's disease (AD). Aluminium does not induce AD pathology *in vivo* in any species, including humans.

The hypothesis that exposure of the elderly population in some regions to high levels of aluminium in drinking-water may exacerbate or accelerate AD is not supported by available data.

It has also been hypothesized that particular exposures, either occupational or via drinking-water, may be associated with non-specific impaired cognitive function. The data in support of this hypothesis are currently inadequate.

There is insufficient health-related evidence to justify revisions to existing WHO Guidelines for aluminium exposure in healthy, non-occupationally exposed humans. As an example, there is an inadequate scientific basis for setting a health-based standard for aluminium in drinking-water.

202

11.1.2 Subpopulations at special risk

In people of all ages with impaired renal function, aluminium accumulation has been shown to cause the clinical syndrome of encephalopathy, vitamin-D-resistant osteomalacia and microcytic anaemia. The sources of aluminium are haemodialysis fluid and aluminium-containing pharmaceutical agents (e.g., phosphate binders). Intestinal absorption can be exacerbated by the use of citrate-containing products. Patients with renal failure are thus at risk of neurotoxicity from aluminium.

Iatrogenic aluminium exposure poses a hazard to patients with chronic renal failure and to premature infants. Every effort should be made to limit such exposure in these groups.

11.1.3 Occupationally exposed populations

Workers having long-term, high-level exposure to fine aluminium particulates may be at increased risk of adverse health effects. However, there are insufficient data from which to develop, with any degree of certainty, occupational exposure limits with regards to the adverse effects of aluminium.

Exposure to stamped pyrotechnic aluminium powder, usually coated with mineral oil lubricants, has caused pulmonary fibrosis (aluminosis), whereas exposure to other forms of aluminium has not been proved to cause pulmonary fibrosis. Most reported cases involved exposure to other potentially fibrogenic agents.

Irritant-induced asthma has been shown to be associated with inhalation of aluminium sulfate, aluminium fluoride and potassium aluminium tetrafluoride, and found to occur within the complex environment of primary aluminium production, especially in potrooms.

11.1.4 Environmental risk

Aluminium-bearing solid phases in the environment are relatively insoluble, particularly at circumneutral pH values, resulting in low concentrations of dissolved aluminium in most natural waters.

In acidic or poorly buffered environments subjected to strong acidifying inputs, concentrations of aluminium can increase to levels resulting in adverse effects on both aquatic organisms and terrestrial plants. However, there exist large species, strain and life-history stage differences in sensitivity to this metal.

The detrimental biological effects from elevated concentrations of inorganic monomeric aluminium can be mitigated in the presence of organic acids, fluorides, silicate and high levels of calcium and magnesium.

A substantial reduction in species richness is associated with the mobilization of the more toxic forms of aluminium in acid-stressed waters. This loss of species diversity is reflected at all trophic levels.

11.2 Recommendations

11.2.1 *Public health protection*

a)   Strategies should be developed to limit exposure for patients with severly impaired renal function who are exposed to aluminium from pharmaceutical products.

b)   For patients with end-stage renal failure treated by dialysis, exposure to aluminium should be limited by treatment of the water and elimination of aluminium contamination of the chemicals used to prepare dialysis fluid. It is suggested that dialysis fluids should contain less than 15 µg aluminium/litre.

11.2.2 *Recommendations for protection of the environment*

a)   Soil and water acidification can mobilize aluminium and have detrimental effects on aquatic and terrestrial lifeforms. Actions that cause enhanced acidification, e.g., emissions of SO_2, NO_x and NH_3, should continue to be restricted.

b)   When waters are limed to mitigate aluminium toxicity to fish, it should be done in such a manner that sufficient time is available for establishment of equilibrium between the aluminium species before the water reaches the most biologically sensitive or valuable parts of the system.

12. FURTHER RESEARCH

In order to improve the scientific database on aluminium for the assessment of the risks to human health, thus decreasing the present level of uncertainty, the Task Group considered that additional research in several areas was essential.

12.1 Bioavailability and kinetics

(a) Future studies should address the issue of whether aluminium in drinking-water is more bioavailable than that from other sources such as food, consumer products and food additives paying particular attention to the study of factors that can modify aluminium uptake by the body. This question is best answered by studies in humans using ^{26}Al although appropriately designed animal experiments would provide useful data.

(b) Once aluminium has gained access to the brain, at what rate is it mobilized or excreted? Is the brain a "one-way sink for aluminium"? These questions can only be addressed successfully in an animal model where serial cortical biopsies can be performed.

(c) In view of the importance of achieving international concordance of accurate chemical analysis for aluminium in environmental and biological samples, it is recommended that the development of expert reference laboratories and systems of quality control should be facilitated and supported.

12.2 Toxicological data

(a) It is thought unlikely that further studies of parenteral aluminium exposure to normal animals will improve the database significantly. There is, however, a need for well-designed animal studies focusing on neurotoxicity and reproductive and developmental end-points using protocols developed for the assessment of dose-response relationships for exposures by either the oral or inhalation routes.

(b) Research in experimental animals on the factors related to the development of Alzheimer's disease (AD) is hampered by the lack of a suitable model. However, aged primates or transgenic mice bearing the human APP gene with familial AD point mutation could potentially be used for this purpose (with some reservations). The advantage of these models is that total aluminium intake can be controlled during the relevant portion of the animal's life span (about 3-10 years and 1-2 years for primates and mice, respectively).

(c)   There is a requirement for further studies to determine the effects of diminished renal function on aluminium toxicokinetics. Such studies should be designed to assess the impact of early-stage renal disease (varying degrees) and age-related decreases in renal function on aluminium retention and toxicity.

12.3 Research on the relationship between aluminium exposure and Alzheimer's disease

(a)   Further studies of aluminium levels in bulk tissues from brains of patients with AD are unlikely to be of value in resolving the current controversy or enable the distinction to be made between a pathogenic factor and an epiphenomenon.

(b)   The knowledge base is unlikely to be advanced significantly by further ecological retrospective studies of exposure to aluminium in drinking-water and AD. Rather, prospective studies of matched cohorts of elderly people from stable populations living in areas with high and low levels of aluminium in drinking-water are required, with special attention to known confounding factors. Exposure should preferably be assessed through monitoring of aluminium in the tap water of all cohort members. Although as an outcome measure it is preferable to compare the pathological configuration of AD to reference populations, this may be impractical, and standardized clinical assessments have to be relied on using carefully considered criteria for the diagnosis of Alzheimer-type dementia.

(c)   As Alzheimer-type neuropathology is almost universal in older Down's syndrome subjects, and as decline in cognitive function, as assessed by decline in activities of daily living skills, is relatively common (25-35), a point study of rates of cognitive impairment in Down's syndrome patients over 40 years of age from high and low water aluminium areas might be performed relatively quickly and with small numbers of subjects. Unbiased subject recruitment would, however, present problems.

(d) If the hypothesis that higher drinking-water aluminium levels are an accelerating or exacerbating factor for AD is correct, a neuropathological assessment of elderly subjects dying of an unrelated cause requiring routine postmortem examination (e.g., passengers in road traffic accident) ought to reveal a greater burden of Alzheimer's pathology in those from areas with high aluminium levels in drinking-water than those from areas with low aluminium levels.

12.4 Occupational exposure

The possible adverse effects of occupational aluminium exposure on the health of workers should be a specific priority for future research.

13. PREVIOUS EVALUATIONS BY INTERNATIONAL BODIES

At the Thirty-third Meeting of the Joint FAO/WHO Expert Committee on Food Additives and Food Contaminants, a provisional tolerable weekly intake (PTWI) of 7.0 mg/kg body weight was recommended. This value included the intake of aluminium from its use as a food additive (FAO/WHO, 1989).

On the basis of non-health-related criteria, a WHO Drinking-Water Guideline of 0.2 mg/litre has been proposed (WHO, 1993). No health-based guideline was recommended.

The carcinogenic risk from aluminium and its compounds has not been evaluated by the International Agency for Research on Cancer (IARC). However, that there is sufficient evidence that certain exposures occurring during aluminium production cause cancer in humans. Most epidemiological studies suggest pitch volatiles to be the causative agent (IARC, 1987).

Regulatory standards for aluminium and some aluminium compounds established by national bodies in several countries and the European Union are summarized in the legal file of the International Register of Potentially Toxic Chemicals (IRPTC, 1993).

REFERENCES

Abernathy AR, Larson GL, & Mathews RC (1984) Heavy metals in the surficial sediments of Fontana Lake, North Carolina. Water Res, **18**(3): 351-354.

Abrahamsen G, Stuanes AO, & Tveite B (1994) Long-term experiments with acid rain in Norwegian forest ecosystems. Berlin, Heidelberg, New York, Springer-Verlag, pp 297-331.

Abramson MJ, Wlodarczyk JH, Saunders NA, & Hensley MJ (1989) Does aluminum smelting cause lung disease? Am Rev Respir Dis, **139**: 1042-1057.

Adler AJ & Berlyne GM (1985) Duodenal aluminum absorption in the rat: effect of vitamin D. Am J Physiol, **249**: G/209-G/213.

Albers PH & Camardese MB (1993a) Effects of acidification on metal accumulation by aquatic plants and invertebrates. 1. Constructed wetlands. Environ Toxicol Chem, **12**: 959-967.

Albers PH & Camardese MB (1993b) Effects of acidification on metal accumulation by aquatic plants and invertebrates. 2. Wetlands, ponds and small lakes. Environ Toxicol Chem, **12**: 969-976.

Alberts JJ, Leyden DE, & Patterson TA (1976) Distribution of total Al, Cd, Co, Cu, Ni and Zn in the tongue of the ocean and the northwestern Atlantic Ocean. Mar Chem, **4**: 51-56.

Alderman FR & Gitelman HJ (1980) Improved electrothermal determination of aluminum in serum by atomic absorption spectroscopy. Clin Chem, **26**: 258-260.

Alfrey AC (1978) Dialysis encephalopathy syndrome. Annu Rev Med, **29**: 93-98.

Alfrey AC (1980) Aluminum metabolism in uremia. Neurotoxicology, **1**: 43-53.

Alfrey AC, Mishell JM, Burks J, Contiguglia SR, Rudolph H, Lewin E, & Holmes JH (1972) Syndrome of dyspraxia and multifocal seizures associated with chronic hemodialysis. Trans Am Soc Artif Intern Organs, **18**: 257-261.

Alfrey AC, Legendre GR, & Kaehny WD (1976) The dialysis encephalopathy syndrome: Possible aluminum intoxication. N Engl J Med, **294**: 184-188.

Alfrey AC, Hegg A, & Craswell P (1980) Metabolism and toxicity of aluminium in renal failure. Am J Clin Nutr, **33**: 1509-1516.

Alfrey AC, Sedman A, & Chan YL (1985) The compartmentalization and metabolism of aluminum in uremic rats. J Lab Clin Med, **105**: 227-233.

Allen VG & Fontenot JP (1984) Influence of aluminium as sulfate, chloride and citrate on magnesium and calcium metabolism in sheep. J Anim Sci, **59**: 798-804.

Allen VG, Horn FP, & Fontenot JP (1986) Influence of ingestion of aluminium, citric acid and soil on mineral metabolism of lactating beef cows. J Anim Sci, **62**: 1396-1403.

Altmann P, Dhanesha U, Hamon C, Cunningham J, Blair J, & Marsh F (1989) Disturbance of cerebral function by aluminium in haemodialysis patients without overt aluminium toxicity. Lancet, **2**: 7-12.

Amundsen CE, Hanssen JE, Semb A, & Steinnes E (1992) Long-range atmospheric transport of trace elements to southern Norway. Atmos Environ, **A26**(7): 1309-1324.

Andersen JR (1987) Graphite furnace atomic absorption spectrometric screening method for the determination of aluminium in haemodialysis concentrates. J Anal Atmos Spectrom, **2**: 257-259.

Andorn MC, Britton RS, & Bacon BR (1990) Evidence that lipid peroxidation and total iron are increased in Alzheimer's brain. Neurobiol Aging, **11**: 316.

Andreoli SP, Bergstein JM, & Sherrard DJ (1984) Aluminum intoxication from aluminum-containing phosphate binders in children with azotemia not undergoing dialysis. N Engl J Med, **310**: 1079-1084.

Arieff AI, Cooper JD, Armstrong D, & Lazarowitz VC (1979) Dementia, renal failure, and brain aluminum. Ann Int Med, **90**: 741-747.

Aston RJ, Sadler K, Milner AGP, & Lynam S (1987) The effects of pH and related factors on stream invertebrates. Leatherhead, Central Electricity Generating Board, Technology Planning and Research Division, Central Electricity Research Laboratories (Report No. TPRD/L/2792/N84).

ATSDR (1992) Toxicological profile for aluminum and compounds. Atlanta, Georgia, Agency for Toxic Substances and Disease Registry, 136 pp (TP-91/01).

Bache BW (1980) The acidification of soils. In: Hutchinson TC & Havas M ed. Effects of acid precipitation on terrestrial ecosystems. New York, London, Plenum Press, pp 183-202.

Bache BW (1986) Aluminium mobilization in soils and waters. J Geol Soc (Lond), **143**: 699-706.

Baker JP & Schofield CL (1982) Aluminum toxicity to fish in acidic waters. Water Air Soil Pollut, **18**: 289-309.

Banks WA & Kastin AJ (1985) Aluminum alters the permeability of the blood-brain barrier to some non-peptides. Neuropharmacology, **24**: 407-412.

Banks WA, Kastin AJ, Fasold MB, Barrera CM, & Augereau G (1988a) Studies of the slow bidirectional transport of iron and transferrin across the blood-brain barrier. Brain Res Bull, **21**: 881-885.

Banks WA, Kastin AJ, & Fasold MB (1988b) Differential effect of aluminum on the blood-brain barrier transport of peptides, technetium and albumin. J Pharmacol Exp Ther, **244**: 579-585.

Bartlett RJ & Riego DC (1972a) Toxicity of hydroxy aluminum in relation to pH and phosphorus. Soil Sci, **114**(3): 194-200.

Bartlett RJ & Riego DC (1972b) Effect of chelation on the toxicity of aluminum. Plant Soil, **37**: 419-423.

Bast-Pettersen R, Drablos PA, Goffeng LO, Thomassen Y, & Torres CG (1994) Neuropsychological deficit among elderly workers in aluminium production. Am J Ind Med, **25**: 649-662.

Baxter MJ, Burrell JA, Crews HM, & Massey RC (1988) The effects of fluoride on the leaching of aluminium saucepans during cooking. Food Addit Contam, **5**: 651-656.

Beavington F & Cawse PA (1979) The deposition of trace elements and major nutrients in dust and rainwater in northern Nigeria. Sci Total Environ, **13**: 263-274.

Benett RW, Persaud TVN, & Moore KL (1975) Experimental studies on the effects of aluminum on pregnancy and fetal development. Anat Anz, **138**: 365-378.

Bengtsson B-E (1978) Use of a harpacticoid copepod in toxicity tests. Mar Pollut Bull, **9**(9): 238-241.

Benninger LK & Wells JT (1993) Sources of sediment to the Neuse River estuary, North Carolina. Mar Chem, **43**: 137-156.

Berdén M, Clarke N, Danielsson LG, & Sparén A (1994) Aluminium speciation: variations caused by the choice of analytical method and by sample storage. Water Air Soil Pollut, **72**: 213-233.

Berg DJ & Burns TA (1985) The distribution of aluminum in the tissues of three fish species. J Freshw Ecol, **3**: 113-120.

Berggren D (1992) Speciation and mobilization of aluminium and cadmium in podzols and cambisols of S. Sweden. Water Air Soil Pollut, **62**: 125-156.

Bergkvist B (1987) Leaching of metals from forest soils as influenced by tree species and management. For Ecol Manage, **22**: 29-56.

Berlyne GM, Yagil R, Ben-Ari J, Weinberger G, Knopf E, & Danovitch GM (1972) Aluminium toxicity in rats. Lancet, **1**: 564-567.

Bernuzzi V, Desor D, & Lehr PR (1986) Effects of prenatal aluminium exposure on neuromotor maturation in the rat. Neurobehav Toxicol Teratol, **8**: 115-119.

Bernuzzi V, Desor D, & Lehr PR (1989a) Effects of postnatal aluminium lactate exposure on neuromotor maturation in the rat. Bull Environ Contam Toxicol, **42**: 451-455.

Bernuzzi V, Desor D, & Lehr PR (1989b) Developmental alterations in offspring of female rats orally intoxicated by aluminum chloride or lactate during gestation. Teratology, **40**: 21-27.

Berrill M, Hollett L, Margosian A, & Hudson J (1985) Variation in tolerance to low environmental pH by the crayfish *Orconectes rusticus, O. propinquus,* and *Cambarus robustus.* Can J Zool, **63**: 2586-2589.

Bertholf RL, Wills MR, & Savory J (1984) Quantitative study of aluminum binding to human serum albumin and transferrin by chelex competitive binding assay. Biochem Biophys Res Commun, **125**: 1020-1024.

Bettinelli M, Baroni U, Fontana F, & Poisetti P (1985) Evaluation of the L'vov platform and matric modification for the determination of aluminium in serum. Analyst, **110**: 19-22.

Bhamra RK & Costa M (1992) Trace elements aluminum, arsenic, cadmium, mercury, and nickel. In: Lippmann M ed. Environmental toxicants: Human exposures and their health effects. New York, Van Nostrand Reinhold Company, pp 575-632.

Biesinger KE & Christensen GM (1972) Effects of various metals on survival, growth, reproduction, and metabolism of *Daphnia magna.* J Fish Res Board Can, **29**: 1691-1700.

Birchall JD (1991) The role of silicon in aluminium toxicity. In: Lord Walton of Detchant ed. Alzheimer's disease and the environment. London, Royal Society of Medicine Services Ltd, pp 70-77 (Round Table Series No. 26).

Bird SC, Brown SJ, & Vaughan E (1990) The influence of land management on stream water chemistry. In: Edwards RW, Gee AS, & Stoner JH ed. Acid waters in Wales. Dordrecht, Boston, London, Kluwer Academic Publishers, pp 241-253.

Blotcky AJ, Claassen JP, Roman FR, Rack EP, & Badakhsh S (1992) Determination of aluminum by chemical and instrumental neutron activation analysis in biological standard reference material and human brain tissue. Anal Chem, **64**: 2910-2913.

Blume H-P & Brümmer G (1991) Prediction of heavy metal behavior in soil by means of simple field tests. Ecotoxicol Environ Saf, **22**: 164-174.

Böhler-Sommeregger K & Lindemayr H (1986) Contact sensitivity to aluminium. Contact Dermatitis, **15**: 278-281.

Booth CE, McDonald DG, Simons BP, & Wood CM (1988) Effects of aluminum and low pH on net ion fluxes and ion balance in the brook trout (*Salvelinus fontinalis*). Can J Fish Aquat Sci, **45**: 1563-1574.

Borg H (1987) Trace metals and water chemistry of forest lakes in northern Sweden. Water Res, **21**(1): 65-72.

Boult S, Collins DN, White KN, & Curtis CD (1994) Metal transport in a stream polluted by acid mine drainage - the Afon Goch, Anglesey, UK. Environ Pollut, **84**: 279-284.

Bouman AA, Platenkamp AJ, & Posma FD (1986) Determination of aluminium in human tissues by flameless atomic absorption spectroscopy and comparison of reference values. Ann Clin Biochem, **23**: 97-101.

Boxman AW, Krabbendam H, Bellemakers MJS, & Roelofs JGM (1991) Effects of ammonium and aluminium on the development and nutrition of *Pinus nigra* in hydroculture. Environ Pollut, **73**: 119-136.

Brady DJ, Edwards DG, Asher CJ, & Blamey FPC (1993) Calcium amelioration of aluminium toxicity effects on root hair development in soybean [*Glycine max* (L.) Merr.]. New Phytol, **123**: 531-538.

Bräunlich H, Fleck C, Kersten L, Stein G, Laske V, Müller A, & Keil E (1986) Renal effects of aluminium in uraemic rats and rats with intact kidney function. J Appl Toxicol, **6**: 55-59.

Brezonik PL, Mach CE, Downing G, Richardson N, & Brighman M (1990) Effects of acidification on minor and trace metal chemistry in Little Rock Lake, Wisconsin. Environ Toxicol Chem, **9**: 871-885.

Bringmann G & Kühn R (1959) [The toxic effects of wastewater on aquatic bacteria, algae, and small crustacea.] Gesundheits-Ingenieur, **80**(4): 115-120 (in German).

Brown DJA (1983) Effect of calcium and aluminum concentrations on the survival of brown trout (*Salmo trutta*) at low pH. Bull Environ Contam Toxicol, **30**: 582-587.

Bruland KW (1983) Trace elements in sea-water. In: Riley JP & Chester R ed. Chemical oceanography. New York, London, Academic Press, vol 8, pp 157-220.

Brumbaugh WG & Kane DA (1985) Variability of aluminum concentrations in organs and whole bodies of smallmouth bass (*Micropterus dolimieui*). Environ Sci Technol, **19**: 828-831.

Buckler DR, Mehrle PM, Cleveland L, & Dwyer FJ (1987) Influence of pH on the toxicity of aluminium and other inorganic contaminants to east coast striped bass. Water Air Soil Pollut, **35**: 97-106.

Budavari S ed. (1989) The Merck index: An encyclopedia of chemicals, drugs and biologicals, 11th ed. Rahway, New Jersey, Merck & Co., pp 54-60.

Buergel PM & Soltero RA (1983) The distribution and accumulation of aluminum in rainbow trout following a whole-lake alum treatment. J Freshw Ecol, **2**(1): 37-44.

Bugiani O & Ghetti B (1982) Progressing encephalomyelopathy with muscular athropy, induced by aluminum powder. Neurobiol Aging, **3**: 209-222.

Bull KR & Hall JR (1986) Aluminium in the rivers Esk and Duddon, Cumbria, and their tributaries. Environ Pollut, **B12**: 165-193.

Buratti M, Caravelli G, Calzaferri G, & Colombi A (1984) Determination of aluminium in body fluids by solvent extraction and atomic absorption spectroscopy with electro-thermal atomization. Clin Chim Acta, **141**: 253-259.

Burnatowska-Hledin MA & Mayor GH (1984) The effects of aluminum loading on selected tissue calcium and magnesium concentrations in rats. Biol Trace Elem Res, **6**: 531-535.

Burnel D, Hutin MF, Netter P, Kessler M, Huriet C, & Gaucher A (1982) Intérêt du dosage de l'aluminium osseux par polarographie impulsionelle. Pathol Biol, **30**: 27-32.

Burton TM & Allan JW (1986) Influence of pH, aluminum, and organic matter on stream invertebrates. Can J Fish Aquat Sci, **43**: 1285-1289.

Bush AI, Pettingell WH, Multhaup G, Paradis MD, Vonsattel J-P, Gusella JF, Beyreuther K, Masters CL, & Tanzi RE (1994) Rapid induction of Alzheimer Aβ amyloid formation by zinc. Science, **265**: 1464-1467.

Caines LA, Watt AW, & Wells DE (1985) The uptake and release of some trace metals by aquatic bryophytes in acidified waters in Scotland. Environ Pollut, **B10**: 1-18.

Cakir A, Sullivan TW, & Struwe FJ (1977) Effect of supplemental aluminum on the value of fertilizer phosphates in turkey diets. Poult Sci, **56**: 544-549.

Cam JM, Luck VA, Eastwood JB, & De Wardener HE (1976) The effect of aluminium hydroxide orally on calcium, phosphorus and aluminium in normal subjects. Clin Sci Mol Med, **51**: 407-414.

Cann CE, Prussin SG, & Gordan GS (1979) Aluminum uptake by the parathyroid glands. J Clin Endocrinol Metab, **49**: 543-545.

Carrière D, Fischer KL, Peakall DB, & Anghern P (1986) Effects of dietary aluminum sulphate on reproductive success and growth of ringed turtle doves (*Streptopelia risoria*). Can J Zool, **64**: 1500-1505.

Cawse PA (1974) A survey of atmospheric trace elements in the U.K. (1972-73). Harwell, United Kingdom Atomic Energy Authority , 84 pp (Report No. AERE-R 7669).

Cawse PA (1987) Trace and major elements in the atmosphere at rural locations in Great Britain, 1972-1981. In: Coughtrey PJ, Martin MH, & Unsworth MH ed. Pollutant transport and fate in ecosystems. Oxford, London, Blackwell Scientific Publications, pp 89-112 (British Ecological Society Special Publication No. 6).

Chadwick DJ & Whelan J (1992) Aluminium in biology and medicine. New York, Chichester, Brisbane, Toronto, John Wiley and Sons, 138 pp (Ciba Foundation Symposium No. 169).

Chainy GBN, Sahoo A, & Swain C (1993) Effect of aluminum on lipid peroxidation of cerebral hemisphere of chick. Bull Environ Contam Toxicol, **50**: 85-91.

Chan YL, Alfrey AC, Posen S, Lissner D, Hills E, Dunstan CR, & Evans RA (1983) Effect of aluminum on normal and uremic rats: tissue distribution, vitamin D metabolites, and quantitative bone histology. Calcif Tissue Int, **35**: 344-351.

Chan JC, Jacob M, Brown S, Savory J, & Wills MR (1988) Aluminum metabolism in rats: effects of vitamin D, dihydrotachysterol, 1,25-dihydroxyvitamin D and phosphate binders. Nephron, **48**: 61-64.

Channon SM, Arfeen S, & Ward MK (1988) Long-term accumulation of aluminium in patients with renal failure. Trace Elem Med, **5**: 154-157.

Chappuis P, Duhaux L, Paolaggi F, De Vernejoul MC, & Rousselet F (1988) Analytical problems encountered in determining aluminum status from hair in controls and hemodialyzed patients. Clin Chem, **34**: 2253-2255.

Chen W, Monnat RJ, Chen M, & Mottet K (1978) Aluminum induced pulmonary granulomatosis. Hum Pathol, **9**: 705-712.

Chenery EM (1955) A preliminary study of aluminium and the tea bush. Plant Soil, **VI**(2): 174-200.

Cherroret G, Bernuzzi V, Desor D, Hutin M-F, Burnel D, & Lehr PR (1992) Effects of postnatal aluminum exposure on choline acetyltransferase activity and learning abilities in the rat. Neurotoxicol Teratol, **14**: 259-264.

Chester R & Bradshaw GF (1991) Source control on the distribution of particulate trace metals in the North Sea atmosphere. Mar Pollut Bull, **22**(1): 30-36.

Chou L & Wollast R (1989) Distribution and geochemistry of aluminium in the Mediterranean Sea. Water Pollut Res Rep, **13**: 232-240.

Chow WM (1992) Behaviour of aluminium and its ecological significance in natural waters. In: Schulhof P ed. IWSA International Workshop on Aluminium in Drinking Water, Hong Kong, 15-17 January 1992. Oxford, London, Blackwell Scientific Publications, pp 1-10.

Christie H, Mackay RJ, & Fisher AM (1963) Pulmonary effects of inhalation of aluminum by rats and hamsters. Ind Hyg J, **24**: 47-56.

Christophersen N & Seip HM (1982) A model for streamwater chemistry at Birkenes, Norway. Water Resour Res, **18**(4): 977-996.

Clark KL & Hall RJ (1985) Effects of elevated hydrogen ion and aluminum concentrations on the survival of amphibian embryos and larvae. Can J Zool, **63**: 116-123.

Clark KL & Lazerte BD (1985) A laboratory study of the effects of aluminum and pH on amphibian eggs and tadpoles. Can J Fish Aquat Sci, **42**: 1544-1551.

Clarkson DT (1967) Aluminium tolerance in species within the genus *Agrostis*. J Ecol, **54**: 167-178.

Clayton DB (1989) Water polution at Lowermoore North Cornwall: Report of the Lowermoor incident health advisory committee. Truro, United Kingdom, Cornwall District Health Authority, 22 pp.

Clayton RM, Sedowofia SKA, Rankin JM, & Manning A (1992) Long-term effects of aluminium on the fetal mouse brain. Life Sci, **51**: 1921-1928.

Clemmensen O & Knudsen HE (1980) Contact sensitivity to aluminium in a patient hyposensitized with aluminium precipitated grass pollen. Contact Dermatitis, **6**: 305-308.

Cleveland L, Little EE, Hamilton SJ, Buckler DR, & Huhn JB (1986) Interactive toxicity of aluminum and acidity to early life stages of brook trout. Trans Am Fish Soc, **115**: 610-620.

Cleveland L, Little EE, Wiedmeyer RH, & Buckler DR (1989) Chronic no-observed-effect concentrations of aluminum for brook trout exposed in low-calcium, dilute acidic water. In: Lewis TE ed. Environmental chemistry and toxicology of aluminum. Proceedings of the 194th Annual Meeting of the American Chemical Society, New Orleans (LA), 30 August-4 September 1987. Chelsea, Michigan, Lewis Publishers Inc., pp 229-246.

Cleveland L, Buckler DR, & Brumbaugh WG (1991) Residue dynamics and effects of aluminum on growth and mortality in brook trout. Environ Toxicol Chem, **10**: 243-248.

Colomina MT, Gomez M, Domingo JL, Llobet JM, & Corbella J (1992) Concurrent ingestion of lactate and aluminum can result in development toxicity in mice. Res Commun Chem Pathol Pharmacol, **77**: 95-106.

Colomina MT, Gomez M, Domingo JL, Llobet JM, & Corbella J (1994) Lack of maternal and developmental toxicity in mice given high doses of aluminium hydroxide and ascorbic acid during gestation. Pharmacol Toxicol, **74**: 236-239.

Commisaris RL, Cordon JJ, Sprague S, Keiser J, Mayov G, & Rich R (1982) Behavioral changes in rats after chronic aluminium and parathyroid hormone administration. Neurobehav Toxicol Teratol, **4**: 403-410.

Connor DJ, Jope RS, & Harrell LE (1988) Chronic, oral aluminum administration to rats: Cognition and cholinergic parameters. Pharmacol Biochem Behav, **31**: 467-474.

Coriat A-M & Gillard RD (1986) Beware the cups that cheer. Nature (Lond), **321**: 570.

Corrin B (1963) Aluminium pneumoconiosis. II. Effect on the rat lung of intratracheal injections of stamped aluminium powders containing different lubricating agents and of a granular aluminium powder. Br J Ind Med, **20**: 268-276.

Cosby BJ, Wright RF, Hornberger GM, & Galloway JN (1985) Modeling the effects of acid deposition: estimation of long-term water quality responses in a small forested catchment. Water Resour Res, **21**(11): 1591-1601.

Cosby BJ, Whitehead PG, & Neale R (1986) A preliminary model of long-term changes in stream acidity in southwestern Scotland. J Hydrol, **84**: 381-401.

Cournot-Witmer G, Zinngraff J, Plachot JJ, Escaig F, Lefevre R, Boumati P, Bourdeau A, Garabédian M, Galle P, Bourdon R, Drüeke T, & Balsan S (1981) Aluminium localization in bone from hemodialyzed patients: Relationship to matrix mineralization. Kidney Int, **20**: 375-385.

Courtijn E, Vandecasteele C, Yu ZQ, Nagels M, & Dams R (1987) Determination and speciation of aluminium in acidified surface waters. In: Witters H & Vanderborght O ed. Ecophysiology of acid stress in aquatic organisms: Proceedings of an International Symposium, Antwerp, 13-16 January 1987. Antwerp, Belgian Royal Zoological Society, pp 33-44.

Courtijn E, Vandecasteele C, & Dams R (1990) Speciation of aluminium in surface water. Sci Total Environ, 90: 191-202.

Cranmer JM, Wilkins JD, Cannon DJ, & Smith L (1986) Fetal-placental-maternal uptake of aluminum in mice following gestational exposure: Effect of dose and route of administration. Neurotoxicology, 7: 601-608.

Crapper DR & Dalton AJ (1973a) Alterations in short term retention, conditioned avoidance response acquisition and motivation following aluminum induced neurofibrillary degeneration. Physiol Behav, 10: 925-933.

Crapper DR & Dalton AJ (1973b) Aluminum induced neurofibrillary degeneration, brain electrical activity and alterations in acquisition and retention. Physiol Behav, 10: 935-945.

Crapper DR, Krishnan SS, & Dalton AJ (1973) Brain aluminum distribution in Alzheimer's disease and experimental neurofibrillary degeneration. Science, 180: 511-513.

Crapper DR, Krishnan SS, & Quittkat S (1976) Aluminum, neurofibrillar degeneration and Alzheimer's disease. Brain, 99: 67-80.

Crapper DR, Quittkat S, Krishnan SS, Dalton AJ, & De Boni U (1980) Intranuclear aluminum content in Alzheimer's disease, dialysis encephalopathy and experimental aluminum encephalopathy. Acta Neuropathol, 50: 19-24.

Crapper McLachlan DR (1986) Aluminum and Alzheimer's disease. Neurobiol Aging, 7: 525-532.

Crapper McLachlan DR & Farnell BJ (1986) Cellular mechanisms of aluminium toxicity. Ann Ist Super Sanita, 22: 697-702.

Crapper McLachlan DR, Dam TV, Farnell BJ, & Lewis PN (1983) Aluminum inhibition of ADP-ribosylation *in vivo* and *in vitro*. Neurobehav Toxicol Teratol, 5: 645-647.

Crapper McLachlan DR, Lukiw WJ, & Kruck TPA (1989) New evidence for an active role of aluminum in Alzheimer's disease. Can J Neurol Sci, 16: 490-497.

Crapper McLachlan DR, Dalton AJ, Kruck TPA, Bell MY, Smith WL, Kalow W, & Andrews DF (1991) Intramuscular desferrioxamine in patients with Alzheimer's disease. Lancet, 337: 1304-1308.

Cronan CS, Kelly JM, Schofield CL, & Goldstein RA (1987) Aluminium geochemistry and tree toxicity in forests exposed to acidic deposition. In: Perry R ed. Acid rain: Scientific and technical advances. London, Selper, pp 649-656.

Cuenca G & Herrera R (1987) Ecophysiology of aluminium in terrestrial plants, growing in acid and aluminium-rich tropical soils. In: Witters H & Vanderborght O ed. Ecophysiology of acid stress in aquatic organisms: Proceedings of an International Symposium, Antwerp, 13-16 January 1987. Antwerp, Belgian Royal Zoological Society, pp 57-73.

Cummins CP (1986) Effects of aluminium and low pH on growth and development in *Rana temporaria* tadpoles. Oecologia, 69: 248-252.

Dabeka RW & McKenzie AD (1990) Aluminium levels in Canadian infant formulae and estimation of aluminium intakes from formulae by infants 0-3 months old. Food Addit Contam, 7(2): 275-282.

Dahlgren RA & Ugolini FC (1989) Aluminum fractionation of soil solutions from unperturbed and tephra-treated spodosols, Cascade Range, Washington, USA. Soil Sci Soc Am J, 53: 559-566.

Dalziel TRK, Morris R, & Brown DJA (1986) The effects of low pH, low calcium concentrations and elevated aluminium concentrations on sodium fluxes in brown trout, *Salmo trutta* L. Water Air Soil Pollut, **30**: 569-577.

Dalziel TRK, Morris R, & Brown DJA (1987) Sodium uptake inhibition in brown trout, *Salmo trutta* exposed to elevated aluminium concentrations at low pH. In: Witters H & Vanderborght O ed. Ecophysiology of acid stress in aquatic organisms: Proceedings of an International Conference, Antwerp, 13-16 January 1987. Antwerp, Belgian Royal Zoological Society, pp 421-434.

Dantzman CL & Breland HL (1969) Chemical status of some water sources in south central Florida. Soil Crop Sci Soc Fla Proc, **29**: 18-28.

Day JP, Barker J, Evans LJA, Perks J, Seabright PJ, Ackrill P, Lilley JS, Drumm PV, & Newton GWA (1991) Aluminium absorption studied by ^{26}Al tracer. Lancet, **337**: 1345.

Day JP, Barker J, King SJ, Miller RV, Templar J, Lilley JS, Drumm PV, Newton GWA, Fifield LK, Stone JOH, Allan GL, Edwardson JA, Moore PB, Ferrier IN, Priest ND, Newton D, Talbot RJ, Brock JH, Sanchez L, Dobson CB, Itzhaki RF, Radunovic A, & Bradbury MWB (1994) Biological chemistry of aluminium studied using ^{26}Al and accelerator mass spectrometry. Nucl Instrum Methods Phys Res, **B92**: 463-468.

Dean JR (1989) Ion chromatographic determination of aluminium with ultraviolet spectrophotometric detection. Analyst, **114**: 165-168.

De Boni U, Seger M, & Crapper McLachlan DR (1980) Functional consequences of chromatin bound aluminum in cultured human cells. In: Liss L ed. Aluminum neurotoxicity. Park Forest, South Illinois, Pathotox Publishers, Inc., pp 65-81.

De La Campa MRF, Garcia MED, & Sanz-Medel A (1988) Room-temperature liquid phosphorimetry of the aluminium-ferron chelate in micellar media. Determination of aluminium. Anal Chim Acta, **212**: 235-243.

Delonay AJ, Little EE, Woodward DF, Brumbauch WG, Farag AM, & Rabeni CF (1993) Sensitivity of early-life-stage golden trout to low pH and elevated aluminum. Environ Toxicol Chem, **12**: 1223-1232.

Den Dooren De Jong LE (1971) Tolerance of *Azotobacter* for metallic and non-metallic ions. Antonie van Leeuwenhoek, **37**: 119-124.

De Villiers PR (1962) The chemical composition of the water of the Orange River at Vioolsdrif, Cape Province. Ann Geol Opname Repub S Afr, **1**: 197-208.

De Vuyst P, Dumortier P, Rickaert F, Van De Weyer R, Lenclud C, & Yernault JC (1986) Occupational lung fibrosis in an aluminium polisher. Eur J Respir Dis, **68**: 131-140.

De Vuyst P, Dumortier P, Schandené L, Estenne M, Verhest A, & Yernault JC (1987) Sarcoid-like lung granulomatosis induced by aluminum dust. Am Rev Respir Dis, **135**: 493-497.

DIN (1993) [German standard procedures for testing water, sewage water and sludge: Physical, chemical, biological and bacterial procedures.] Society of German Chemists, Expert Group on Water Chemistry and German Institute for Standardization (DIN), Standardization Committee for Water (NAW), vol II, pp E9/1-11, E22/1-21 (DIN 38 406, Sections 9 and 22) (in German).

Dinman BD (1983) Aluminium, alloys and compounds. In: Parmeggiani L ed. Encyclopedia of occupational health and safety. Geneva, International Labour Organisation, vol 1, pp 131-135.

Dinman BD (1988a) Aluminium in the lung: the pyropowder conundrum. J Occup Med, **29**(11): 869-876.

Dinman BD (1988b) Alumina-related pulmonary disease. J Occup Med, **30**: 328-335.

Di Paolo JA & Casto BC (1979) Quantitative studies of *in vitro* morphological transformation of Syrian hamster cells by inorganic metal salts. Cancer Res, **39**: 1008-1013.

Dobbs AJ, French P, Gunn AM, Hunt DTE, & Winnard DA (1989) Aluminum speciation and toxicity in upland waters. In: Lewis TE ed. Environmental chemistry and toxicology of aluminum. Proceedings of the 194th Annual Meeting of the American Chemical Society, New Orleans, LA, 30 August-4 September 1987. Chelsea, Michigan, Lewis Publishers Inc., pp 209-228.

Doese M (1938) [Industrial medicine studies on injury to health caused by aluminium, in particular lung disease from aluminium dust.] Arch Gewerbepathol, **8**: 501-531 (in German).

Domingo JL (1995) Reproductive and developmental toxicity of aluminium: A review. Neurotoxicol Teratol, **17**(4): 515-521.

Domingo JL, Paternain JL, Llobet JM, & Corbella J (1987a) Effects of oral aluminum administration on perinatal and postnatal development in rats. Res Commun Chem Pathol Pharmacol, **57**: 129-132.

Domingo JL, Llobet JM, Gomez M, Tomas JM, & Corbella J (1987b) Nutritional and toxicological effects of short-term ingestion of aluminum by the rat. Res Commun Chem Pathol Pharmacol, **56**: 409-419.

Domingo JL, Paternain JL, Llobet JM, & Corbella J (1987c) The effects of aluminium ingestion on reproduction and postnatal survival in rats. Life Sci, **41**: 1127-1131.

Domingo JL, Gomez M, Bosque MA, & Corbella J (1989) Lack of teratogenicity of aluminum hydroxide in rats. Life Sci, **45**: 243-247.

Donald JM, Golub MS, Gershwin ME, & Keen CL (1989) Neurobehavioral effects in offspring of mice given excess aluminum in diet during gestation and lactation. Neurotoxicol Teratol, **11**: 345-351.

Dorfman D (1977) Tolerance of *Fundulus heteroclitus* to different metals in salt waters. Bull NJ Acad Sci, **22**(2): 21-23.

Drew RT, Gupta BN, Bend JR, & Hook GER (1974) Inhalation studies with a glycol complex of aluminum-chloride-hydroxide. Arch Environ Health, **28**: 321-326.

Driscoll CT (1984) A procedure for the fractionation of aqueous aluminum in dilute acidic waters. Int J Environ Anal Chem, **16**: 267-283.

Driscoll CT, Baker JP, Bisogni JJ, & Schofield CL (1980) Effect of aluminium speciation on fish in dilute acidified waters. Nature (Lond), **284**: 161-164.

Driscoll CT, Johnson NM, Likens GE, & Feller MC (1988) Effects of acidic deposition on the chemistry of headwater streams: a comparison between Hubbard Brook, New Hampshire, and Jamieson Creek, British Columbia. Water Resour Res, **24**(2): 195-200.

Driscoll CT, Wyskowski BJ, Destaffan P, & Newton RM (1989) Chemistry and transfer of aluminum in a forested watershed in the Adirondack region of New York, USA. In: Lewis TE ed. Environmental chemistry and toxicology of aluminum. Proceedings of the 194th Annual Meeting of the American Chemical Society, New Orleans, LA, 30 August-4 September 1987. Chelsea, Michigan, Lewis Publishers Inc., pp 83-105.

Duce RA, Hoffman GL, & Zoller WH (1975) Atmospheric trace metals at remote northern and southern hemisphere sites: pollution or natural? Science, **187**: 59-61.

Dunemann L & Schwedt G (1984) [Element species analysis in soil solutions by gel chromatography and chemical reaction detectors.] Fresenius Z Anal Chem, **317**: 394-399 (in German).

Eaton JG, Swenson WA, McCormick JH, Simonson TD, & Jensen KM (1992) A field and laboratory investigation of acid effects on largemouth bass, rock bass, black crappie, and yellow perch. Trans Am Fish Soc, **121**: 644-658.

Ecelbarger CA & Greger JL (1991) Dietary citrate and kidney function affect aluminum, zinc, and iron utilization in rats. J Nutr, **121**: 1755-1762.

Ecker F-J, Hirai E, & Chohji T (1990) The release of heavy metals from snowpacks on the Japan Sea side of Japan. Environ Pollut, **65**: 141-153.

Edwardson JA (1992) Alzheimer's disease and brain mineral metabolism. In: Munro H & Schlierf G ed. Nutrition of the elderly. New York, Raven Press, pp 193-202 (Nestlé Nutrition Workshop Series, Volume 29).

Edwardson JA, Candy JM, Ince PG, McArthur FK, Morris CM, Oakley AE, Taylor GA, & Bjertness E (1992) Aluminium accumulation, beta-amyloid deposition and neurofibrillary changes in the central nervous system. In: Aluminium in biology and medicine. New York, Chichester, Brisbane, Toronto, John Wiley and Sons, pp 165-185 (Ciba Foundation Symposium No. 169).

Edwardson JA, Moore PB, Ferrier IN, Lilley JS, Newton GWA, Barker J, Templar J, & Day JP (1993) Effect of silicon on gastrointestinal absorption of aluminium. Lancet, **342**(7): 211-212.

Eisenreich SJ (1980) Atmospheric input of trace metals to Lake Michigan. Water Air Soil Pollut, **13**: 287-301.

Elinder CG, Ahrengart L, Lidums V, Pettersson E, & Sjögren B (1991) Evidence of aluminium accumulation in aluminium welders. Br J Ind Med, **48**: 735-738.

Ellen G, Egmond E, Van Loon JW, Sahertian ET, & Tolsma K (1990) Dietary intakes of some essential and non-essential trace elements, nitrate, nitrite and N-nitrosamines by Dutch adults estimated in a 24-hour duplicate portion study. Food Addit Contam, **7**: 207-221.

Elliot HL, Dryburgh F, Fell GS, Sabet S, & MacDougall AI (1978) Aluminium toxicity during regular haemodialysis. Br Med J, **1**: 1101-1103.

Ellis HA, McCarthy JH, & Herrington J (1979) Bone aluminium in haemodialysed patients and in rats injected with aluminium chloride: relationship to impaired bone mineralisation. J Clin Pathol, **32**: 832-844.

Ermolenko LV & Dedkov YM (1988) Photometric determination of aluminum in water with the sulfonitrazo DAF reagent. J Anal Chem (USSR), **43**: 815-820.

Exley C, Tollervey A, Gray G, Roberts S, & Birchall JD (1993) Silicon, aluminium and the biological availability of phosphorus in algae. Proc R Soc (Lond), **B253**: 93-99.

Fairman B, Sanz-Medel A, Gallego M, Quintela MJ, Jones P, & Benson R (1994) Method comparison for the determination of labile aluminium species in natural waters. Anal Chim Acta, **286**: 401-409.

FAO/WHO (1989) Aluminium. In: Evaluation of certain food additives and contaminants. Thirty-third report of the Joint FAO/WHO Expert Committee on Food Additives. Geneva, World Health Organization, pp 28-31 (WHO Technical Report Series No. 776).

Farag AM, Woodward DF, Little EE, Steadman B, & Vertucci FA (1993) The effects of low pH and elevated aluminum on yellowstone cutthroat trout (*Oncorhynchus clarki bouvieri*). Environ Toxicol Chem, **12**: 719-731.

Farnell BJ, Crapper McLachlan DR, Baimbridge K, De Boni U, Wong L, & Wood PL (1985) Calcium metabolism in aluminum encephalopathy. Exp Neurol, **88**: 68-83.

Feely RA, Sackett WM, & Harris JE (1971) Distribution of particulate aluminum in the Gulf of Mexico. J Geophys Res, **76**(24): 5893-5902.

Feth JH, Rogers SM, & Roberson CE (1964) Chemical composition of snow in the northern Sierra Nevada and other areas. Washington, DC, US Department of Interior, Geological Survey, 39 pp (Geological Survey-Water Supply Paper No. 1535-J).

Fileman CF, Althaus M, Law RJ, & Haslam I (1991) Dissolved and particulate trace metals in surface waters over the Dogger Bank, Central North Sea. Mar Pollut Bull, **22**(5): 241-244.

Filipek LH, Nordstrom DK, & Ficklin WH (1987) Interaction of acid mine drainage with waters and sediments of West Squaw Creek in the West Shasta mining district, California. Environ Sci Technol, **21**: 388-396.

Finberg L, Dweck HS, Holmes F, Kretchmer N, Mauer AM, Reynolds JW, & Suskind RM (1986) Aluminum toxicity in infants and children. Pediatrics, **78**: 1150-1154.

Finelli VN, Que Hee SS, & Niemeier RW (1981) Influence of exposure to aluminium chloride and fluoride dusts on some biochemical and physiological parameters in rats. In: Brown SS & Davies DS ed. Organ-directed toxicity chemical indices and mechanisms (IUPAC). New York, Pergamon Press, pp 291-295.

Fischer T & Rystedt I (1982) A case of contact sensitivity to aluminium. Contact Dermatitis, **8**: 343.

Fisher DW, Gambell AW, Likens GE, & Bormann FH (1968) Atmospheric contributions to water quality of streams in the Hubbard Brook Experimental Forest, New Hampshire. Water Resour Res, **4**: 1115-1126.

Fivelstad S & Leivestad H (1984) Aluminium toxicity to Atlantic salmon (*Salmo salar* L.) and brown trout (*Salmo trutta* L.): mortality and physiological response. Oslo, Norway, Institute of Fresh Water Ecology, pp 69-77 (Research Report No. 61).

Flaten TP (1990) Geographical associations between aluminium in drinking water and death rates with dementia (including Alzheimer's disease), Parkinson's disease and amyotrophic lateral sclerosis in Norway. Environ Geochem Health, **12**: 152-167.

Flaten TP, Glattre E, Viste A, & Søreide O (1991) Mortality from dementia among gastro-duodenal ulcer patients. J Epidemiol Community Health, **45**: 203-206.

Fleming RF & Lindstrom RM (1987) Precise determination of aluminum by instrumental neutron activation. J Radioanal Nucl Chem, **113**: 35-42.

Flendrig JA, Kruis H, & Das HA (1976) Aluminium and dialysis dementia. Lancet, **1**: 1235.

Flora SJS, Dhawan M, & Tandon SK (1991) Effects of combined exposure to aluminium and ethanol on aluminium body burden and some neuronal, hepatic and haematopoietic biochemical variables in the rat. Hum Exp Toxicol, **10**: 45-48.

Folsom BR, Popescu NA, & Wood JM (1986) Comparative study of aluminum and copper transport and toxicity in an acid-tolerant freshwater green alga. Environ Sci Technol, **20**: 616-620.

Forbes WF, McAiney CA, Hayward LM, & Agwani N (1994) Geochemical risk factors for mental functioning, based on the Ontario longitudinal study of aging (LSA): II. The role of pH. Can J Aging, **13**: 249-267.

Foy CD & Gerloff GC (1972) Response of *Chlorella pyrenoidosa* to aluminum and low pH. J Phycol, **8**: 268-271.

Fraga CG, Oteiza PI, Golub MS, Gershwin ME, & Keen CL (1990) Effects of aluminum on brain lipid peroxidation. Toxicol Lett, **51**: 213-219.

France RL & Stokes PM (1987) Influence of manganese, calcium, and aluminum on hydrogen ion toxicity to the amphipod *Hyalella azteca*. Can J Zool, **65**: 3071-3078.

Franceschetti S, Bugiani O, Panzica F, Tagliavini F, & Avanzini G (1990) Changes in excitability of CA1 pyramidal neurons in slices prepared from $AlCl_3$-treated rabbits. Epilepsy Res, **6**: 39-48.

Frank WB, Haupin WE, Dawless RK, Granger DA, Wei MW, Calhoun KJ, & Bonney TB (1985) Aluminum. In: Gerhartz W, Yamamoto YS, Campbell FT, Pfefferkorn R, & Rounsaville JF ed. Ullmann's encyclopedia of industrial chemistry - Volume A1: Abrasives to aluminium oxide, 5th revised ed. Weinheim, Verlag Chemie, pp 459-480.

Frecker MF (1991) Dementia in Newfoundlands: Identification of a geographical isolate? J Epidemiol Community Health, **45**: 307-311.

Freda J & McDonald DG (1990) Effects of aluminum on the leopard frog, *Rana pipiens*: life stage comparisons and aluminum uptake. Can J Fish Aquat Sci, **47**: 210-216.

Freda J & McDonald DG (1993) Toxicity of amphibian breeding ponds in the Sudbury region. Can J Fish Aquat Sci, **50**: 1497-1503.

Freeman RA (1973) Recovery of rainbow trout from aluminum poisoning. Trans Am Fish Soc, **102**(1): 152-154.

Freeman RA & Everhart WH (1971) Toxicity of aluminum hydroxide complexes in neutral and basic media to rainbow trout. Trans Am Fish Soc, **100**(4): 644-658.

Frick KG & Herrmann J (1990) Aluminum accumulation in a lotic mayfly at low pH - a laboratory study. Ecotoxicol Environ Saf, **19**: 81-88.

Froment DH, Buddington B, Miller NL, & Alfrey AC (1989a) Effect of solubility on the gastrointestinal absorption of aluminum from various aluminum compounds in the rat. J Lab Clin Med, **114**: 237-242.

Froment DPH, Molitoris BA, Buddington B, Miller N, & Alfrey AC (1989b) Site and mechanism of enhanced gastrointestinal absorption of aluminum by citrate. Kidney Int, **36**: 978-984.

Frost L, Johansen P, Pedersen S, Veien N, Aabel Östergaard P, & Nielsen MH (1985) Persistant subcutaneous nodules in children hyposensitized with aluminium-containing allergen extracts. Allergy, **40**: 368-372.

Fulton B, Jaw S, & Jeffery EH (1989) Bioavailability of aluminum from drinking water. Fundam Appl Toxicol, **12**: 144-150.

Furrer G (1993) New aspects on the chemistry of aluminum in soils. Aquat Sci, **55**(4): 281-290.

Gajdusek DC & Salazar AM (1982) Amyotrophic lateral sclerosis and parkinsonian syndromes in high incidence among the Auyu and Jakai people of West New Guinea. Neurology, **32**: 107-126.

Galceran T, Finch J, Bergfeld M, Coburn JW, Martin K, Teitelbaum S, & Slatopolsky E (1987) Biological effects of aluminum on normal dogs: studies on the isolated perfused bone. Endocrinology (Baltimore), **121**: 406-413.

Ganrot PO (1986) Metabolism and possible health effects of aluminum. Environ Health Perspect, **65**: 363-441.

Garcia RP, Liu YM, Garcia MED, & Sanz-Medel A (1991) Solid-surface room-temperature phosphorescence optosensing in continuous flow systems: an approach for ultratrace metal ion determination. Anal Chem, **63**: 1759-1763.

Gardinier PE, Ottaway JM, Fell GS, & Halls DJ (1981) Determination of aluminium in blood plasma or serum by electrothermal atomic absorption spectrometry. Anal Chim Acta, **128**: 57-66.

Gardinier PE, Schierl R, & Kreutzer K (1987) Aluminium speciation in soil solutions as studied by size exclusion chromatography. Plant Soil, **103**: 151-154.

Garruto RM, Fukatsu R, Yanagihara R, Gajdusek DC, Hook G, & Fiori CE (1984) Imaging of calcium and aluminum in neurofibrillary tangle-bearing neurons in parkinsonism-dementia of Guam. Proc Natl Acad Sci (USA), **81**: 1875-1879.

Gascon C, Planas D, & Moreau G (1987) The interaction of pH, calcium and aluminium concentrations on the survival and development of wood frog (*Rana sylvatica*) eggs and tadpoles. In: Witters H & Vanderborght O ed. Ecophysiology of acid stress in aquatic organisms: Proceedings of an International Symposium, Antwerp, 13-16 January 1987. Antwerp, Belgian Royal Zoological Society, pp 189-199.

Genter RB & Amyot DJ (1994) Freshwater benthic algal population and community changes due to acidity and aluminum-acid mixtures in artificial streams. Environ Toxicol Chem, **13**(3): 369-380.

Gitelman HJ, Alderman FR, Kurs-Lasky M, & Rockette HE (1995) Serum and urinary aluminium levels of workers in the aluminium industry. Ann Occup Hyg, **39**: 181-191.

Goate AM, Chartier-Harlin MC, Mullan M, Brown J, Crawford F, Fidani L, Guiffral L, Haynes A, & Hardy JA (1991) Segregation of a mis-sense mutation in the amyloid precursor protein gene with familial Alzheimer disease. Nature (Lond), **349**: 704-706.

Godbold DL, Dictus K, & Hüttermann A (1988a) Influence of aluminium and nitrate on root growth and mineral nutrition of Norway spruce (*Picea abies*) seedlings. Can J For Res, **18**: 1167-1171.

Godbold DL, Fritz E, & Hüttermann A (1988b) Aluminum toxicity and forest decline. Proc Natl Acad Sci (USA), **85**: 3888-3892.

Goenaga X & Williams DJA (1988) Aluminium speciation in surface waters from a Welsh upland area. Environ Pollut, **52**: 131-149.

Goenaga X & Williams DJA (1990) Determination of aluminium speciation in acid waters. In: Edwards RW, Gee AS, & Stoner JH ed. Acid waters in Wales. Dordrecht, Boston, London, Kluwer Academic Publishers, pp 189-201.

Goenaga X, Bryant R, & Williams DJA (1987) Influence of sorption processes on aluminum determinations in acidic waters. Anal Chem, **59**: 2673-2678.

Golub MS, Gershwin ME, Donald JM, Negri S, & Keen CL (1987) Maternal and developmental toxicity of chronic aluminum exposure in mice. Fundam Appl Toxicol, **8**: 346-357.

Golub MS, Donald JM, Gershwin ME, & Keen CL (1989) Effects of aluminum ingestion on spontaneous motor activity of mice. Neurotoxicol Teratol, **11**: 231-235.

Golub MS, Keen CL, & Gershwin ME (1992) Neurodevelopmental effect of aluminum in mice: Fostering studies. Neurotoxicol Teratol, **14**: 177-182.

Golub MS, Han B, Keen CL, & Gershwin ME (1993) Developmental patterns of aluminium in mouse brain and interactions between dietary aluminium excess and manganese deficiency. Toxicology, **81**: 33-47.

Golub MS, Han B, Keen CL, & Gershwin ME (1994) Auditory startle in Swiss Webster mice fed excess aluminium in diet. Neurotoxicol Teratol, **16**: 423-425.

Golub MS, Han B, Keen CL, Gershwin ME, & Tarara RP (1995) Behavioral performance of Swiss Webster mice exposed to excess dietary aluminum during development or during development and as adults. Toxicol Appl Pharmacol, **133**: 64-72.

Gomez M, Domingo JL, Llobet JM, Tomas JM, & Corbella J (1986) Short-term oral toxicity study of aluminium in rats. Arch Pharmacol Toxicol, **12**: 145-151.

Gomez M, Bosque MA, Domingo JL, Llobet JM, & Corbella J (1990) Evaluation of the maternal and developmental toxicity of aluminum from high doses of aluminum hydroxide in rats. Vet Hum Toxicol, **32**: 545-548.

Gomez M, Domingo JL, & Llobet JM (1991) Developmental toxicity evaluation of oral aluminum in rats: Influence of citrate. Neurotoxicol Teratol, **13**: 323-328.

Good PF, Perl DP, Bierer LM, & Schmeidler J (1992) Selective accumulation of aluminium and iron in the neurofibrillary tangles of Alzheimer's disease: a laser microprobe (LAMMA) study. Ann Neurol, **31**: 286-292.

Goodman WG (1984) Short-term aluminum administration in the rat: reductions in formation without osteomalacia. J Lab Clin Med, **103**: 749-757.

Goodman WG (1986) Experimental aluminum-induced bone disease: Studies *in vivo*. Kidney Int, **18**(suppl): S32-S36.

Goodman WG (1990) Pathophysiologic mechanisms of aluminum toxicity: Aluminum-induced bone disease. In: de Broe ME & Coburn JW ed. Aluminum and renal failure. Dordrecht, Boston, London, Kluwer Academic Publishers, pp 87-108.

Goodman WG, Henry DA, Horst R, Nudelman RK, Alfrey AC, & Coburn JW (1984a) Parenteral aluminum administration in the dog: II. Induction osteomalacia and effects on vitamin D metabolism. Kidney Int, **25**: 370-375.

Goodman WG, Gilligan J, & Horst R (1984b) Short-term aluminum administration in the rat: effects on bone formation and relationship with renal osteomalacia. J Clin Invest, **73**: 171-181.

Göransson A & Eldhuset TD (1987) Effects of aluminium on growth and nutrient uptake of *Betula pendula* seedlings. Physiol Plant, **69**: 193-199.

Grahn O (1980) Fishkills in two moderately acid lakes due to high aluminum concentration. In: Drabløs D & Tollan A ed. Ecological impact of acid precipitation: Proceedings of an International Conference. Sandefjord, Norway, 11-14 March 1980. Oslo-Ås, SNSF, pp 310-311.

Grant LD, Elias R, Goyer R, Nicholson W, & Olem H (1990) Indirect health effects associated with acidic deposition. Washington, DC, National Acid Precipitation Assessment Program, 173 pp (NAPAP Report No. 23).

Graves AB, White E, Koepsell TD, Reifler BV, Van Belle G, & Larson EB (1990) The association between aluminum-containing products and Alzheimer's disease. J Clin Epidemiol, **43**: 35-44.

Greger JL & Baier MJ (1983a) Excretion and retention of low or moderate levels of aluminium by human subjects. Food Chem Toxicol, **21**: 473-477.

Greger JL & Baier MJ (1983b) Effect of dietary aluminum on mineral metabolism of adult males. Am J Clin Nutr, **38**: 411-419.

Greger JL & Powers CF (1992) Assessment of exposure to parenteral and oral aluminum with and without citrate using a desferrioxamine test in rats. Toxicology, **76**: 119-132.

Greger JL, Bula EN, & Gum ET (1985a) Mineral metabolism of rats fed moderate levels of various aluminum compounds for short periods of time. J Nutr, **115**: 1708-1716.

Greger JL, Goetz W, & Sullivan D (1985b) Aluminium levels in foods cooked and stored in aluminium pans, trays and foil. J Food Prot, **48**: 772-777.

Greger JL, Gum ET, & Bula EN (1986) Mineral metabolism of rats fed various levels of aluminum hydroxide. Biol Trace Elem Res, **9**: 67-77.

Gross P, De Treville RTP, Cralley LJ, Grandquist WT, & Pundsack FL (1970) The pulmonary response to fibrous dusts of diverse compositions. Am Ind Hyg Assoc J, **31**: 125-132.

Gross P, Harley RA, & Detreville RTP (1973) Pulmonary reaction to metallic aluminum powders. Arch Environ Health, **26**: 227-236.

Guieu C, Martin JM, Thomas AJ, & Elbaz-Poulichet F (1991) Atmospheric versus river inputs of metals to the Gulf of Lions: Total concentrations, partitioning and fluxes. Mar Pollut Bull, **22**(4): 176-183.

Gundersen P & Rasmussen L (1990) Nitrification in forest soils: effects from nitrogen deposition on soil acidification and aluminum release. Rev Environ Contam Toxicol, **113**: 1-45.

Gundersen DT, Bustaman S, Seim WK, & Curtis LR (1994) pH, hardness, and humic acid influence aluminum toxicity to rainbow trout (*Oncorhynchus mykiss*) in weakly alkaline waters. Can J Fish Aquat Sci, **51**: 1345-1355.

Gunn JM & Noakes DLG (1987) Latent effects of pulse exposure to aluminum and low pH on size, ionic composition, and feeding efficiency of lake trout (*Salvelinus namaycush*) alevins. Can J Fish Aquat Sci, **44**: 1418-1424.

Gupta SK, Waters DH, & Gwilt PR (1986) Absorption and disposition of aluminium in the rat. J Pharm Sci, **75**: 586-589.

Guy SP, Jones D, Mann DMA, & Itzhaki RF (1991) Human neuroblastoma cells treated with aluminium express an epitope associated with Alzheimer's disease neurofibrillary tangles. Neurosci Lett, **121**: 166-168.

Hackett C (1962) Stimulative effects of aluminium on plant growth. Nature (Lond), **195**(4840): 471-472.

Hackett C (1964) Ecological aspects of the nutrition of *Deschampsia flexuosa* (L.) Trin: I. The effect of aluminium, manganese and pH on germination. J Ecol, **52**: 159-167.

Hackett C (1967) Ecological aspects of the nutrition of *Deschampsia flexuosa* (L.) Trin: III. Investigation of phosphorus requirement and response to aluminium in water culture, and a study of growth in soil. J Ecol, **55**: 831-840.

Hahn PHB & Guenter W (1986) Effect of dietary fluoride and aluminum on laying hen performance and fluoride concentration in blood, soft tissue, bone, and egg. Poult Sci, **65**: 1343-1349.

Hall RJ, Likens GE, Fiance SB, & Hendrey GR (1980) Experimental acidification of a stream in the Hubbard Brook Experimental Forest, New Hampshire. Ecology, **61**(4): 976-989.

Hall RJ, Driscoll CT, Likens GE, & Pratt JM (1985) Physical, chemical, and biological consequences of episodic aluminum additions to a stream. Limnol Oceanogr, **30**(1): 212-220.

Hall RJ, Driscoll CT, & Likens GE (1987) Importance of hydrogen ions and aluminium in regulating the structure and function of stream ecosystems: an experimental test. Freshw Biol, **18**: 17-43.

Harriman R, Morrison BRS, Caines LA, Collen P, & Watt AW (1987) Long-term changes in fish populations of acid streams and lochs in Galloway, south west Scotland. Water Air Soil Pollut, **32**: 89-112.

Häsänen E & Huttunen S (1989) Acid deposition and the element composition of pine tree rings. Chemosphere, **18**(9/10): 1913-1920.

Häsänen E, Lipponen M, Minkkinen P, Kattainen R, Markkanen K, & Brjukhanov P (1990) Elemental concentrations of aerosol samples from the Baltic Sea area. Chemosphere, **21**(3): 339-347.

Haugen AA, Becher G, & Bjørseth A (1983) Biological monitoring of occupational exposure to polycyclic aromatic hydrocarbons (PAHs) in an aluminium plant (Abstract). Eur J Cancer Clin Oncol, **19**: 1287.

Havas M (1985) Aluminum bioaccumulation and toxicity to *Daphnia magna* in soft water at low pH. Can J Fish Aquat Sci, **42**: 1741-1748.

Havas M & Hutchinson TC (1982) Aquatic invertebrates from the Smoking Hills, N.W.T.: effect of pH and metals on mortality. Can J Fish Aquat Sci, **39**: 890-903.

Havas M & Likens GE (1985) Toxicity of aluminum and hydrogen ions to *Daphnia catawba, Holopedium gibberum, Chaoborus punctipennis,* and *Chironomus anthrocinus* from Mirror Lake, New Hampshire. Can J Zool, **63**: 1114-1119.

Havens KE (1990) Aluminum binding to ion exchange sites in acid-sensitive versus acid-tolerant cladocerans. Environ Pollut, **64**: 133-141.

Havens KE (1991) Littoral zooplankton responses to acid and aluminum stress during short-term laboratory bioassays. Environ Pollut, **73**: 71-84.

Havens KE (1993) Acid and aluminum effects on the survival of littoral macro-invertebrates during acute bioassays. Environ Pollut, **80**: 95-100.

Havens KE & Heath RT (1989) Acid and aluminum effects on freshwater zooplankton: an *in situ* mesocosm study. Environ Pollut, **62**: 195-211.

Helliwell S, Batley GE, Florence TM, & Lumsden BG (1983) Speciation and toxicity of aluminium in a model fresh water. Environ Technol Lett, **4**: 141-144.

Hellou J, Fancey LL, & Payne JF (1992a) Concentrations of twenty-four elements in bluefin tuna *Thunnus thynnus* from the northwest Atlantic. Chemosphere, **24**(2): 211-218.

Hellou J, Warren WG, Payne JF, Belkhode S, & Lobel P (1992b) Heavy metals and other elements in three tissues of cod, *Gadus morhua* from the northwest Atlantic. Mar Pollut Bull, **24**(9): 452-458.

Helmboldt O, Hudson LK, Misra C, Wefers K, Stark H, & Danner M (1985) Aluminum compounds, inorganic. In: Gerhartz W, Yamamoto YS, Campbell FT, Pfefferkorn R, & Rounsaville JF ed. Ullmann's encyclopedia of industrial chemistry - Volume A1: Abrasives to aluminum oxide, 5th revised ed. Weinheim, Verlag Chemie, pp 527-541.

Hem JD & Roberson CE (1967) Form and stability of aluminum hydroxide complexes in dilute solution. In: Chemistry of aluminum in natural water. Washington, DC, US Department of Interior, Geological Survey (Geological Survey-Water Supply Paper No. 1827-A).

Henriksen A, Skogheim OK, & Rosseland BO (1984) Episodic changes in pH and aluminium-speciation kill fish in a Norwegian salmon river. Vatten, **40**: 255-260.

Henriksen A, Lien L, Traaen TS, Sevaldrud IS, & Brakke DF (1988a) Lake acidification in Norway: present and predicted fish status. Ambio, **18**(6): 314-321.

Henriksen A, Lien L, Traaen TS, Sevaldrud IS, & Brakke DF (1988b) Lake acidification in Norway - present and predicted chemical status. Ambio, **17**(4): 259-266.

Henriksen A, Wathne BM, Røgeberg EJS, Norton SA, & Brakke DF (1988c) The role of stream substrates in aluminium mobility and acid neutralization. Water Res, **22**(8): 1069-1073.

Henry HL & Norman AW (1985) Interactions between aluminium and the actions and metabolism of vitamin D_3 in the chick. Calcif Tissue Int, **37**: 484-490.

Henry DA, Goodman WG, Nudelman RK, Didomenico NC, Alfrey AC, Slatopolsky E, Stanley TM, & Coburn JW (1984) Parenteral aluminum administration in the dog: I. Plasma kinetics, tissue levels, calcium metabolism, and para-thyroid hormone. Kidney Int, **25**: 362-369.

Herbert A, Sterling G, Abraham J, & Corrin B (1982) Desquamative interstitial pneumonia in an aluminum welder. Hum Pathol, **13**: 694-699.

Herrmann J (1987) Sodium levels of lotic mayfly nymphs being exposed to aluminium at low pH. A preliminary report. Ann Soc R Zool Belg, **117**: 181-188.

Herrmann J & Andersson KG (1986) Aluminium impact on respiration of lotic mayflies at low pH. Water Air Soil Pollut, **30**: 703-709.

Herzog P, Schmitt KF, Grendhal T, Van der Linden J, & Holtermüller KH (1982) VI.5. Evaluation of serum and urine electrolyte changes during therapy with a magnesium-aluminum containing antacid: results of a prospective study. In: Halter F ed. Antacids in the eighties: Symposium on Antacids, Hamburg, June 1980. München, Urban & Schwarzenberg, pp 123-135.

Hickie BE, Hutchinson NJ, Dixon DG, & Hodson PV (1993) Toxicity of trace metal mixtures to alevin rainbow trout (*Oncorhynchus mykiss*) and larval fathead minnow (*Pimephales promelas*) in soft, acidic water. Can J Fish Aquat Sci, **50**: 1348-1355.

Hicks JS, Hackett DS, & Sprague GL (1987) Toxicity and aluminium concentration in bone following dietary administration of two sodium aluminium phosphate formulations in rats. Food Chem Toxicol, **25**(7): 533-538.

Hjortsbert U, Orbaek P, Arborelius M Jr, & Karlsson J-E (1994) Upper airway irritation and small airways hyperreactivity due to exposure to potassium aluminium tetrafluoride flux: an extended case report. Occup Environ Med, **51**: 706-709.

Hodsman AB, Sherrard DJ, Alfrey AC, Ott S, Brickman AS, Miller NL, Maloney NA, & Coburn JW (1982) Bone aluminum and histomorphometric features of renal osteodystrophy. J Clin Endocrinol Metab, **54**: 539-546.

Hodsman AB, Anderson C, & Leung FY (1984) Accelerated accumulation of aluminum by osteoid matrix in vitamin D deficiency. Miner Electrolyte Metab, **10**: 309-315.

Höhr D, Abel J, & Wilhelm M (1989) Renal clearance of aluminium: studies in the isolated perfused rat kidney. Toxicol Lett, **45**: 165-174.

Hoke RA, Giesy JP, & Kreis RG (1992) Sediment pore water toxicity identification in the lower Fox River and Green Bay, Wisconsin, using the microtox assay. Ecotoxicol Environ Saf, **23**: 343-354.

Hörnström E, Ekström C, & Duraini MO (1984) Effects of pH and different levels of aluminium on lake plankton in the Swedish west coast area. Oslo, Norway, Institute of Fresh Water Ecology, pp 115-127 (Research Report No. 61).

Horst WJ, Wagner A, & Marschner H (1982) Mucilage protects root meristems from aluminium injury. Z Pflanzenphysiol Bd, **105**: 435-444.

Hosovski E, Mastelica Z, Sunderic D, & Radulovic D (1990) Mental abilities of workers exposed to aluminium. Med Lav, **81**: 119-123.

Huang JW, Grunes DL, & Kochian LV (1992a) Aluminum effects on the kinetics of calcium uptake into cells of the wheat root apex: Quantification of calcium fluxes using a calcium-selective vibrating microelectrode. Planta, **188**: 414-421.

Huang JW, Shaff JE, Grunes DL, & Kochian LV (1992b) Aluminum effects on calcium fluxes at the root apex of aluminum-tolerant and aluminum-sensitive wheat cultivars. Plant Physiol, **98**: 230-237.

Hudson LK, Misra C, & Wefers K (1985) Aluminum oxide. In: Gerhartz W, Yamamoto YS, Campbell FT, Pfefferkorn R, & Rounsaville JF ed. Ullmann's encyclopedia of industrial chemistry - Volume A1: Abrasives to aluminum oxide, 5th revised ed. Weinheim, Verlag Chemie, pp 557-594.

Huett DO & Menary RC (1980) Aluminium distribution in freeze-dried roots of cabbage, lettuce and kikuyu grass by energy-dispersive x-ray analysis. Aust J Plant Physiol, **7**: 101-111.

Hunn JB, Cleveland L, & Little EE (1987) Influence of pH and aluminum on developing brook trout in a low calcium water. Environ Pollut, **43**: 63-73.

Hunter JB, Ross SL, & Tannahill J (1980) Aluminium pollution and fish toxicity. J Water Pollut Control Fed, **79**: 413-420.

Hussein AS, Cantor AH, & Johnson TH (1988) Use of high levels of dietary aluminum and zinc for inducing pauses in egg production of Japanese quail. Poult Sci, **67**: 1157-1165.

Hussein AS, Cantor AH, & Johnson TH (1989a) Effect of dietary aluminum on calcium and phosphorus metabolism and performance of laying hens. Poult Sci, **68**: 706-714.

Hussein AS, Cantor AH, & Johnson TH (1989b) Comparison of the use of dietary aluminum with the use of feed restriction for force-molting laying hens. Poult Sci, **68**: 891-896.

Hutchinson NJ & Sprague JB (1986) Toxicity of trace metal mixtures to American flagfish (*Jordanella floridae*) in soft, acidic water and implications for cultural acidification. Can J Fish Aquat Sci, **43**: 647-655.

Hydes DJ (1977) Dissolved aluminium concentration in sea water. Nature (Lond), **268**: 136-137.

Hydes DJ (1979) Aluminum in seawater: control by inorganic processes. Science, **205**: 1260-1262.

Hydes DJ (1983) Distribution of aluminium in waters of the north east Atlantic 25°N to 35°N. Geochim Cosmochim Acta, **47**: 967-973.

Hydes DJ & Kremling K (1993) Patchiness in dissolved metals (Al, Cd, Co, Cu, Mn, Ni) in North Sea surface waters: seasonal differences and influence of suspended sediment. Cont Shelf Res, **13**(10): 1083-1101.

Hydes DJ & Liss PS (1977) The behaviour of dissolved aluminium in estuarine and coastal waters. Estuar Coast Mar Sci, **5**: 755-769.

IARC (1987) Cadmium and cadmium compounds. In: Overall evaluations of carcinogenicity: An updating of IARC Monographs, Volumes 1 to 42. Lyon, International Agency for Research on Cancer, pp 139-142 (IARC Monographs on the Evaluation of the Carcinogenic Risk of Chemicals to Humans, Supplement 7).

Ingersoll CG, Gulley DD, Mount DR, Mueller ME, Fernandez JD, Hockett JR, & Bergman HL (1990) Aluminum and acid toxicity to two strains of brook trout (*Salvelinus fontinalis*). Can J Fish Aquat Sci, **47**: 1641-1648.

IPAI (1993) Statistical summary - Volume 5. London, International Primary Aluminium Institute, 36 pp.

IRPTC (1993) IRPTC legal file 1986. Geneva, International Register of Potentially Toxic Chemicals, United Nations Environment Programme.

Irvine KN, Drake JJ, & James W (1992) Particulate trace element concentrations and loadings associated with erosion of pervious urban land. Environ Technol, **13**: 231-237.

Ittel TH, Gruber E, Heinrichs A, Handt S, Hofstädter F, & Sieberth HG (1992) Effect of fluoride on aluminum-induced bone disease in rats with renal failure. Kidney Int, **41**: 1340-1348.

Jacobs RW, Duong T, Jones RE, Trapp GA, & Scheibel AB (1989) A re-examination of aluminium in Alzheimer's disease: Analysis by energy dispersive x-ray microprobe and flameless atomic absorbtion spectrophotometry. Can J Neurol Sci, **16**: 498-503.

Jacqmin H, Commenges D, Letenneur L, Barberger-Gateau P, & Dartigues JF (1994) Components of drinking water and risk of cognitive impairment in the elderly. Am J. Epidemiol, **139**: 48-57.

Jäger DE, Wilhelm M, Witte G, & Ohnesorge FK (1991) Intestinal absorption of aluminium: studies in the isolated perfused rat intestinal preparation. J Trace Elem Electrolytes Health Dis, **5**(2): 81-85.

Jagoe CH, Haines TA, & Buckler DR (1987) Abnormal gill development in Atlantic salmon (*Salmo salar*) fry exposed to aluminium at low pH. In: Witters H & Vanderborght O ed. Ecophysiology of acid stress in aquatic organisms: Proceedings of an International Symposium, Antwerp, 13-16 January 1987. Antwerp, Belgian Royal Zoological Society, pp 375-386.

James BR & Riha SJ (1989) Aluminum leaching by mineral acids in forest soils: I. Nitric-sulfuric acid differences. Soil Sci Soc Am J, **53**: 259-264.

Jederlinic PJ, Abraham JL, Churg A, Himmelstein JS, Epler GR, & Gaensler EA (1990) Pulmonary fibrosis in aluminum oxide workers. Am Rev Respir Dis, **142**: 1179-1184.

Johnson GVM & Jope RS (1987) Aluminum alters cyclic AMP and cyclic GMP levels but not presynaptic cholinergic markers in rat brain *in vivo*. Brain Res, **403**: 1-6.

Johnson NM, Driscoll CT, Eaton JS, Likens GE, & McDowell WH (1981) 'Acid rain' dissolved aluminum and chemical weathering at the Hubbard Brook Experimental Forest, New Hampshire. Geochim Cosmochim Acta, **45**: 1421-1437.

Johnson MG, Culp LR, & George SE (1986) Temporal and spatial trends in metal loadings to sediments of the Turkey Lakes, Ontario. Can J Fish Aquat Sci, **43**: 754-762.

Johnson GVW, Cogdill KW, & Jope RS (1990) Oral aluminum alters *in vitro* protein phosphorylation and kinase activities in rat brain. Neurobiol Aging, **11**: 209-216.

Johnson GVW, Watson AL Jr, Lartius R, Uemura E, & Jope RS (1992) Dietary aluminum selectively decreases MAP-2 in brains of developing and adult rats. Neurotoxicology, **13**: 463-474.

Jones P (1991) The investigation of aluminium speciation in natural and potable waters using short-column ion chromatography. Int J Environ Anal Chem, **44**: 1-10.

Jones KC & Bennett BG (1985) Exposure commitment assessments of environmental pollutants. London, University of London, King's College, Monitoring and Assessment Research Centre, 33 pp (MARC Technical Report 33).

Jones BF, Kennedy VC, & Zellweger GW (1974) Comparison of observed and calculated concentrations of dissolved Al and Fe in stream water. Water Resour Res, **10**(4): 791-793.

Jope RS & Johnson GVW (1992) Neurotoxic effects of dietary aluminium. In: Aluminium in biology and medicine. New York, Chichester, Brisbane, Toronto, John Wiley and Sons, pp 254-267 (Ciba Foundation Symposium No. 169.

Jorhem L & Haegglund G (1992) Aluminium in foodstuffs and diets in Sweden. Z Lebensm.unters Forsch, **194**: 38-42.

Joslin JD, Kelly JM, Wolfe MH, & Rustad LE (1988) Elemental patterns in roots and foliage of mature spruce across a gradient of soil aluminium. Water Air Soil Pollut, **40**: 375-390.

Jouhanneau P, Lacour B, Raisbeck G, Yiou F, Banide H, Brown E, & Drüeke T (1993) Gastrointestinal absorption of aluminium in rats using ^{26}Al and accelerator mass spectrometry. Clin Nephrol, **40**(4): 244-248.

Kabra SG & Narayanan R (1988) Aluminium phosphide: worse than Bhopal. Lancet, **1**: 1333.

Kada T, Hirano K, & Shirasu Y (1980) Screening of environmental chemical mutagens by the rec(-) assay system with *Bacillus subtilis*. In: Hollaender A & de Serres FJ ed. Chemical mutagens: Principles and methods for their detection. New York, London, Plenum Press, pp 149-173.

Kaehny WD, Hegg AP, & Alfrey AC (1977a) Gastrointestinal absorption of aluminum from aluminum- containing antacids. N Engl J Med, **296**: 1389-1390.

Kaehny WD, Alfrey AC, Holman RE, & Shorr WJ (1977b) Aluminium transfer during hemodialysis. Kidney Int, **12**: 361-365.

Kanematsu N, Hara M, & Kada T (1980) Rec assay and mutagenicity studies on metal compounds. Mutat Res, **77**: 109-116.

Kappel LC, Youngberg H, Ingraham RH, Hembry FG, Robinson DL, & Cherney JH (1983) Effects of dietary aluminum on magnesium status of cows. Am J Vet Res, **44**: 770-773.

Karlik SJ, Eichhorn GL, & Crapper McLachlan DR (1980) Molecular interactions of aluminum with DNA. Neurotoxicology, **1**: 83-88.

Karlsson-Norrgren L, Dickson W, Ljungberg O, & Runn P (1986a) Acid water and aluminium exposure: gill lesions and aluminium accumulation in farmed brown trout, *Salmo trutta* L. J Fish Dis, **9**: 1-9.

Karlsson-Norrgren L, Björklund I, Ljungberg O, & Runn P (1986b) Acid water and aluminium exposure: experimentally induced gill lesions in brown trout, *Salmo trutta* L. J Fish Dis, **9**: 11-25.

Katz AC, Frank DW, Sauerhoff MW, Zwicker GM, & Freudenthal RI (1984) A 6-month dietary toxicity study of acidic sodium aluminium phosphate in beagle dogs. Food Chem Toxicol, **22**: 7-9.

Kerr DNS & Ward MK (1988) Aluminum intoxication: History of its clinical recognition and management. In: Sigel H & Sigel A ed. Metal ions in biological systems - Volume 24: Aluminum and its role in biology. New York, Basel, Marcel Dekker, Inc., pp 217-258.

Kersten M, Dicke M, Kriews M, Naumann K, Schmidt D, Schulz M, Schwikowski M, & Steiger M (1988) Distribution and fate of heavy metals in the North Sea. In: Salomons W ed. Pollution of the North Sea: An assessment. Berlin, Heidelberg, New York, Springer Verlag, pp 300-347.

Khangarot BS & Ray PK (1989) Investigation of correlation between physicochemical properties of metals and their toxicity to the water flea *Daphnia magna* Straus. Ecotoxicol Environ Saf, **18**: 109-120.

Kim YS, Lee MH, & Wisniewski HM (1986) Aluminum induced reversible change in permeability of the blood-brain barrier to [^{14}C]sucrose. Brain Res, **377**: 286-291.

King RG, Sharp JA, & Boura ALA (1983) The effects of Al^{3+}, Cd^{2+} and Mn^{2+} on human erythrocyte choline transport. Biochem Pharmacol, **32**: 3611-3617.

Kinraide TB, Ryan PR, & Kochian LV (1992) Interactive effects of Al^{3+}, H^+, and other cations on root elongation considered in terms of cell-surface electrical potential. Plant Physiol, **99**: 1461-1468.

Klaprat DA, Brown SB, & Hara TJ (1988) The effect of low pH and aluminum on the olfactory organ of rainbow trout, *Salmo gairdneri.* Environ Biol Fish, **22**(1): 69-77.

Klein GL (1991) The aluminum content of parenteral solutions: Current status. Nutr Rev, **49**: 74-79.

Knutti R & Zimmerli B (1985) [Investigation of the daily portions of Swiss food establishments: III. Lead, cadmium, mercury, nickel and aluminium. Mitt Geb Lebensm.hyg, **76**: 206-232 (in German).

Kobayashi K, Yumoto S, Nagai H, Hosoyama Y, Imamura M, Masuzawa S, Koizumi Y, & Yamashita H (1990) ^{26}Al tracer experiment by accelerator mass spectrometry and its application to the studies for amyotrophic lateral sclerosis and Alzheimer's disease. I. Proc Jpn Acad, **B66**: 189-192.

Koga A (1967) Iron, aluminium and manganese concentrations in waters discharged from Wairakei drillholes. N Z J Sci, **10**: 979-987.

Kongerud J (1991) Occupational exposure and asthma: An epidemioligic study of aluminium potroom workers. Nor J Occup Med, **2**(suppl): 1-192.

Kongerud J & Samuelsen SO (1991) A longitudinal study of respiratory symptoms in aluminium potroom workers. Am Rev Respir Dis, **144**: 10-16.

Kongerud J, Groennesby JK, & Magnus P (1990) Respiratory symptoms and lung function of aluminium potroom workers. Scand J Work Environ Health, **16**: 270-277.

Kopp JF & Kroner RC (1970) Trace metals in the waters of the United States. Washington, DC, US Department of Interior, Federal Water Pollution Control Administration (Report No. 9208-4).

Kremling K (1985) The distribution of cadmium, copper, nickel, manganese, and aluminium in surface waters of the open Atlantic and European shelf area. Deep-Sea Res, **32**(5): 531-555.

Krueger GL, Morris TK, Suskind RR, & Widner EM (1984) The health effects of aluminum compounds in mammals. CRC Crit Rev Toxicol, **13**: 1-24.

Kupchella L & Syty A (1980) Determination of nickel, manganese, copper and aluminium in chewing gum by nonflame atomic absorption spectrometry. J Agric Food Chem, **28**: 1035-1036.

Lamb DS & Bailey GC (1981) Acute and chronic effects of alum to midge larva (*Diptera: Chironomidae*). Bull Environ Contam Toxicol, **27**: 59-67.

Landolt W, Guecheva M, & Bucher JB (1989) The spatial distribution of different elements in and on the foliage of Norway spruce growing in Switzerland. Environ Pollut, **56**: 155-167.

Landsberg JP, McDonald B, & Watt F (1992) Absence of aluminium in neuritic plaque cores in Alzheimer's disease. Nature (Lond), **360**: 65-68.

Lantzy RJ & MacKenzie FT (1979) Atmospheric trace metals: global cycles and assessment of man's impact. Geochim Cosmochim Acta, **43**: 511-525.

Lawrence GB, Fuller RD, & Driscoll CT (1986) Spatial relationships of aluminum chemistry in the streams of the Hubbard Brook Experimental Forest, New Hampshire. Biogeochemistry, **2**: 115-135.

Lawrence GB, Fuller RD, & Driscoll CT (1987) Release of aluminum following whole-tree harvesting at the Hubbard Brook Experimental Forest, New Hampshire. J Environ Qual, **16**(4): 383-390.

Lawrence GB, Driscoll CT, & Fuller RD (1988) Hydrologic control of aluminum chemistry in an acidic headwater stream. Water Resour Res, **24**(5): 659-669.

Lazerte BD (1984) Forms of aqueous aluminum in acidified catchments of central Ontario: a methodological analysis. Can J Fish Aquat Sci, **41**: 766-776.

Leblondel G & Allain P (1980) Blood and brain aluminium concentrations in mice after intraperitoneal injection of different aluminium compounds. Res Commun Chem Pathol Pharmacol, **27**: 579-586.

Lee CR (1972) Interrelationships of aluminum and manganese on the potato plant. Agron J, **64**: 546-549.

Lee YH (1985) Aluminium speciation in different water types. Ecol Bull, **37**: 109-119.

Lee RE & Von Lehmden DJ (1973) Trace metal pollution in the environment. J Air Pollut Control Assoc, **23**(10): 853-857.

Leharne S, Charlesworth D, & Chowdhry B (1992) A survey of metal levels in street dusts in an inner London neighbourhood. Environ Int, **18**: 263-270.

Leinonen KP (1989) The influence of soil preparation on the levels of aluminium, manganese, iron, copper, zinc, cadmium and mercury in *Vaccinium myrtillus*. Chemosphere, **18**(7/8): 1581-1587.

Leivestad H, Jensen E, Kjartansson H, & Xingfu L (1987) Aqueous speciation of aluminium and toxic effects on Atlantic salmon. In: Witters H & Vanderborght O ed. Ecophysiology of acid stress in aquatic organisms: Proceedings of an International Symposium, Antwerp, 13-16 January 1987. Antwerp, Belgian Royal Zoological Society, pp 387-398.

Léonard A & Gerber GB (1988) Mutagenicity, carcinogenicity, and teratogenicity of aluminum. Mutat Res, **196**: 247-257.

Lewis CW & Macias ES (1980) Composition of size-fractionated aerosol in Charleston, West Virginia. Atmos Environ, **14**: 185-194.

Lide DR (1991) CRC handboook of chemistry and physics: A ready-reference book of chemical and physical data, 71st ed. Boca Raton, Florida, CRC Press, pp 4/3, 4/41-4/42.

Lindemann J, Holtkamp E, & Herrmann R (1990) The impact of aluminium on green algae isolated from two hydrochemically different headwater streams, Bavaria, Germany. Environ Pollut, **67**: 61-77.

Lione A (1983) The prophylactic reduction of aluminium intake. Food Chem Toxicol, **21**: 103-109.

Liss L & Thornton DJ (1986) The rationale for aluminum absorption control in early stages of Alzheimer disease. Neurobiol Aging, **7**: 552-554.

Litaor MI (1987) Aluminum chemistry: fractionation, speciation, and mineral equilibria of soil interstitial waters of an alpine watershed, Front Range, Colorado. Geochim Cosmochim Acta, **51**: 1285-1295.

Ljunggren KG, Lidums V, & Sjögren B (1991) Blood and urine levels of aluminium among workers exposed to aluminium flakes. Br J Ind Med, **48**: 106-109.

Llobet JM, Domingo JL, Gomez M, Tomas JM, & Corbella J (1987) Acute toxicity studies of aluminium compounds: antidotal efficacy of several chelating agents. Pharmacol Toxicol, **60**: 280-283.

Longstreth WT, Rosenstock L, & Heyer NJ (1985) Potroom palsy? Neurologic disorder in three aluminum smelter workers. Arch Int Med, **145**: 1972-1975.

Losno R, Colin JL, Le Bris N, Bergametti G, Jickells T, & Lim B (1993) Aluminium solubility in rainwater and molten snow. J Atmos Chem, **17**: 29-43.

Lovell MA, Ehmann WD, & Markesbery WR (1993) Laser microprobe analysis of brain aluminium in Alzheimer's disease. Ann Neurol, **33**: 36-42.

Lükewille A & Van Breemen N (1992) Aluminium precipitates from groundwater of an aquifer affected by acid atmospheric deposition in the Senne, northern Germany. Water Air Soil Pollut, **63**: 411-416.

Lydersen E, Björnstad HE, Salbu B, & Pappas AC (1987) Trace element speciation in natural waters using hollow-fiber ultrafiltration. In: Ladner L ed. Speciation of metals in water, sediments and soil systems: Lecture notes in earth sciences. Berlin, Heidelberg, New York, Springer Verlag, vol 11, pp 58-97.

Lydersen E, Salbu B, Poleo ABS, & Muniz IP (1990) The influence of temperature on aqueous aluminium chemistry. Water Air Soil Pollut, **51**: 203-215.

Lydersen E, Poleo ABS, Nandrup Pettersen M, Riise G, Salbu B, Kroglund F, & Rosseland BO (1994) The importance of "in situ" measurements to relate toxicity and chemistry in dynamic aluminium freshwater systems. J Ecol Chem, **3**: 357-365.

McCahon CP, Pascoe D, & McKavanagh C (1987) Histochemical observations on the salmonids *Salmo salar* L. and *Salmo trutta* L. and the ephemeropterans *Baetis rhodani*(Pict.) and *Ecdyonurus venosus* (Fabr.) following a simulated episode of acidity in an upland stream. Hydrobiologia, **153**: 3-12.

McCormack KM, Ottosen LD, Sanger VL, Sprague S, Mayor GH, & Hook JB (1979) Effect on prenatal administration of aluminum and parathyroid hormone on fetal development in the rat. Proc Soc Exp Biol Med, **161**: 74-77.

McDermott JR, Smith A, Ward MK, Parkinson IS, & Kerr DNS (1978) Brain-aluminium concentration in dialyses encephalopathy. Lancet, **1**: 901-904.

McDermott JR, Smith I, Iqbal K, & Wisniewski HM (1979) Brain aluminum in aging and Alzheimer disease. Neurology, **29**: 809-814.

Mach CE & Brezonik PL (1989) Trace metal research at Little Rock Lake, Wisconsin: background data, enclosure experiments, and the first three years of acidification. Sci Total Environ, **87/88**: 269-285.

MacKenzie FT, Stoffyn M, & Wollast R (1978) Aluminum in seawater: control by biological activity. Science, **199**: 680-682.

Mackie GL (1989) Tolerances of five benthic invertebrates to hydrogen ions and metals (Cd, Pb, Al). Arch Environ Contam Toxicol, **18**: 215-223.

McLachlan DRC (1989) Aluminium neurotoxicity: Criteria for assigning a role in Alzheimer's disease. In: Lewis TE ed. Environmental chemistry and toxicology of aluminium. Chelsea, Michigan, Lewis Publishers Inc., pp 299-315.

McLachlan DRC (in press) Aluminium and the risk for Alzheimer's disease. Environmetrics.

McLachlan DR & Massiah J (1992) Aluminum ingestion: A risk factor for Alzheimer's disease? Chapter 4. In: Isaacson RL & Jensen KF ed. The vulnerable brain and environmental risks - Volume 2. Toxins in food. New York, London, Plenum Press, chapter 4, pp 49-60.

McLachlan DR, Bergeron C, Smith JE, Boomer D, & Rifat SL (1996) Risk for neuropathologically confirmed Alzheimer's disease and residual aluminium in municipal drinking water employing weighted residential histories. Neurology, **46**(2): 401-405.

McLaughlin AIG, Kazantzis G, King E, Teare D, Porter RJ, & Owen R (1962) Pulmonary fibrosis and encephalopathy associated with the inhalation of aluminium dust. Br J Ind Med, **19**: 253-263.

McMillan TM, Freemont AJ, Herxheimer A, Denton J, Taylor AP, Pazianas M, Cummin ARC, & Eastwood JB (1993) Camelford water poisoning accident: serial neuropsychological assessments and further observations on bone aluminium. Hum Exp Toxicol, **12**: 37-42.

Madigosky SR, Alvarez-Hernandez X, & Glass J (1991) Lead, cadmium, and aluminum accumulation in the red swamp crayfish *Procambarus clarkii* G. collected from roadside drainage ditches in Louisiana. Arch Environ Contam Toxicol, **20**: 253-258.

Madigosky SR, Alvarez-Hernandez X, & Glass J (1992) Concentrations of aluminum in gut tissue of crayfish (*Procambarus clarkii*), purged in sodium chloride. Bull Environ Contam Toxicol, **49**: 626-632.

Malley DF & Chang PSS (1985) Effects of aluminum and acid on calcium uptake by the crayfish *Orconectes virilis*. Arch Environ Contam Toxicol, **14**: 739-747.

Malley DF, Chang PSS, & Moore CM (1987) Changes in the aluminum content of tissues of crayfish held in the laboratory and in experimental field enclosures. Can Tech Rep Fish Aquat Sci, **1480**: 54-68.

Manna GK & Das RK (1972) Chromosome aberration in mice induced by aluminum chloride. Nucleus, **15**: 180-186.

Mantyh PW, Ghilardi JR, Rogers S, Demaster E, Clark JA, Stimson ER, & Maggio JE (1993) Aluminum, iron, and zinc ions promote aggregation of physiological concentrations of β-amyloid peptide. J Neurochem, **61**: 1171-1174.

Markesbery WR, Ehmann WD, Hossain TIM, Alauddin M, & Goodin DT (1981) Instrumental neutron activation analysis of brain aluminum in Alzheimer disease and aging. Ann Neurol, **10**: 511-516.

Marsden SNE, Parkinson IS, Ward MK, Ellsi HA, & Kerr DNS (1979) Evidence for aluminium accumulation in renal failure. Proc Eur Dial Transplant Assoc, **16**: 588-596.

Martin RB (1986) The chemistry of aluminium as related to biology and medicine. Clin Chem, **32**: 1797-1806.

Martin RB (1992) Aluminium speciation in biology. In: Aluminium in biology and medicine. New York, Chichester, Brisbane, Toronto, John Wiley and Sons, pp 5-25 (Ciba Foundation Symposium No. 169).

Martyn CN, Osmond C, Edwardson JA, Barker DJP, Harris EC, & Lacey RF (1989) Geographical relation between Alzheimer's disease and aluminium in drinking water. Lancet, **1**: 59-62.

Marzin DR & Phi HV (1985) Study of the mutagenicity of metal derivatives with *Salmonelia typhimurium* TA102. Mutat Res, **155**: 49-51.

Mason CF & MacDonald SM (1988) Metal contamination in mosses and otter distribution in a rural Welsh river receiving mine drainage. Chemosphere, **17**(6): 1159-1166.

Mauras Y & Allain P (1985) Automatic determination of aluminum in biological samples by inductively coupled plasma emission spectrometry. Anal Chem, **57**: 1706.

Mauras Y, Allain P, & Riberi P (1982) Etude de l'absorption digestive de l'hydrocarbonate d'aluminium chez l'individu sain. Thérapie, **37**: 598-600.

Mayor GH, Keiser JA, Makdani D, & Ku PK (1977) Aluminum absorption and distribution: Effect of parathyroid hormone. Science, **197**: 1187-1189.

Meding B, Augustsson A, & Hansson C (1984) Short communications. Patch test reactions to aluminium. Contact Dermatitis, **10**: 107.

Mersch J, Guérold F, Rousselle P, & Pihan J-C (1993) Transplanted aquatic mosses for monitoring trace metal mobilization in acidified streams of the Vosges Mountains, France. Bull Environ Contam Toxicol, **51**: 255-259.

Mesco ER, Kachen C, & Timiras PS (1991) Effects of aluminium on tau proteins in human neuroblastoma cells. Mol Chem Neuropathol, **14**(3): 199-212.

Meyer FA & Kasper W (1942) [Examination of the effects of aluminium on the lung.] Dtsch Arch Klin Med, **189**: 471-495 (in German).

Michel P, Commenges D, Dartigues JF, Gagnon M, Barberger-Gateau P, Letenneur L, & Paquid Research Group (1991) Study of the relationship between aluminium concentration in drinking water and risk of Alzheimer's disease. In: Iqbal K, McLachlan DRC, Winblad B, & Wisniewski HM ed. Alzheimer's disease: Basic mechanisms, diagnosis and therapeutic strategies. New York, John Wiley, pp 387-391.

Miller RR, Churg AM, Hutcheon M, & Lam S (1984) Pulmonary alveolar proteinosis and aluminum dust exposure. Am Rev Respir Dis, **130**: 312-315.

Mitchell J, Manning GB, Molyneux M, & Lane RE (1961) Pulmonary fibrosis in workers exposed to finely powdered aluminium. Br J Ind Med, **18**: 10-20.

Mizuno N & Yoshida H (1993) Effects of exchangeable aluminium on the reduction of potato scab. Plant Soil, **155/156**: 505-508.

Monteagudo FSE, Isaacson LC, Wilson G, Hickman R, & Folb PI (1988) Aluminium exretion by the distal tubule of the pig kidney. Nephron, **49**: 245-250.

Moomaw JC, Nakamura MT, & Sherman GD (1959) Aluminium in some Hawaiian plants. Pac Sci, **13**: 335-341.

Mühlenberg W (1990) [High aluminium levels in wells of the southern sandy health-land of lower Saxony by acid precipitation: Interpretation from hygienic and ecological points of view.] Öffentl Gesundh.wes, **52**: 1-8 (in German with English summary).

Mulder J, Van Breemen N, Rasmussen L, & Driscoll CT (1989) Aluminum chemistry of acidic sandy soils with various inputs of acidic deposition in the Netherlands and in Denmark In: Lewis TE ed. Environmental chemistry and toxicology of aluminum. Proceedings of the 194th Annual Meeting of the American Chemical Society, New Orleans, LA, 30 August-4 September 1987. Chelsea, Michigan, Lewis Publishers Inc., pp 171-169.

Muller G, Bernuzzi V, Desor D, Hutin M-F, Burnel D, & Lehr PR (1990) Developmental alterations in offspring of female rats orally intoxicated by aluminum lactate at different gestation periods. Teratology, **42**: 253-261.

Muller G, Hutin MF, Burnel D, & Lehr PR (1992) Aluminum transfer through milk in female rats intoxicated by aluminum chloride. Biol Trace Elem Res, **34**: 79-87.

Muller G, Burnel D, Gery A, & Lehr PR (1993) Element variations in pregnant and nonpregnant female rats orally intoxicated by aluminium lactate. Biol Trace Elem Res, **39**: 211-219.

Muniz IP & Leivestad H (1980) Toxic effects of aluminium on the brown trout, *Salmo trutta* L. In: Drabløs D & Tollan A ed. Ecological impact of acid precipitation: Proceedings of an International Conference, Sandefjord, Norway, 11-14 March 1980. Oslo-Ås, SNSF, pp 320-321.

Muramoto S (1981) Influence of complexans (NTA, EDTA) on the toxicity of aluminum chloride and sulfate to fish at high concentrations. Bull Environ Contam Toxicol, **27**: 221-225.

Nagy S & Nikdel S (1986) Tin, iron and aluminum contents of commercially canned single-strength grapefruit juice stored at varying temperatures. J Agric Food Chem, **34**: 588-593.

Nalewajko C & Paul B (1985) Effects of manipulations of aluminum concentrations and pH on phosphate uptake and photosynthesis of planktonic communities in two Precambrian shield lakes. Can J Fish Aquat Sci, **42**: 1946-1953.

Neal C (1988) Aluminium solubility relationships in acid waters: a practical example of the need for a radical reappraisal. J Hydrol, **104**: 141-159.

Neal C & Williams RJ (1988) Towards establishing aluminium hydroxy silicate solubility relationships for natural waters. J Hydrol, **97**: 347-352.

Neal C, Whitehead P, Neale R, & Cosby J (1986) Modelling the effects of acidic deposition and conifer afforestation on stream acidity in the British uplands. J Hydrol, **86**: 15-26.

Neal C, Reynolds B, Stevens PA, Hornung M, & Brown SJ (1990) Dissolved inorganic aluminium in acidic stream and soil waters in Wales. In: Edwards RW, Gee AS, & Stoner JH ed. Acid waters in Wales. Dordrecht, Boston, London, Kluwer Academic Publishers, pp 173-188.

Neal C, Reynolds B, Smith CJ, Hill S, Neal M, Conway T, Ryland GP, Jeffrey H, Robson AJ, & Fisher R (1992) The impact of conifer harvesting on stream water pH, alkalinity and aluminium concentrations for the British uplands: an example for an acidic and acid sensitive catchment in mid-Wales. Sci Total Environ, **126**: 75-87.

Neri LC & Hewitt D (1991) Aluminium, Alzheimer's disease, and drinking water. Lancet, **338**: 390.

Neville CM & Campbell PGC (1988) Possible mechanisms of aluminum toxicity in a dilute, acidic environment to fingerlings and older life stages of salmonids. Water Air Soil Pollut, **42**: 311-327.

NFA (1993) The 1992 Australian market basket survey - A total diet survey of pesticides and contaminants. Canberra, Australian National Food Authority, 96 pp.

Nieboer E, Gibson BL, Oxman AD, & Kramer JR (1995) Health effects of aluminium: A Critical review with emphasis in drinking water. Environ Rev, **3**: 29-85.

Nilsson SI & Bergkvist B (1983) Aluminium chemistry and acidification processes in a shallow podzol on the Swedish westcoast. Water Air Soil Pollut, **20**: 311-329.

NIOSH (1984) Aluminium and compounds: Method 7300. In: NIOSH manual. Cincinnati, Ohio, National Institute for Occupational Safety and Health, vol 5, p 173/1.

Nishioka H (1975) Mutagenic activities of metal compounds in bacteria. Mutat Res, **31**: 185-189.

Nordal KP, Dahl E, Thomassen Y, Brodwall EK, & Halse J (1988) Seasonal variations in serum aluminium concentrations. Pharmacol Toxicol, **62**: 80-83.

Norrgren L & Degerman E (1993) Effects of different water qualities on the early development of Atlantic salmon and brown trout exposed *in situ*. Ambio, **22**(4): 213-218.

Norton SA (1971) Geochemical cycles involving flora, lake water and bottom sediments. Orono, Maine, University of Maine, Water Resources Research Center (NTIS PB-206 197).

Nyholm NEI (1981) Evidence of involvement of aluminum in causation of defective formation of eggshells and of impaired breeding in wild passerine birds. Environ Res, **26**: 363-371.

Oberly TJ, Piper CE, & McDonald DS (1982) Mutagenicity of metal salts in the L5178Y mouse lymphoma assay. J Toxicol Environ Health, **9**: 367-376.

O'Donnell TV, Welford B, & Coleman ED (1989) Potroom asthma: New Zealand experience and follow-up. Am J Ind Med, **15**: 43-49.

Ogilvie DM & Stechey DM (1983) Effects of aluminum on respiratory responses and spontaneous activity of rainbow trout, *Salmo gairdneri*. Environ Toxicol Chem, **2**: 43-48.

Ohtawa M, Seko M, & Takayama F (1983) Effect of aluminum ingestion on lipid peroxidation in rats. Chem Pharm Bull, **31**: 1415-1418.

OMEE (1995) Drinking water surveillance programme - Province of Ontario. Toronto, Canada, Ontario Ministry of Environment and Energy.

Ondov JM, Zoller WH, & Gordon GE (1982) Trace element emissions on aerosols from motor vehicles. Environ Sci Technol, **16**(6): 318-328.

Ondreicka R, Ginter E, & Kortus J (1966) Chronic toxicity of aluminium in rats and mice and its effects on phosphorus metabolism. Br J Ind Med, **23**: 305-312.

Ormerod SJ, Allinson N, Hudson D, & Tyler SJ (1986) The distribution of breeding dippers (*Cinclus cinclus* (L.); Aves) in relation to stream acidity in upland Wales. Freshw Biol, **16**: 501-507.

Ormerod SJ, Boole P, McCahon CP, Weatherley NS, Pascoe D, & Edwards RW (1987a) Short-term experimental acidification of a Welsh stream: comparing the biological effects of hydrogen ions and aluminium. Freshw Biol, **17**: 341-356.

Ormerod SJ, Weatherly NS, French P, Blake S, & Jones WM (1987b) The physiological response of brown trout *Salmo trutta* to induced episodes of low pH and elevated aluminium in a Welsh hill-stream In: Witters H & Vanderborght O ed. Ecophysiology of acid stress in aquatic organisms: Proceedings of an International Symposium, Antwerp, 13-16 January 1987. Antwerp, Belgian Royal Zoological Society, pp 435-447.

Ormerod SJ, Bull KR, Cummins CP, Tyler SJ, & Vickery JA (1988) Egg mass and shell thickness in dippers *Cinclus cinclus* in relation to stream acidity in Wales and Scotland. Environ Pollut, **55**: 107-121.

Ormerod SJ, Donald AP, & Brown SJ (1989) The influence of plantation forestry on the pH and aluminium concentration of upland Welsh streams: a re-examination. Environ Pollut, **62**: 47-62.

Ormerod SJ, Weatherley NS, Merrett WJ, Gee AS, & Whitehead PG (1990) Restoring acidified streams in upland Wales: a modelling comparison of the chemical and biological effects of liming and reduced sulphate deposition. Environ Pollut, **64**: 67-85.

Ott SM, Feist E, Andress DL, Liu CC, Sherrard DJ, Alfrey AC, Slatopolsky E, & Howard GA (1987) Development and reversibility of aluminum-induced bone lesions in the rat. J Lab Clin Med, **109**: 40-47.

Ottley CJ & Harrison RM (1993) Atmospheric dry deposition flux of metallic species to the North Sea. Atmos Environ, **27A**(5): 685-695.

Panasenkov YV (1987) Determination of the effect of aluminium sulphate on natural microbial coenoses in experiment. J Hyg Epidemiol Microbiol Immunol, **31**(3): 279-286.

Parent L & Campbell PGC (1994) Aluminum bioavailability to the green alga *Chlorella pyrenoidosa* in acidified synthetic soft water. Environ Toxicol Chem, **13**(4): 587-598.

Parker DR & Bertsch PM (1992a) Identification and quantification of the "Al_{13}" tridecameric polycation using ferron. Environ Sci Technol, **26**(5): 908-914.

Parker DR & Bertsch PM (1992b) Formation of the "Al_{13}" tridecameric polycation under diverse synthesis conditions. Environ Sci Technol, **26**(5): 914-916.

Paternain JL, Domingo JL, Llobet JM, & Corbella J (1988) Embryotoxic and teratogenic effects of aluminum nitrate in rats upon oral administration. Teratology, **38**: 253-257.

Pennington JAT & Schoen SA (1995) Estimates of dietary exposure to aluminium. Food Addit Contam, **12**(1): 119-128.

Perl DP, Gajdusek DC, Garruto RM, Yanagihara RT, & Gibbs CJ (1982) Intraneuronal aluminum accumulation in amyotrophic lateral sclerosis and parkinsonism-dementia of Guam. Science, **217**: 1053-1055.

Petit TL, Biedermann GB, & McMullen PA (1980) Neurofibrillary degeneration, dying back and learning-memory deficits after aluminum administration, implications for brain aging. Exp Neurol, **67**: 152-162.

Petrich SM & Reish DJ (1979) Effects of aluminium and nickel on survival and reproduction in polychaetous annelids. Bull Environ Contam Toxicol, **23**: 698-702.

Pettersen JC, Hackett DS, & Zwicker GM (1990) Twenty-six week toxicity study with kasal (basic sodium aluminum phosphate) in beagle dogs. Environ Geochem Health, **12**: 121-123.

Pigott GH & Ishmael J (1981) An assessment of the fibrogenic potential of two refractory fibres by intraperitoneal injection in rats. Toxicol Lett, **8**: 153.

Pigott GH, Gaskell BA, & Ishmael J (1981) Effects of long term inhalation of alumina fibres in rats. Br J Exp Pathol, **62**: 323-331.

Pillay KKS & Thomas CC (1971) Determination of the trace element levels in atmospheric pollutants by neutron activation analysis. J Radioanal Chem, **7**: 107-118.

Pitchai R, Subramanian R, Selvapathy P, & Elangovan R (1992) Aluminium content of drinking water in Madras. Water Supply, **10**(4): 83-86.

Plankey BJ & Patterson HH (1987) Kinetics of aluminum-fulvic acid complexation in acidic waters. Environ Sci Technol, **21**: 595-601.

Platts MM, Owen G, & Smith S (1984) Water purification and the incidence of fractures in patients receiving home haemodialysis supervised by a single centre: evidence for "safe" upper limit of aluminium in water. Br Med J, **288**: 969-972.

Poléo ABS, Lydersen E, Rosseland BO, Kroglund F, Salbu B, Vogt RD, & Kvellestad A (1994) Increased mortality of fish due to changing Al-chemistry of mixing zones between limed streams and acidic tributaries. Water Air Soil Pollut, **75**: 339-351.

Priest ND (1990) The distribution and behaviour of heavy metals in the skeleton and body: studies with bone-seeking radionuclides. In: Priest ND & Van de Vyver F ed. Trace metals and fluoride in bones and teeth. Boca Raton, Florida, CRC Press, pp 83-139.

Priest ND (1993) The bioavailability and metabolism of aluminium compounds in man. Proc Nutr Soc, **52**: 231-240.

Priest ND (1994) A human volunteer feeding study using aluminium-26 labelled aluminium citrate, aluminium hydroxide and aluminium hydroxide in the presence of citrate. Harwell, Oxfordshire, AEA Technology (Report No. AEA-TPD-268).

Priest ND, Newton, D, & Talbot RJ (1991) Metabolism of aluminium-26 and gallium-67 in a volunteer following their injections as citrates. Harwell, Oxfordshire, AEA Technology (Report No. AEA-EE-0106).

Priest N, Newton D, & Talbot R (1992) Metabolism of Al-26 and Ga-67 following injection as citrates. In: Gitelman HJ ed. Proceedings of the Second International Conference on Aluminium and Health. Washington, DC, Alumunium Association, pp 7-10.

Priest ND, Talbot RJ, & Austin JG (1995a) The bioavailability in young adults of aluminium ingested in drinking water. Harwell, Oxfordshire, AEA Technology (Report No. AEA-TPD-269).

Priest ND, Newton D, Day JP, Talbot RJ, & Warner AJ (1995b) Human metabolism of aluminium-26 and gallium-67 injected as citrates. Hum Exp Toxicol, **14**(3): 287-293.

Priest N, Newton D, & Talbot R (1996) Studies on the metabolism of injected and ingested aluminium using ^{26}Al. In: Proceedings of the Third International Conference on Aluminium and Health, Miami, Florida. Washington, DC, Aluminium Association, pp 30-34.

Provan SD & Yokel RA (1988) Aluminum uptake by the in situ rat gut preparation. J Pharmacol Exp Ther, **245**: 928-931.

Quarles LD (1991) Paradoxical toxic and trophic osseous actions of aluminum: Potential explanations. Miner Electrolyte Metab, **17**: 233-239.

Quarles LD, Dennis VW, Gitelman HJ, Harrelson JM, & Drezner MK (1985) Aluminum deposition at the osteoid-bone interface. J Clin Invest, **75**: 1441-1447.

Quarles LD, Gitelman HJ, & Drezner MK (1988) Induction of bone formation in the beagle: a novel effect of aluminum. J Clin Invest, **81**: 1056-1066.

Quarles LD, Gitelman HJ, & Drezner MK (1989) Aluminium-induced de novo bone formation in the beagle: a parathyroid hormone-dependent event. J Clin Invest, **83**: 1644-1650.

Quarles LD, Murphy G, Vogler JB, & Drezner MK (1990) Aluminum-induced neo-osteogenesis: a generalized process affecting trabecular networking in the axial skeleton. J Bone Miner Metab, **5**: 625-635.

Que Hee SS & Boyle JR (1988) Simultaneous multielemental analysis of some environmental and biological samples by inductively coupled plasma atomic emission spectrometry. Anal Chem, **60**: 1033-1042.

Rabe A, Lee MH, Shek J, & Wisniewski HM (1982) Learning deficit in immature rabbits with aluminum-induced neurofibrillary changes. Exp Neurol, **76**: 441-446.

Rahn KA (1981) Atmospheric, riverine and oceanic sources of seven trace constituents to the Arctic Ocean. Atmos Environ, **15**(8): 1507-1516.

Rao KSJ & Divakar S (1993) Spectroscopic studies on the effects of aluminum ion on calf-thymus DNA. Bull Environ Contam Toxicol, **50**: 92-99.

Recker RR, Blotcky AJ, Leffler JA, & Rack EP (1977) Evidence for aluminum absorption from the gastrointestinal tract and bone deposition by aluminum carbonate ingestion with normal renal function. J Lab Clin Med, **90**: 810-815.

Reich PB, Oleskyn J, & Tjoelker MG (1994) Relationship of aluminium and calcium to net CO_2 exchange among diverse Scots pine provenances under pollution stress in Poland. Oecologia, **97**: 82-92.

Reynolds B, Stevens PA, Adamson JK, Hughes S, & Roberts JD (1992) Effects of clearfelling on stream and soil water aluminium chemistry in three UK forests. Environ Pollut, **77**: 157-165.

Rifat SL, Eastwood MR, Crapper McLachlan DR, & Corey PN (1990) Effect of exposure of miners to aluminium powder. Lancet, **336**: 1162-1165.

Robertson JA, Felsenfeld AJ, Haygood CC, Wilson P, Clarke C, & Llach F (1983) Animal model of aluminum-induced osteomalacia: Role of chronic renal failure. Kidney Int, **23**: 327-335.

Rodriguez M, Felsenfeld AJ, & Llach F (1990) Aluminum administration in the rat separately affects the osteoblast and bone mineralization. J Bone Miner Res, 5: 59-68.

Röllin HB, Theodorou P, & Kilroe-Smith TA (1991a) Deposition of aluminium in tissues of rabbits exposed to inhalations of low concentration of Al_2O_3 dust. Br J Ind Med, **48**: 389-391.

Röllin HB, Theodorou P, & Kilroe-Smith TA (1991b) The effect of exposure to aluminium on concentrations of essential metals in serum of foundry workers. Br J Ind Med, **48**: 243-246.

Ronneberg A & Langmark F (1992) Epidemiologic evidence of cancer in aluminium reduction plant workers. Am J Ind Med, **22**: 573-590.

Rosa IV, Henry PR, & Ammermann CB (1982) Interrelationship of dietary phosphorus, aluminium and iron on performance and tissue mineral composition in lambs. J Anim Sci, **1982**: 1231-1240.

Rosseland BO & Skogheim OK (1984) A comparative study on salmonid fish species in acid aluminium-rich water. II. Physiological stress and mortality of one- and two-year-old fish. Oslo, Norway, Institute of Fresh Water Ecology, pp 186-194 (Research Report No. 61).

Rosseland BO & Staurnes M (1994) Physiological mechanisms for toxic effects and resistance to acidic water: an ecophysiological and ecotoxicological approach. In: Steinberg CEW & wright RF ed. Acidification of freshwater ecosystems: Implications for the future. New York, Chichester, Brisbane, Toronto, John Wiley and Sons, pp 228-246.

Rosseland BO, Eldhuset TD, & Staurnes M (1990) Environmental effects of aluminium. Environ Geochem Health, **12**(1-2): 17-27.

Rosseland BO, Blakar IA, Bulger A, Kroglund F, Kvellstad A, Lydersen E, Oughton DH, Salbu B, Staurnes M, & Vogt R (1992) The mixing zone between limed and acidic river waters: complex aluminium chemistry and extreme toxicity for salmonids. Environ Pollut, **78**(1/3): 3-8.

Roy AK, Sharma A, & Talukder G (1988) Some aspects of aluminum toxicity in plants. Bot Rev, **54**(2): 145-178.

Roy AK, Talukder G, & Sharma A (1990) Effects of aluminium sulphate on human leukocyte chromosomes *in vitro*. Mutat Res, **244**: 179-184.

Roy AK, Sharma A, & Talukder G (1991a) Effects of aluminum salts on bone marrow chromosomes in rats *in vivo*. Cytobios, **66**: 105-112.

Roy AK, Talukder G, & Sharma A (1991b) Similar effects *in vivo* of two aluminum salts on the liver, kidney, bone, and brain of *Rattus norvegicus*. Bull Environ Contam Toxicol, **47**: 288-295.

Rueter JG, O'Reilly KT, & Petersen RR (1987) Indirect aluminum toxicity to the green alga *Scenedesmus* through increased cupric ion activity. Environ Sci Technol, **21**(5): 435-438.

Ryther J, Losordo TM, Furr AK, Parkinson TF, Gutenman WH, Pakkala IS, & Lisk DJ (1979) Concentration of elements in marine organisms cultured in seawater flowing through coal-fly ash. Bull Environ Contam Toxicol, **23**: 207-210.

Sackett W & Arrhenius G (1962) Distribution of aluminum species in the hydrosphere. I. Aluminum in the ocean. Geochim Cosmochim Acta, **26**: 955-968.

Saia AN, Slagsvold P, Bergh H, & Laksesvela B (1977) High fluorine water to weather sheep maintained in pens. Nord Vet Med, **29**: 172-180.

Saia B, Cortese S, Piazza G, Camposampietro A, & Clonfero E (1981) Chest x-ray findings among aluminium production plant workers. Med Lav, **4**: 323-329.

St George-Hyslop P, Haines J, Rogaev E, Mortilla M, Vaula G, Pericak-Vance M, Foncin JF, Montesi M, Bruni A, Sorbi S, Raincro I, Pinessi I, Pollen D, Polinski R, Nee I, Kennedy J, Macciardi F, Rogaeva E, Liang Y, Alexandrova N, Lukiw W, Schlumpf K, Tanzi R, Tsuda T, Farrer L, Cantu J-M, Duara R, Amaducci L, Bergamini I, Gusella J, Roses A, & Crapper McLachlan D (1992) Genetic evidence for a novel familial Alzheimer disease gene on chromosome 14. Nature (Genet), **2**: 330-334.

Sanin S, Tuncel G, Gaines AF, & Balkas TI (1992) Concentrations and distributions of some major and minor elements in the sediments of the River Göksu and Tasucu Delta, Turkey. Mar Pollut Bull, **24**(3): 167-169.

Santos F, Chan JCM, Yang MS, Savory J, & Wills MR (1987) Aluminum deposition in the central nervous system: Preferential accumulation in the hippocampus in weenling rats. Med Biol, **65**: 53-55.

Sanz-Medel A, Roza RR, Alonson RG, Vallina AN, & Cannata J (1987) Atomic spectrometric methods (atomic absorption and inductively coupled plasma atomic emission) for the determination of aluminium at the parts per billion level in biological fluids. J Anal Atmos Spec, **2**: 177-184.

Saunders A, Strittmatter WJ, Schmechel St George-Hyslop P, Pericak-Vance MA, Joo SH, Rosi BL, Gusella JF, Crapper MacLachlan DR, Alberts MJ, Hulette C, Crain B, Goldgaber D, & Roses AD (1993) Association of apolipoprotein E allelle E4 with late onset familial and sporadic Alzheimer disease. Neurology, **43**: 1467-1472.

Savory J, Nicholson JR, & Wills MR (1987) Is aluminium leaching enhanced by fluoride? Nature (Lond), **327**: 107-108.

Sax NI & Lewis RJSR (1987) Hawley's condensed chemical dictionary, 11th ed. New York, Van Nostrand Reinhold Company, pp 42-51.

Schaller KH & Valentin H (1984) Biological indicators for the assessment of human exposure to industrial chemicals. Luxembourg, Commission of the European Communities, pp 21-29.

Schecher WD & Driscoll CT (1987) An evaluation of uncertainty associated with aluminum equilibrium calculations. Water Resour Res, **23**(4): 525-534.

Schenck RU, Bjorksten J, & Yaeger L (1989) Composition and consequences of aluminum in water, beverages, and other ingestibles. In: Lewis TE ed. Environmental chemistry and toxicology of aluminum. Chelsa, Michigan, Lewis Publishers Inc., pp 247-269.

Schofield CL & Trojnar JR (1980) Aluminum toxicity to brook trout (*Salvelinus fontinalis*) in acidified waters. In: Toribara TY, Miller MW, & Marrow PE ed. Polluted rain: Proceedings of the 12th Rochester International Conference on Environmental Toxicity, Rochester, May 1979. New York, London, Plenum Press, pp 341-366.

Schreeder MT, Favero MS, Hughes JR, Petersen NJ, Bennett PH, & Maynard JE (1983) Dialysis encephalopathy and aluminum exposure: An epidemiologic analysis. J Chronic Dis, **36**: 581-593.

Schwedt G (1989) [Photometric determination of aluminium.] Stuttgart, Wissenschaftliche Verlagsgesellschaft mbH, pp IV/A1/1-4, II/A1/1-3 (in German).

Sedman AB, Alfrey AC, Miller NL, & Goodman WG (1987) Tissue and cellular basis for impaired bone formation in aluminum-related osteomalacia in the pig. J Clin Invest, **79**: 86-92.

Segner H, Marthaler R, & Linnenbach M (1988) Growth, aluminium uptake and mucous cell morphometrics of early life stages of brown trout, *Salmo trutta*, in low pH water. Environ Biol Fish, **21**(2): 153-159.

Seip HM, Müller L, & Naas A (1984) Aluminium speciation: comparison of two spectrophotometric analytical methods and observed concentrations in some acidic aquatic systems in southern Norway. Water Air Soil Pollut, **23**: 81-95.

Seip HM, Christophersen N, & Sullivan TJ (1989) Episodic variations in streamwater aluminum chemistry at Birkenes, southernmost Norway. In: Lewis TE ed. Environmental chemistry and toxicology of aluminum. Proceedings of the 194th Annual Meeting of the American Chemical Society, New Orleans, LA, 30 August-4 September 1987. Chelsea, Michigan, Lewis Publishers Inc., pp 159-169.

Shacklette HT & Boerngen JG (1984) Element concentrations in soils and other surficial materials of the conterminous United States. Washington, DC, US Department of Interior, Geological Survey, 105 pp (Geological Survey Professional Paper No. 1270).

Shaver CG & Riddell AR (1947) Lung changes associated with the manufacture of alumina abrasives. J Ind Hyg Toxicol, **29**: 145-157.

Sheets WD (1957) Toxicity studies of metal-finishing wastes. Sew Ind Wastes, **29**(12): 1380-1384.

Shin R-W, Lee VM-Y, & Trojanowski JQ (1994) Aluminum modifies the properties of Alzheimer's disease $PHF_{(tau)}$ proteins *in vivo* and *in vitro*. J Neurosci, **14**(11): 7221-7233.

Shore D & Wyatt RJ (1983) Aluminum and Alzheimer's disease. J Nerv Ment Dis, **71**: 553-558.

Siddens LK, Seim WK, Curtis LR, & Chapman GA (1986) Comparison of continuous and episodic exposure to acidic, aluminum-contaminated waters of brook trout (*Salvelinus fontinalis*). Can J Fish Aquat Sci, **43**: 2036-2040.

Silvey WD (1967) Occurrence of selected minor elements in the waters of California. Washington, DC, US Department of Interior, Geological Survey, 25 pp (Geological Survey-Water Supply Paper No. 1535-L).

Simons LH, Monaghan PH, & Taggart MS (1953) Aluminum and iron in Atlantic and Gulf of Mexico surface waters. Anal Chem, **25**: 989-990.

Simonsson Bg, Sjöberg A, Rolf C, & Haeger-Aronsen B (1985) Acute and long-term airway hyperreactivity in aluminium-salt exposed workers with nocturnal asthma. Eur J Respir Dis, **66**: 105-118.

Simpson W, Kerr DNS, Hill AVL, & Siddiqui JY (1973) Skeletal changes in patients on regular hemodialysis. Diagn Radiol, **107**: 313-320.

Sjögren B & Elinder CG (1992) Proposal of a dose-response relationship between aluminium welding fume exposure and effect on the central nervous system. Med Lav, **83**(5): 484-488.

Sjögren B & Ulfvarson U (1985) Respiratory symtoms and pulmonary function among welders working with aluminum, stainless steel and railroad tracks. Scand J Work Environ Health, **11**: 27-32.

Sjögren B, Lundberg I, & Lidums V (1983) Aluminium in the blood and urine of industrially exposed workers. Br J Ind Med, **40**: 301-304.

Sjögren B, Lidums V, Hakansson M, & Hedstrom L (1985) Exposure and urinary excretion of aluminum during welding. Scand J Work Environ Health, **11**: 39-43.

Sjögren B, Elinder CG, Lidums V, & Chang G (1988) Uptake and urinary excretion of aluminum among welders. Int Arch Occup Environ Health, **60**: 77-79.

Sjögren B, Gustavsson P, & Hogstedt C (1990) Neuropsychiatric symptoms among welders exposed to neurotoxic metals. Br J Ind Med, **47**: 704-707.

Sjögren B, Ljunggren KG, Almkvist O, Frech W, & Basun H (1994a) Aluminosis and dementia. Lancet, **344**(8930): 1154.

Sjögren B, Iregren A, Frech W, Hagman M, Johansson L, Tesarz M, & Wennberg A (1994b) [Effects on the nervous system among welders exposed to aluminum or manganese.] Solna, Sweden, National Institute of Occupational Health, 27 pp (Work and Health Scientific Publication Series) (in Swedish with English summary).

Sjöström J (1994) Aluminium and sulphate in acidic soils and groundwaters on the Swedish west coast. Water Air Soil Pollut, **75**: 127-139.

Skalsky HL & Carchman RA (1983) Aluminum homeostasis in man. J Am Coll Toxicol, **2**: 405-423.

Skogheim OK & Rosseland BO (1986) Mortality of smolt of Atlantic salmon, *Salmo salar* L., at low levels of aluminium in acidic softwater. Bull Environ Contam Toxicol, **37**: 258-265.

Skogheim OK, Rosseland BO, & Sevaldrud IH (1984) Deaths of spawners of Atlantic salmon (*Salmo salar* L.) in River Ogna, SW Norway, caused by acidified aluminium-rich water. Oslo, Norway, Institute of Fresh Water Ecology, pp 195-202 (Research Report No. 61).

Slanina P, Falkeborn Y, Frech W, & Cedergren A (1984) Aluminium concentrations in the brain and bone of rats fed citric acid, aluminium citrate or aluminium hydroxide. Food Chem Toxicol, **22**: 391-397.

Slanina P, Frech W, Bernhardson A, Cedergren A, & Mattsson P (1985) Influence of dietary factors on aluminium absorption and retention in the brain and bone rats. Acta Pharmacol Toxicol, **56**: 331-336.

Slanina P, Frech W, Ekström L-G, Lööf L, Slorach S, & Cedergren A (1986) Dietary citric acid enhances absorption of aluminium in antacids. Clin Chem, **32**: 539-541.

Smith LF (1995) Public health role, aluminium and Alzheimer's disease. Environmetrics, **6**: 277-286.

Solomon PR, Koota D, & Pendlebury WW (1990) Disrupted retention of the classically conditioned nictitating membrane response in the aluminum-intoxicated rabbit using electrical stimulation of the brain as a conditioned stimulus. Neurobiol Aging, **11**: 523-528.

Sorenson JRJ, Campbell IR, Tepper LB, & Lingg RD (1974) Aluminum in the environment and human health. Environ Health Perspect, **8**: 3-95.

Söyseth V, Kingerud J, Ekstrand J, & Boe J (1994) Relation between exposure to fluoride and bronchial responsiveness in aluminium potroom workers with work-related asthma-like symptoms. Thorax, **49**: 984-989.

Sparling DW (1991) Acid precipitation and food quality: effects of dietary Al, Ca, and P on bone and liver characteristics in American black ducks and mallards. Arch Environ Contam Toxicol, **21**: 281-288.

Stacy BD, King EJ, Harrison CV, Nagelschmidt G, & Nelson S (1959) Tissue changes in rats' lungs caused by hydroxides, oxides and phosphates of aluminium and iron. Pathol Bacteriol, **77**: 417-426.

Stanley RA (1974) Toxicity of heavy metals and salts to eurasian watermilfoil (*Myriophyllum spicatum* L.). Arch Environ Contam Toxicol, **2**(4): 331-341.

Stanton MF (1974) Fiber carcinogenesis: is asbestos the only hazard? (editorial). J Natl Cancer Inst, **52**: 633.

Staurnes M, Blix P, & Reite OB (1993) Effects of acid water and aluminum on parr-smolt transformation and seawater tolerance in Atlantic salmon, *Salmo salar*. Can J Fish Aquat Sci, **50**: 1816-1827.

Steinegger A, Rickenbacher U, & Schlatter C (1990) Aluminium. In: Hutzinger O ed. The handbook of environmental chemistry. Berlin, Heidelberg, New York, Springer Verlag, vol 3, part E, pp 155-184.

Steinhagen WH, Cavender FL, & Cockrell BY (1978) Six month inhalation exposures of rats and guinea pigs to aluminum chlorhydrate. J Environ Pathol Toxicol, **1**: 267-277.

Stern AJ, Perl DP, Monoz-Garcia D, Good PF, Abraham C, & Selkoe DJ (1986) Investigation of silicon and aluminum content in isolated senile plaque cores by laser microprobe mass analysis (LAMMA). J Neuropathol Exp Neurol, **45**: 361.

Sternweis PC & Gilman AG (1982) Aluminum: A requirement for activation of the regulatory component of adenylate cyclase by fluoride. Proc Natl Acad Sci (USA), **79**: 4888-4891.

Stoffyn M (1979) Biological control of dissolved aluminum in seawater: experimental evidence. Science, **203**: 651-653.

Stoffyn M & MacKenzie FT (1982) Fate of dissolved aluminum in the oceans. Mar Chem, **11**: 105-127.

Stokinger HE (1987) The metals. In: Clayton GD & Clayton FE ed. Patty's industrial hygiene and toxicology, 3rd revised ed. - Volume 2A: Toxicology. New York, Chichester, Brisbane, Toronto, John Wiley and Sons, pp 1493-1505.

Stone CJ, McLaurin DA, Steinhagen WH, Cavender FL, & Haseman JK (1979) Tissue deposition patterns after chronic inhalation exposures of rats and guinea pigs to aluminum chlorhydrate. Toxicol Appl Pharmacol, **49**: 71-76.

Stoner JH, Gee AS, & Wade KR (1984) The effects of acidification on the ecology of streams in the Upper Tywi catchment in west Wales. Environ Pollut, **A35**: 125-157.

Strong MJ & Garruto RM (1991a) Neuron-specific thresholds of aluminum toxicity *in vitro*: A comparative analysis of dissociated fetal rabbit hippocampal and motor neuron-enriched cultures. Lab Invest, **65**: 243-249.

Strong MJ & Garruto RM (1991b) Chronic aluminum-induced motor neuron degeneration: Clinical, neuropathological and molecular biological aspects. Can J Neurol Sci, **18**: 428-431.

Strong MJ, Wolff AV, Wakayama I, & Garruto RM (1991) Aluminum-induced chronic myelopathy in rabbits. Neurotoxicology, **12**: 9-22.

Subramanian V, Jha PK, & Van Grieken R (1988) Heavy metals in the Ganges estuary. Mar Pollut Bull, **19**(6): 290-293.

Talbot RJ, Newton D, Priest ND, Austin JG, & Day JP (1995) Inter-subject variability in the metabolism of aluminium following intravenous injection as citrate. Hum Exp Toxicol, **14**(7): 595-599.

Tarkka T, Yli-Mäyry N, Mannermaa RM, Majamaa K, & Oikarinen J (1993) Specific non-enzymatic glycation of the rat histone H1 nucleotide binding site *in vitro* in the presence of AlF_4^-. A putative mechanism for impaired chromatin function. Biochim Biophys Acta, **1180**: 294-298.

Taylor GJ (1991) Current views of the aluminum stress response: the physiological basis of tolerance. Curr Top Plant Biochem Physiol, **10**: 57-93.

Taylor GJ (1995) Overcoming barriers to understanding the cellular basis of aluminium resistance. Plant Soil, **171**(1): 89-103.

Taylor GJ & Foy CD (1985) Mechanisms of aluminum tolerance in *Triticum aestivum* L. (wheat): I. Differential pH induced by winter cultivars in nutrient solutions. Am J Bot, **72**(5): 695-701.

Teraoka H (1981) Distribution of 24 elements in the internal organs of normal males and metallic workers in Japan. Arch Environ Health, **36**: 155-165.

Teraoka H, Morii F, & Kobayashi J (1981) The concentrations of 24 elements in foodstuffs and the estimate of their daily intake. J Jpn Soc Food Nutr, **34**: 221-239.

Thompson JJ & Houk RS (1986) Inductively coupled plasma mass spectrometric detection for multielement flow injection analysis and elemental speciation by reversed-phase liquid chromatography. Anal Chem, **58**: 2541-2548.

Thompson GW & Medve RJ (1984) Effects of aluminum and manganese on the growth of ectomycorrhizal fungi. Appl Environ Microbiol, **48**(3): 556-560.

Thomson SM, Burnett DC, Bergmann JD, & Hixson CJ (1986) Comparative inhalation hazards of aluminum and brass powders using bronchopulmonary lavage as an indicator of lung damage. J Appl Toxicol, **6**: 197-209.

Thorne BM, Cook A, Donohoe T, Lyon S, Medeiros DM, & Moutzoukis C (1987) Aluminum toxicity and behavior in the weanling Long-Evans rat. Bull Psychon Soc, **25**: 129-132.

Thornton DJ, Liss L, & Lott JA (1983) Effect of ethanol on the uptake and distribution of aluminum in rats. Clin Chem, **29**: 1281.

Tipping E & Backes CA (1988) Organic complexation of Al in acid waters: model-testing by titration of a streamwater sample. Water Res, **22**(5): 593-595.

Tipping E, Woof C, Backes CA, & Ohnstad M (1988a) Aluminium speciation in acidic natural waters: testing of a model for Al-humic complexation. Water Res, **22**(3): 321-326.

Tipping E, Woof C, Walters PB, & Ohnstad M (1988b) Conditions required for the precipitation of aluminium in acidic natural waters. Water Res, **22**(5): 585-592.

Tipping E, Backes CA, & Hurley MA (1988c) The complexation of protons, aluminium and calcium by aquatic humic substances: a model incorporating binding-site heterogeneity and macroionic effects. Water Res, **22**(5): 597-611.

Tipping E, Backes CA, & Hurley MA (1989a) Modeling the interactions of Al species, protons and Ca^{2+} with humic substances in acid waters and soils In: Lewis TE ed. Environmental chemistry and toxicology of aluminum. Proceedings of the 194th Annual Meeting of the American Chemical Society, New Orleans, LA, 30 August-4 September 1987. Chelsea, Michigan, Lewis Publishers Inc., pp 59-82.

Tipping E, Ohnstad M, & Woof C (1989b) Adsorption of aluminium by stream particulates. Environ Pollut, **57**: 85-96.

Tipton IH & Cook MJ (1963) Trace elements in human tissue: Part II. Adult subjects from the United States. Health Phys, **9**: 103-145.

Townsend MC, Enterline PE, Sussman NB, Bonney TB, & Rippey LL (1985) Pulmonary function in relation to total dust exposure at a bauxite refinery and alumina-based chemical products plant. Am Rev Respir Dis, **132**: 1174-1180.

Trapp GA (1983) Plasma aluminum is bound to transferrin. Life Sci, **33**: 311.

Tyler G (1994) Plant uptake of aluminium from calcareous soils. Experientia (Basel), **50**: 701-703.

Ulfvarson U (1981) Survey of air contaminants from welding. Scand J Work Environ Health, **7**(suppl 2): 1-28.

UK MAFF (1993) Aluminium in food - 39th report of the Steering Group on Chemical Aspects of Food Surveillance. London, UK Ministry of Agriculture, Fisheries and Food, 52 pp.

US Bureau of Mines (1967) Potential sources of aluminium. Washington, DC, US Government Printing Office, pp 3-4.

Valdivia R, Ammerman CB, Wilcox CJ, & Henry PR (1978) Effect of dietary aluminum on animal performance and tissue mineral levels in growing steers. J Anim Sci, **47**: 1351-1356.

Valdivia R, Ammermann CB, Henry PR, Feaster JP, & Wilcox CJ (1982) Effect of dietary aluminium and phosphorus on performance, phosphorus utilization and tissue mineral composition in sheep. J Anim Sci, **55**: 402-410.

Vallyathan V, Bergeron WN, Robichaux PA, & Craighead JE (1982) Pulmonary fibrosis in an aluminum arc welder. Chest, **81**: 372-374.

Van Bennekom AJ & Jager JE (1978) Dissolved aluminium in the Zaire river plume. Neth J Sea Res, **12**(3/4): 358-367.

Van Benschoten JE & Edzwald JK (1990) Measuring aluminum during water treatment: methodology and application. J Am Water Works Assoc, **82**: 71-78.

Van Broeckhoven C, Backhovens H, Cruts M, De Winter G, Bruyland M, Cras P, Martin J-J (1992) Mapping of a gene predisposing to early onset Alzheimer's disease to chromosome 14q24.3. Nature (Genet), **2**: 335-339.

Van de Vyver F & Visser WJ (1990) Aluminium accumulation in bone. In: Priest ND & Van de Vyver F Trace metals and fluoride in bones and teeth. Boca Raton, Florida, CRC Press, pp 41-81.

Van der Voet GB (1992) Intestinal absorption of aluminium. In: Aluminium in biology and medicine. New York, Chichester, Brisbane, Toronto, John Wiley and Sons, pp 109-122 (Ciba Foundation Symposium No. 169).

Van der Voet GB & De Wolff FA (1984) A method of studying the intestinal absorption of aluminium in the rat. Arch Toxicol, **55**: 168-172.

Van der Voet GB, De Haas EJM, & De Wolff FA (1985) Monitoring of aluminum in whole blood, plasma, serum, and water by a single procedure using flameless atomic absorption spectrophotometry. J Anal Toxicol, **9**: 97-100.

Van Duijn CM, Stijnen T, & Hofman A (1991) Risk factors for Alzheimer's disease: overview of the EURODEM collaborative re-analysis of case-control studies. Int J Epidemiol, **20**(2): S/4-S/12.

Varo P & Koivistoinen P (1980) Mineral element composition of Finnish foods: XII. General discussion and nutritional evaluation. Acta Agric Scand, **22**(suppl): 165-171.

Veien NK, Hattel T, Justesen O, & Noerholm A (1986) Aluminium allergy. Contact Dermatitis, **15**: 295-297.

Vogt KA, Dahlgren R, Ugolini F, Zabowski D, Moore EE, & Zasoski R (1987) Aluminum, Fe, Ca, Mg, K, Mn, Cu, Zn, and P in above- and below-ground biomass. II. Pools and circulation in a subalpine *Abies amabilis* stand. Biogeochemistry, **4**: 295-311.

Vorbrodt AW, Dobrogowska DH, & Lossinsky AS (1994) Ultracytochemical studies of the effects of aluminum on the blood-brain barrier of mice. J Microchem Cytochem, **42**(2): 203-212.

Wade K & Banister AJ (1973) The chemistry of aluminium, gallium, indium and thallium: Comprehensive inorganic chemistry. Oxford, New York, Pergamon Press, chapter 12, pp 993-1036.

Wagatsuma T (1983) Characterization of absorption sites for aluminum in the roots. Soil Sci Plant Nutr, **29**(4): 499-515.

Walker WJ, Cronan CS, & Patterson HH (1988) A kinetic study of aluminum adsorption by aluminosilicate clay minerals. Geochim Cosmochim Acta, **52**: 55-62.

Walker WJ, Cronan CS, & Bloom PR (1990) Aluminum solubility in organic soil horizons from northern and southern forested watersheds. Soil Sci Soc Am J, **54**: 369-374.

Wallen IE, Greer WC, & Lasater R (1957) Toxicity to *Gambusia affinis* of certain pure chemicals in turbid waters. Sew Ind Wastes, **29**: 695-711.

Walton J, Hams G, & Wilcox D (1994) Bioavailability of aluminium from drinking water: Co-exposure with foods and beverages. Melbourne, Australia, Urban Water Research Association of Australia, Melbourne Water Corporation, 38 pp (Research Report No. 83).

Walton J, Tuniz C, Fink D, Jacobsen G, & Wilcox D (1995) Uptake of trace amounts of aluminium into the brain from drinking water. Neurotoxicology, **16**: 187-190.

Ward MK (1991) Aluminium toxicity and people with impaired renal function. In: Lord Walton of Detchant ed. Alzheimer's disease and the environment. London, Royal Society of Medicine Services Ltd, pp 106-110 (Round Table Series No. 26).

Ward MK, Feest TG, Ellis HA, Parkinson IS, Kerr DNS, Herrington J, & Goode GL (1978) Osteomalacic dialysis osteodystrophy: Evidence for a water-borne aetiological agent, probably aluminium. Lancet, **1**: 841-845.

Watt WD, Scott CD, & White WJ (1983) Evidence of acidification of some Nova Scotian rivers and its impact on Atlantic salmon, *Salmo salar*. Can J Fish Aquat Sci, **40**: 462-473.

Weatherley NS, Ormerod SJ, Thomas SP, & Edwards RW (1988) The response of macroinvertebrates to experimental episodes of low pH with different forms of aluminium, during a natural spate. Hydrobiologia, **169**: 225-232.

Weatherley NS, Rogers AP, Goenaga X, & Ormerod SJ (1990) The survival of early life stages of brown trout (*Salmo trutta* L.) in relation to aluminium speciation in upland Welsh streams. Aquat Toxicol, **17**: 213-230.

Wedrychowski A, Schmidt WN, & Hnilica LS (1986) The *in-vivo* cross-linking of proteins and DNA by heavy metals. J Biol Chem, **261**: 3370.

Wefers K & Bell GM (1972) Oxides and hydroxides of aluminum. East St. Louis, Illinois, ALCOA (Aluminium Company of America), Research Laboratories (Technical Paper No. 19).

Wettstein A, Aeppli J, Gautschi K, & Peter M (1991) Failure to find a relationship beetwen mnestic skills of octogenarians and aluminium in drinking water. Int Arch Occup Environ Health, **63**: 97-103.

Wheeler DM, Power IL, & Edmeades DC (1993) Effect of various metal ions on growth of two wheat lines known to differ in aluminium tolerance. Plant Soil, **155/156**: 489-492.

White DM, Longstreth WT, Rosenstock L, Claypoole KHJ, Brodkin CA, & Townes BD (1992) Neurologic syndrome in 25 workers from an aluminum smelting plant. Arch Intern Med, **152**: 1443-1448.

Whitehead PG, Bird S, Hornung M, Cosby J, Neal C, & Paricos P (1988) Stream acidification trends in the Welsh uplands: a modelling study of the Llyn Brianne catchments. J Hydrol, **101**: 191-212.

Whitehead PG, Musgrove TJ, & Cosby BJ (1990) Hydrochemical modelling of acidification in Wales. In: Edwards RW, Gee AS, & Stoner JH ed. Acid waters in Wales. Dordrecht, Boston, London, Kluwer Academic Publishers, pp 255-277.

WHO (1993) Guidelines for drinking-water quality, 2nd ed. - Volume 1: Recommendations. Geneva, World Health Organization, pp 39-40.

Wicklung Glynn A, Norrgren L, & Malmborg O (1992) The influence of calcium and humic substances on aluminium accumulation and toxicity in the minnow, *Phoxinus phoxinus*, at low pH. Comp Biochem Physiol, **102C**(3): 427-432.

Wild A ed. (1988) Russell's soil conditions and plant growth, 11th ed. Harlow, Longman Scientific & Technical.

Wilhelm M & Idel H (1995) [Aluminium in drinking water: a risk factor for Alzheimer's disease?] Forum Städte-Hyg, **46**: 255-258 (in German with English summary).

Wilhelm M, Passlick J, Busch T, Szydlik M, & Ohnesorge FK (1989) Scalp hair as an indicator of aluminium exposure: comparison to bone and plasma. Hum Toxicol, **8**: 5-9.

Wilhelm M, Jäger E, & Ohnesorge FK (1990) Aluminium toxicokinetics. Pharmacol Toxicol, **66**: 4-9.

Wilhelm M, Zhang X-J, Hafner D, & Ohnesorge FK (1992) Single-dose toxicokinetics of aluminum in the rat. Arch Toxicol, **66**: 700-705.

Wilhelm M, Lombeck I, Kouros B, Wuthe J, & Ohnesorge FK (1995) [Duplicate study on the dietary intake of some metals/metalloids by German children: Part II. Aluminium, cadmium and lead.] Zent.bl Hyg, **197**: 357-368 (in German with English summary).

Wills MR & Savory J (1983) Aluminium poisoning: Dialysis encephalopathy, osteomalacia, and anaemia. Lancet, **2**: 29-33.

Wills MR & Savory J (1989) Aluminum and chronic renal failure: Sources, absorption, transport, and toxicity. CRC Crit Rev Clin Lab Sci, **27**: 59-107.

Wilson RW, Bergman HL, & Wood CM (1994a) Metabolic costs and physiological consequences of acclimation to aluminum in juvenile rainbow trout (*Oncorhynchus mykiss*): 1. Acclimation specificity, resting physiology, feeding, and growth. Can J Fish Aquat Sci, **51**: 527-535.

Wilson RW, Bergman HL, & Wood CM (1994b) Metabolic costs and physiological consequences of acclimation to aluminum in juvenile rainbow trout (*Oncorhynchus mykiss*): 1. Gill morphology, swimming performance, and aerobic scope. Can J Fish Aquat Sci, **51**: 536-544.

Windom HL (1981) Comparison of atmospheric and riverine transport of trace elements to the continental shelf environment. In: Eisma MB ed. River inputs to the ocean systems: Proceedings of the UNEP/IOC/SCDR Workshops, Rome, 1981. New York, United Nations, pp 360-369.

Wischik CM, Harrington CR, Mukaetova-Ladinska EB, Novak M, Edwards PC, & McArthur FK (1992) Molecular characterization and measurement of Alzheimer's disease pathology: implications for genetic and environmental aetiology. In: Aluminium in biology and medicine. New York, Chichester, Brisbane, Toronto, John Wiley and Sons, pp 268-302 (Ciba Foundation Symposium No. 169).

Wisniewski HM & Kozlowski PB (1982) Evidence for blood-brain barrier changes in senile dementia of the Alzheimer type (SDAT). Ann NY Acad Sci, **396**: 119-129.

Wisniewski HM & Rabe A (1992) Differences between aluminum encephalopathy and Alzheimer's disease. In: Gitelman HJ ed. Proceedings of the Second International Conference on Aluminum and Health. Washington, DC, Aluminium Association, pp 193-194.

Wisniewski HM & Wen GY (1992) Aluminium and Alzheimer's disease. In: Aluminium in biology and medicine. New York, Chichester, Brisbane, Toronto, John Wiley and Sons, pp 142-164 (Ciba Foundation Symposium No. 169).

Wisniewski HM, Sturman JA, & Shek JW (1982) Chronic model of neurofibrillary changes induced in mature rabbits by metallic aluminum. Neurobiol Aging, **3**: 11-22.

Wisser LA, Heinrichs BS, & Leach RM (1990) Effect of aluminum on performance and mineral metabolism in young chicks and laying hens. J Nutr, **120**: 493-498.

Witters HE (1986) Acute acid exposure of rainbow trout, *Salmo gairdneri* Richardson: effects of aluminium and calcium on ion balance and haematology. Aquat Toxicol, **8**: 197-210.

Witters H, Vangenechten JHD, Van Puymbroeck S, & Vanderborght OLJ (1984) Interference of aluminium and pH on the Na-influx in an aquatic insect *Corixa punctata* (Illig.). Bull Environ Contam Toxicol, **32**: 575-579.

World Bureau of Metal Statistics (1994) World bauxite production. World Met Stat, **47**: 6.

Wood CM & McDonald DG (1987) The physiology of acid/aluminium stress in trout. Ann Soc Zool Belg, **117**(suppl 1): 399-410.

Wood DJ, Cooper C, Stevens J, & Edwardson J (1988) Bone mass and dementia in hip fracture patients from areas with different aluminium concentrations in water supplies. Age Ageing, **17**: 415-419.

Wren CD, MacCrimmon HR, & Loescher BR (1983) Examination of bioaccumulation and biomagnification of metals in a Precambrian shield lake. Water Air Soil Pollut, **19**: 277-291.

Wyttenbach A, Bajo S, Tobler L, & Keller T (1985) Major and trace element concentrations in needles of *Picea abies*: levels, distribution functions, correlations and environmental influences. Plant Soil, **85**: 313-325.

Yagi M, Mizukawa K, Kajino M, Tatumi S, Akiyama M, & Ando M (1992) Behaviour of aluminium in water purification process at purification plants in the River Yodo system. Water Supply, **10**(4): 65-75.

Yeats PA & Bewers JM (1982) Discharge of metals from the St Lawrence River. Can J Earth Sci, **19**: 982-992.

Yen-Koo HC (1992) The effect of aluminum on conditioned avoidance response (CAR) in mice. Toxicol Ind Health, **8**: 1-7.

Yokel RA (1983) Repeated systemic aluminum exposure effects on classical conditioning of the rabbit. Neurobehav Toxicol Teratol, **5**: 41-46.

Yokel RA (1984) Toxicity of aluminum exposure during lactation to the maternal and suckling rabbit. Toxicol Appl Pharmacol, **75**: 35-43.

Yokel RA (1985) Toxicity of gestational aluminum exposure to the maternal rabbit and offspring. Toxicol Appl Pharmacol, **79**: 121-133.

Yokel RA (1987) Toxicity of aluminum exposure to the neonatal and immature rabbit. Fundam Appl Toxicol, **9**: 795-806.

Yokel RA & McNamara PJ (1985) Aluminum bioavailability and deposition in adult and immature rabbits. Toxicol Appl Pharmacol, **77**: 344-352.

Yokel RA & McNamara PJ (1989) Elevated aluminium persists in serum and tissues of rabbits after a 6-hour infusion. Toxicol Appl Pharmacol, **99**: 133-138.

Yukawa M, Suzuki-Yasumoto M, Amano K, & Terai M (1980) Distribution of trace elements in the human body determined by neutron activation analysis. Arch Environ Health, **35**: 36-44.

Zelenov KK (1965) Aluminum and titanium in Kava Ijen volcano crater lake (Indonesia). Int Geol Rev, **11**(1): 84-93.

Zietz JR (1985) Aluminum compounds, organic. In: Gerhartz W, Yamamoto YS, Campbell FT, Pfefferkorn R, & Rounsaville JF ed. Ullmann's encyclopedia of industrial chemistry - Volume A1: Abrasives to aluminum oxide, 5th revised ed. Weinheim, Verlag Chemie, pp 543-556.

Zoller WH, Gladney ES, & Duce RA (1974) Atmospheric concentrations and sources of trace metals at the South Pole. Science, **183**: 198-200.

Zwarun AA & Thomas GW (1973) Effect of soluble and exchangeable aluminum on *Pseudomonas stutzeri*. Soil Sci Soc Am Proc, **37**: 386-387.

Zwarun AA, Bloomfield BJ, & Thomas GW (1971) Effect of soluble and exchangeable aluminum on a soil *Bacillus*. Soil Sci Soc Am Proc, **35**: 460-463.

RESUME ET CONCLUSIONS

1. Identité, propriétés chimiques et physiques

L'aluminium est un métal ductile et malléable de couleur blanc argenté. Il appartient au groupe IIIA de la classification périodique et se trouve généralement au degré d'oxydation III dans ses dérivés usuels. Il constitue environ 8% de l'écorce terrestre et c'est l'un des métaux usuels les plus réactifs. En présence d'eau, d'oxygène et d'autres oxydants, il se recouvre d'une couche superficielle d'oxyde qui lui confère une grande résistance à la corrosion. L'oxyde d'aluminium est soluble dans les acides minéraux ainsi que dans les bases fortes, mais il est insoluble dans l'eau. Par contre, le chlorure, le nitrate et le sulfate sont solubles dans l'eau. Les halogénures, l'hydrure et les premiers termes de la série des alkylaluminiums réagissent violemment avec l'eau.

L'aluminium a une forte conductivité thermique et électrique, sa densité est faible et sa résistance à la corrosion élevée. On l'utilise souvent en alliage avec d'autres métaux. Ces alliages sont légers, résistants et faciles à usiner.

2. Méthodes d'analyse

On a mis au point diverses méthodes d'analyse pour la recherche et le dosage de l'aluminium dans les milieux biologiques et les échantillons prélevés dans l'environnement. Les plus fréquemment utilisées sont la spectrométrie d'absorption atomique avec four à électrode de graphite (GF-AAS) et la spectrométrie d'émission atomique avec plasma à couplage inductif (ICP-AES). La principale source d'erreur est la contamination des échantillons, lors du prélèvement et de la préparation de la prise d'essai, par l'aluminium présent dans l'air, les récipients et les réactifs. Selon les traitements préliminaires subis par l'échantillon et les techniques de séparation et de concentration utilisées, les limites de détection vont de 1,9 à 4 µg/litre dans les liquides biologiques et de 0, 005 à 0,5 µg/g de poids sec dans les tissus quand on procède par GF-AAS, et de 5 µg/m^3 d'air ou de 3 µg/litre d'eau quand on procède par ICP-AES.

3. Sources d'exposition humaine et environnementale

De l'aluminium est libéré dans l'environnement tant à la faveur de processus naturels que d'activités humaines. Il est présent sous une forme très concentrée dans les poussières que produisent les exploitations minières et agricoles ainsi que dans les particules produites par la combustion du charbon. Les silicates d'aluminium (argiles), qui sont des constituants majeurs des sols, contribuent pour une large part à la teneur des poussières en silicates. L'appport d'aluminium à l'environnement trouve beaucoup plus son origine dans des processus naturels que dans l'activité humaine. La mobilisation de l'aluminium du fait d'activités humaine est, pour une large part, indirecte et provient de l'émission de substances acidifiantes. D'une façon générale, une diminution du pH entraîne une augmentation de la mobilité et de la biodisponibilité des formes monomères de l'aluminium. La matière première la plus importante pour la production de l'aluminium est la bauxite, qui contient jusqu'à 55 % d'alumine (oxyde d'aluminium). La production mondiale de bauxite a été de 106 millions de tonnes en 1992. Le métal a des usages très variés, dans les industries du bâtiment, de l'automobile et de l'aéronautique, et peut également être utilisé sous la forme d'alliages. Les dérivés de l'aluminium ont également des usages très divers, notamment dans l'industrie du verre, de la céramique et du caoutchouc ainsi que pour la confection de produits destinés à la protection du bois, de produits pharmaceutiques et de tissus imperméables. Les minéraux naturels contenant de l'aluminium, en particulier la bentonite et la zéolite, sont utilisés pour la purification de l'eau, ainsi que dans les sucreries, les brasseries et l'industrie papetière.

4. Transport, distribution et transformation dans l'environnement

L'aluminium est omniprésent dans l'environnement sous forme de silicates, d'oxydes et d'hydroxydes, combiné à d'autres éléments comme le sodium et le fluor ou encore sous forme de complexes organiques. On ne le rencontre pas à l'état natif du fait de sa réactivité. Dans la nature, il n'existe qu'au degré d'oxydation (+3) ; son transport et sa distribution ne dépendent donc que de sa chimie de coordination et des caractéristiques physico-chimiques de l'environnement local. Aux valeurs du pH supérieures à 5,5, les dérivés de l'aluminium d'origine naturelle existent principalement sous forme non dissoute, par exemple sous forme de gibbsite ($Al(OH)_3$) ou d'aluminosilicates, sauf en présence de grandes quantités de matières organiques en solution qui se lient à l'aluminium et peuvent conduire à une augmentation de la teneur en aluminium dissous, dans les cours d'eau et les lacs, par exemple. Plusieurs facteurs influent sur la mobilité de l'aluminium et, par voie de conséquence, sur son transport dans l'environnement. Il s'agit en particulier de la nature des espèces chimiques en cause, des trajectoires d'écoulement, des interactions entre le sol et l'eau et de la composition des matériaux géologiques sous-jacents. La solubilité de l'aluminium en équilibre avec $Al(OH)_3$ en phase solide dépend fortement du pH et de la présence d'agents complexants comme les fluorures, les silicates, les phosphates et les matières organiques. On peut considérer que la chimie de l'aluminium inorganique dans les sols acides et les cours d'eau fait intervenir les processus suivants: solubilité des espèces minérales, échange d'ions et miscibilité à l'eau. Lorsqu'il y a acidification du sol, l'aluminium peut passer en solution et être ainsi transporté dans les cours d'eau. La mobilisation de l'aluminium par précipitation en milieu acide permet aux plantes de fixer une plus grande quantité de cet élément.

5. Concentrations dans l'environnement et exposition humaine

L'aluminium est présent en proportion importante dans un certain nombre de constituants de l'atmosphère, en particulier des poussières arrachées au sol (qu'elles soient d'origine naturelle ou qu'elles résultent de l'activité humaine) et des particules issues de la combustion du charbon. En milieu urbain, la concentration de l'aluminium dans la poussière des rues varie de 3,7 à 11,6 µg/kg. La teneur de l'air en aluminium va de 0,5 ng/m^3 au-dessus de l'Antarctique à plus de 1000 ng/m^3 dans les zones industrialisées.

Dans les eaux douces superficielles ou souterraines, la concentration de l'aluminium peut varier dans des proportions importantes, en fonction de facteurs physico-chimiques et géologiques. L'aluminium peut se trouver en suspension ou en solution. Il peut être lié à des coordinats organiques ou inorganiques ou exister à l'état d'ion libre. En milieu aqueux naturel, les espèces chimiques dans lesquelles l'aluminium est engagé existent à l'état de monomères ou de polymères. La nature de ces espèces dépend du pH et de la concentration en carbone organique dissous, fluorures, sulfates, phosphates et particules en suspension. Au voisinage de la neutralité, la concentration de l'aluminium dissous est généralement assez faible, de l'ordre de 1,0 à 50 µg/litre. Lorsque l'acidité de l'eau augmente, elle peut monter jusqu'à 500-1000 µg/litre. Dans les eaux rendues extrêmement acides par les liquides de drainage de mines, on a mesuré des concentrations d'aluminium en solution qui atteignaient 90 mg/litre.

L'exposition humaine non professionnelle à l'aluminium présent dans l'environnement se produit principalement lors de l'ingestion d'eau ou de nourriture, la nourriture étant essentiellement en cause. L'apport journalier d'aluminium par les aliments et la boisson se situe, chez l'adulte, entre 2,5 et 13 mg, ce qui représente 90 à 95 % de l'apport total. Compte tenu de la valeur-guide internationale actuellement en vigueur, l'apport par l'eau de boisson pourrait se situer aux environs de 0,4 mg par jour, mais il est plus probablement de l'ordre de 0,2 mg. La contribution de la voie d'exposition respiratoire peut atteindre 0,04 mg/jour. Dans certaines circonstances, par exemple en cas d'exposition professionnelle ou lors de l'utlisation d'antiacides, l'exposition pourra être beaucoup plus intense. Par exemple, deux comprimés d'antiacide moyennement dosés peuvent apporter plus de 500 mg d'aluminium. Les études effectuées avec de l'aluminium-26 indiquent que le citrate constitue la forme la plus disponible biologiquement et que sous cette forme, l'aluminium pourrait être absorbé à hauteur de 1%. L'absorption par l'intermédiaire de l'eau de boisson ne représenterait en revanche que 3% de l'apport quotidien total, cette source étant relativement mineure par rapport à l'apport alimentaire. Il n'est pas très facile de déterminer quelle est la quantité effectivement fixée à la suite d'une telle exposition en raison des problèmes d'analyse et d'échantillonnage que cela pose.

6. Cinétique et métabolisme

6.1 Chez l'homme

L'aluminium et ses dérivés sont mal absorbés par l'organisme humain, encore que la vitesse et le taux d'absorption n'aient pas été suffisamment étudiés. Un moyen facile d'évaluer la résorption de l'aluminium consiste à en mesurer la concentration dans l'urine et le sang; on a d'ailleurs constaté une augmentation de la concentration urinaire chez des soudeurs à l'aluminium et des ouvriers travaillant à la production de poudre d'aluminium.

Le mécanisme de résorption de l'aluminium au niveau gastrointestinal n'est pas encore parfaitement élucidé. Les variations observées résultent des propriétés chimiques de cet élément et de la formation de diverses espèces chimiques, sous l'influence du pH, de la force ionique, de la compétition avec d'autres éléments (silicium) ou agents complexants présents dans les voies digestives (des citrates, par ex.).

On a étudié le comportement biologique de l'aluminium et son absorption dans les voies digestives humaines au moyen de l'isotope radioactif Al-26. Des différences interindividuelles importantes ont été mises en évidence. La littérature donne ainsi des taux de résorption de 5×10^{-3} pour le citrate, de $1,04 \times 10^{-4}$ pour l'hydroxyde et de $1,3 \times 10^{-3}$ pour l'hydroxyde ingéré avec du citrate. Une étude de la résorption fractionnée de l'aluminium présent dans l'eau de boisson a donné une valeur de $2,35 \times 10^{-3}$. On en a conclu que les membres de la population générale qui boivent quotidiennement 1,5 litre d'eau contenant 100 µg/litre d'aluminium, absorberaient de la sorte 3% de leur apport total d'aluminium, selon les concentrations présentes dans leur nourriture et leur utilisation éventuelle d'antiacides.

La proportion d'Al^{3+} normalement lié aux protéines chez l'Homme peut atteindre 70-90% chez les malades hémodialysés, avec une augmentation modérée de l'aluminium plasmatique. C'est dans les poumons que l'on peut trouver les taux les plus élevés d'aluminium, parfois présent sous formes de particules inhalées insolubles.

C'est l'urine qui constitue la voie d'excrétion la plus importante de l'aluminium. Après administration par voie orale d'une dose unique d'aluminium, 83% ont été excrétés dans l'urine en l'espace de 13 jours, contre 1,8% dans les matières fécales. La demi-vie de l'aluminium urinaire chez des soudeurs exposés pendant plus de 10 ans s'est révélée être d'au moins 6 mois. Chez des ouvriers à la retraite qui avaient été exposés à de la poudre d'aluminium, le calcul de la demi-vie a donné une valeur comprise entre 0,7 et 8 ans.

6.2   Chez l'animal

La résorption dans les voies digestives est en général inférieure à 1%. Elle dépend principalement de l'espèce chimique en cause et de sa solubilité ainsi que du pH. Les agents complexants organiques comme les citrates, augmentent la résorption. Il peut également y avoir interaction avec le calcium et le système de transport du fer. L'absorption par la voie respiratoire et la voie percutanée n'a pas été étudiée en détail. L'aluminium se répartit dans la plupart des organes en s'accumulant principalement dans les os, du moins lorsque les doses sont fortes. Dans une proportion limitée encore qu'indéterminée, il franchit la barrière hémato-encéphalique et peut parvenir jusqu'au foetus. Il est efficacement éliminé par la voie urinaire. Sa demi-vie plasmatique est d'environ 1 h chez les rongeurs.

7.   Effets sur les mammifères de laboratoire et les systèmes d'épreuve *in vitro*

L'aluminium et ses composés n'ont qu'une faible toxicité aiguë, les valeurs publiées de la DL_{50} par voie orale étant de l'ordre de quelques centaines de mg à 1000 mg d'aluminium par kg de poids corporel et par jour. On n'a pas connaissance de la valeur de la Cl_{50} par inhalation.

Lors des études toxicologiques à court terme qui ont été effectuées sur des rats, des souris ou des chiens avec un eventail suffisant de points d'aboutissement et divers composés de l'aluminium (phosphate sodique, hydroxyde et nitrate) incorporés à la nourriture ou à l'eau de boisson,on n'a constaté que des effets minimes (réduction du gain de poids généralement associée à une moindre consommation de nourriture ou effets histopathologiques modérés aux doses les plus élevées, c'est-à-dire 70 à 300 mg d'aluminium par kg de poids corporel et par jour). Parmi les effets généraux observés après administration parentérale, on peut citer une insuffisance rénale.

On n'a pas eu connaissance de l'existence d'études d'inhalation satisfaisantes. Après administration intratrachéenne d'oxyde d'aluminium, on a observé une fibrose induite par les particules d'oxyde qui était analogue à celle que les études sur la poussière de silice et de charbon ont mise en évidence.

Après avoir gavé des rats avec des rations quotidiennes contenant respectivement 13, 26 ou 52 mg d'aluminium (sous forme de nitrate) par kg de poids corporel, on n'a constaté aucune foetotoxicité manifeste ni effet délétère sur l'ensemble des paramètres génésiques. Toutefois, on a noté un retard de croissance lié à la dose dans la descendance de ces animaux, retard qui s'observait à la dose de 13 mg/kg chez les femelles et à la dose de 26 mg/kg chez les mâles. La dose la plus faible produisant un effet délétère observable (LOAEL) sur le développement, à savoir, une mauvaise ossification, une augmentation de la fréquence des malformations vertébrales et sternébrales, ou encore une réduction du poids des foetus, s'établissait à 13 mg/kg (nitrate d'aluminium). Ces effets n'ont pas été observés après administration d'hydroxyde d'aluminium, à des doses pourtant beaucoup plus fortes. A la dose de 13 mg/kg de nitrate d'aluminium, on a observé une réduction de la croissance postnatale mais on n'a pas cherché à relever la présence éventuelle d'effets toxiques chez les mères. Les études portant sur le développement cérébral ont mis en évidence une diminution de la force d'agrippement dans la descendance de rattes qui avaient reçu 100 mg d'aluminium par kg de poids corporel sous forme de lactate incorporé à leur nourriture, sans présenter elles-mêmes d'effets toxiques.

Rien n'indique que l'aluminium soit cancérogène. Il peut former des complexes avec l'ADN et provoquer la réticulation des protéines et de l'ADN chromosomiques, mais il ne se montre pas mutagène pour les bactéries et n'induit pas de mutations ou de transformations dans des cultures de cellules mammaliennes *in vitro*. Toutefois, des aberrations chromosomiques ont été observées dans les cellules de la moelle osseuse, chez des souris et des rats exposés.

Une somme très importante de faits expérimentaux incite à penser que l'aluminium est neurotoxique chez l'animal d'expérience, encore qu'il y ait des différences considérables entre les espèces. Chez celles qui sont sensibles, les effets toxiques consécutifs à l'administration parentérale d'aluminium se caractérisent par des altérations neurologiques progressives qui conduisent à la mort dans un état de mal épileptique (DL_{50} = 6 µg d'aluminium/g de tissu cérébral sec). Sur le plan morphologique, l'encéphalopathie progressive est associée, au niveau de la moelle épinière, du tronc cérébral et de certaines parties de l'hippocampe, à une atteinte des neurofibrilles dans les neurones de grande taille et de taille moyenne. Ces lésions de dégénérescence neurofibrillaire sont morphologiquement et biochimiquement distinctes de celles que l'on observe dans la maladie d'Alzheimer. Des troubles comportementaux ont été observés, en l'absence d'encéphalopathie ou de lésions du tissu cérébral, chez des animaux ayant reçu des sels solubles d'aluminium (chlorure, lactate, par ex.) dans leur alimentation ou leur eau de boisson à des doses quotidiennes égales ou supérieures à 50 mg d'aluminium par kg de poids corporel.

L'ostéomalacie, sous la forme où elle se manifeste chez l'homme, s'observe régulièrement chez les gros animaux (par exemple, le chien ou le porc) exposés à l'aluminium; une pathologie du même genre s'observe chez les rongeurs. A ce qu'il paraît, ces effets se produisent chez toutes les espèces, y compris l'Homme, à des concentrations d'aluminium de 100 à 200 µg/g de cendres d'os.

8. Effets sur l'Homme

On n'a pas décrit d'effets pathogènes aigus consécutifs à une exposition de la population générale à l'aluminium.

En Angleterre, une population d'environ 20 000 personnes a été exposée pendant au moins 5 jours à des concentrations excessives de sulfate d'aluminium qui avait été déposé accidentellement dans une installation fournissant de l'eau potable. On a fait état à cette occasion de cas de nausée, de vomissements, de diarrhée, d'ulcérations buccales et cutanées, d'éruptions et d'arthralgies. A l'examen, ces symptômes se sont révélés pour la plupart bénins et de brève durée. Aucun effet pathologique durable n'a pu être attribué à des cas précis d'exposition à l'aluminium présent dans l'eau de boisson.

On a émis l'hypothèse que la présence d'aluminium dans l'eau de boisson serait responsable de la survenue ou de l'évolution plus rapide de la maladie d'Alzheimer ou encore de la détérioration des fonctions intellectuelles chez les personnes âgées. On a également avancé que les fumées dégagées lors de la compression de l'aluminium pulvérulent pouvaient également avoir une responsabilité dans la détérioration des fonctions intellectuelles et les pneumopathies observées chez certaines professions.

Une vingtaine d'études épidémiologiques ont été effectuées pour vérifier si la présence d'aluminium dans l'eau de boisson était effectivement un facteur de risque de la maladie d'Alzheimer et deux d'entre elles ont consisté à évaluer l'association entre ce facteur et la détérioration des fonctions intellectuelles. Ces études allaient des enquêtes écologiques aux études cas-témoins. Huit études effectuées sur des populations de Norvège, du Canada, de France, de Suisse et d'Angleterre ont été jugées d'une qualité suffisante pour satisfaire aux critères retenus pour l'évaluation de la relation exposition-effet avec correction pour tenir compte d'au moins quelques facteurs de confusion. Sur les six études consacrées à l'existence éventuelle d'une relation entre l'aluminium de l'eau de boisson et la démence sénile ou la maladie d'Alzheimer, trois seulement ont conclu par l'affirmative. Il est toutefois à noter que chacune de ces études présentait des défauts de conception (par exemple, dans l'évaluation de l'exposition environnementale, pas de prise en compte de l'exposition à l'aluminium de toutes origines, ni de correction pour tenir compte des importants facteurs de confusion que sont le niveau d'instruction, la situation socio-économique et les antécédents familiaux, le recours à des critères de jugement différents pour la maladie d'Alzheimer et le biais de sélection). En général le calcul a donné une valeur de 2 pour le risque relatif, avec un large intervalle de confiance, lorsque la concentration totale de l'aluminium dans l'eau de boisson était égale ou supérieure à 100 µg/litre. Compte tenu des connaissances actuelles sur la maladie d'Alzheimer et de l'ensemble des résultats fournis par ces études épidémiologiques, on a conclu que les données épidémiologiques ne militent pas en faveur de l'existence d'une relation causale entre la maladie d'Alzheimer et la présence d'aluminium dans l'eau de boisson.

Outre les études épidémiologiques précitées qui ont porté sur la relation entre la maladie d'Alzheimer et la présence d'aluminium dans l'eau de boisson, deux autres études ont été consacrées à ce même type de relation chez les populations âgées. Là encore, on a obtenu des résultats contradictoires. La première étude, qui a porté sur 800 octogénaires du sexe masculin qui consommaient une eau contenant jusqu'à 98 µg d'aluminium par litre, n'a pas mis en évidence de relation de cause à effet. La seconde étude, pour laquelle le critère de jugement retenu était "tout signe de détérioration des fonctions mentales", a évalué à 1,72 le risque relatif pour des teneurs en aluminium supérieures à 85 µg/litre chez 250 sujets du sexe masculin. Ces données ne permettent pas de conclure que l'aluminium est à l'origine d'une détérioration des fonctions intellectuelles chez les personnes âgées.

Comme on vient de le voir, les conclusions des travaux relatifs aux effets de l'aluminium sur les fonctions intellectuelles sont contradictoires. La plupart des études ont été effectuées sur des populations de faible effectif et la méthodologie utilisée est discutable, eu égard à l'ampleur de l'effet constaté, à l'appréciation de l'exposition efective et aux facteurs de confusion. Lors d'une étude au cours de laquelle on a comparé la détérioration des fonctions intellectuelles chez des mineurs exposés à une poudre contenant 85% d'aluminium finement pulvérisé et 15% d'oxyde d'aluminium (à titre de prophylaxie contre la silice) à un groupe témoin constitué de mineurs non exposés, les résultats aux tests et le nombre de sujets présentant un déficit dans au moins un test ont mis en évidence un désavantage chez les mineurs exposés. On a constaté l'existence d'une tendance à l'accroissement du risque qui était liée à la dose.

Dans toutes les études relatives à l'exposition professionnelle qui ont été publiées, l'ampleur des effets constatés, la présence de facteurs de confusion, les problèmes posés par l'appréciation de l'exposition effective et le fait qu'on ne peut exclure l'exposition à plusieurs substances, ne permettent guère de conclure que l'aluminium provoque une détérioration des fonctions intellectuelles chez les personnes exposées de par leur profession.

Lors d'études limitées sur des travailleurs exposés à des vapeurs d'aluminium, des syndromes neurologiques et en particulier une détérioration des fonction intellectuelles, des troubles moteurs et des neuropathies périphériques ont été constatés. En comparant un petit groupe de soudeurs d'aluminium à un groupe de soudeurs de fer, on a constaté chez les premiers un léger déficit de l'activité motrice lors de tâches répétitives. Dans une autre étude, une enquête par questionnaire a permis de mettre en évidence une augmentation des symptômes neuropsychiatriques.

Les insuffisants rénaux chroniques qui sont exposés à l'aluminium présent dans les liquides de dialyse et reçoivent des médicaments qui en contiennent, peuvent souffrir de troubles iatrogènes tels qu'encéphalopathies, ostéomalacies résistantes à la vitamine D et anémies microcytaires. Ces syndromes cliniques peuvent être évités en réduisant l'exposition à l'aluminium.

Chez les prématurés, même ceux dont l'insuffisance rénale n'est pas suffisamment grave pour provoquer une augmentation du taux sanguin de créatinine, il peut y avoir accumulation tissulaire d'aluminium, notamment au niveau des os, en cas d'exposition iatrogène à l'aluminium. A partir d'un certain degré d'insuffsance rénale, on peut craindre des convulsions et une encéphalopathie.

L'exposition humaine à l'aluminium est très courante, mais seuls quelques cas d'hypersensibilité ont été signalés à la suite de l'application sur la peau ou de l'administration parentérale de certains composés de l'aluminium.

Des cas de fibrose pulmonaire ont été rapportés chez quelques ouvriers employés à la fabrication d'explosifs et de feux d'artifice et exposés à de très fines poudres d'aluminium comprimées. Dans presque tous les cas, il y avait eu exposition à des particules d'aluminium enrobées d'huile minérale. Ce procédé n'est plus utilisé. D'autres cas de fibrose pulmonaire ont pu être également attribués à la présence d'autres minéraux comme la silice et l'amiante; l'aluminium n'était donc pas seul en cause.

On a pu attribuer l'apparition d'un asthme d'irritation à l'inhalation de composés tels que le sulfate et le fluorure d'aluminium, le tétrafluoraluminate de potassium ainsi qu'au séjour dans l'environnement complexe des ateliers de production de l'aluminium.

On ne dispose pas de données suffisantes pour déterminer dans quelle catégorie de risque cancérogène pour l'Homme se situent l'aluminium et ses dérivés. Quoi qu'il en soit, les études menées sur l'animal n'attribuent aucun pouvoir cancérogène à l'aluminium ou à ses composés.

9. Effets sur les autres êtres vivants au laboratoire ou dans leur milieu naturel

Chez les algues unicellulaires, on observe un effet toxique plus important aux faibles valeurs du pH, lorsque la biodisponibilité de l'aluminium augmente. Elles sont plus sensibles que les autres microorganismes, la plupart des 19 espèces lacustres testées présentant une inhibition totale de la croissance à la concentration de 200 µg/litre d'aluminium total (pH 5,5). Il peut y avoir sélection des souches tolérantes à l'aluminium. Ainsi, on a isolé des algues capables de se développer en présence d'une concentration d'aluminium de

48 µg/litre et d'un pH de 4,6. Dans le cas des invertébrés aquatiques, on a obtenu des valeurs de la Cl_{50} qui vont de 0,48 mg/litre (polychètes) à 59,6 mg/litre (daphnies). En ce qui concerne les poissons, les valeurs vont de 0,095 mg/litre (*Jordanella floridae*) à 235 mg/litre (gambusies). il faut cependant interpréter ces résultats avec prudence du fait que la biodisponibililté de l'aluminium dépend fortement du pH. La grande dispersion des valeurs de la Cl_{50} traduit probablement les variations de la biodisponibilité. L'adjonction d'agents chélatants, comme le NTA ou l'EDTA, réduit la toxicité de l'aluminium pour les poissons.

Les macroinvertébrés réagissent de manière variable à la présence d'aluminium. Lorsque le pH se situe dans les limites normales, la toxicité de l'aluminium augmente à mesure que le pH diminue; toutefois, dans les eaux très acides, l'aluminium peut atténuer l'effet de l'acidité. Certains invertébrés sont très résistants à l'acidité et peuvent abonder dans les eaux acides. On a constaté une augmentation de la dérive des invertébrés dans les cours d'eau où ils sont soumis à un stress dû au pH ou à la présence d'aluminium. Il s'agit là d'une réaction commune à divers facteurs de stress. Lors d'un test, des invertébrés lacustres ont en général survécu à une exposition à l'aluminium mais ont souffert de la diminution des phosphates dans des conditions rendues oligotrophiques par la précipitation de l'aluminium. Les études toxicologiques à court et à long terme effectuées sur les poissons se sont déroulées dans des conditions très diverses et, ce qui est beaucoup plus important, dans des milieux de pH varié. Il ressort des données disponibles que des effets non négligeables ont été observés à des concentrations en aluminium inorganique sous forme de composés monomères ne dépassant pas 25 µg/litre. Toutefois, les relations complexes qui existent entre l'acidité et la biodisponibilité de l'aluminium rendent difficile l'interprétation des données toxicologiques. Lorsque le pH est très bas, c'est-à-dire dans des conditions qui ne sont normalement pas celles qui règnent dans les eaux naturelles, c'est la concentration en ions hydrogène qui constitue le facteur toxique, l'addition d'aluminium ayant tendance à réduire la toxicité. C'est pour un pH compris entre 4,5 et 6,0 que l'aluminium en équililbre exerce son effet toxique maximal. On a également montré que la toxicité augmente avec le pH lorsque celui-ci est alcalin. On explique la toxicité de l'aluminium pour les poissons par le fait qu'ils ne peuvent plus assurer leur osmorégulation ainsi que par des problèmes respiratoires dus à la précipitation de l'aluminium sur le mucus branchial. Le premier de ces effets est associé à des valeurs basses du pH. Ces résultats de laboratoire ont été confirmés par des observation en milieu naturel, notamment dans des conditions d'acidité excessive.

Les oeufs et les larves d'amphibiens souffrent de l'acidité et de la présence d'aluminium, ces deux facteurs étant en interaction. On a fait état d'effets tels que réduction de l'éclosion, éclosion retardée, métamorphose retardée ou à petite taille, et mortalité pour des teneurs en aluminium inférieures à 1 mg/litre.

L'exposition des racines des plantes terrestres à l'aluminium peut réduire la croissance de ces racines, diminuer la fixation des nutriments et provoquer un rabougrissement du végétal. On a cependant montré au laboratoire comme sur le terrain que les végétaux pouvaient manifester une tolérance à l'aluminium.

10. Conclusions

10.1 *Population générale*

Des études sur l'animal ont permis de définir les risques que l'exposition à l'aluminium présente pour le développement neurologique et les fonctions cérébrales. Toutefois, il n'apparaît pas que l'aluminium menace la santé des personnes en bonne santé qui ne sont pas soumises à une exposition professionnelle.

Rien n'indique que l'aluminium puisse jouer un rôle important dans l'étiologie de la maladie d'Alzheimer et en tout état de cause, il ne provoque chez aucune espèce animale ou chez l'Homme des pathologies de type Alzheimer.

On ne dispose pas de données suffisantes pour donner corps à l'hypothèse selon laquelle l'exposition à l'aluminium des personnes vivant dans des régions où l'eau a une forte teneur en cet élément pourrait exacerber la maladie d'Alzheimer ou en accélérer l'évolution.

On ne dispose pas d'éléments d'appréciation suffisants, sur le plan sanitaire, pour entreprendre une révision des valeurs-guides de l'OMS concernant l'exposition à l'aluminium des personnes en bonne santé non exposées professionnellement. Par exemple, il n'existe pas de base scientifique suffisante pour que l'on puisse établir une norme de concentration de l'aluminium dans l'eau de boisson.

10.2 *Sous-groupes de population exposés à un risque particulier*

On a montré que chez des sujets de tous âges atteints d'insuffisance rénale, l'accumulation d'aluminium provoquait un syndrome clinique d'encéphalopathie, une ostéomalacie résistante à la vitamine D et une anémie microcytaire. Cet aluminium peut provenir du liquide d'hémodialyse ou de produits pharmaceutiques qui en contiennent (par exemple les capteurs d'ions phosphate). La prise de produits contenant des citrates peut provoquer une exacerbation de l'absorption intestinale. Les insuffisants rénaux sont donc exposés au risque de neurotoxicité aluminique.

L'exposition iatrogène à l'aluminium constitue une menace pour les insuffisants rénaux chroniques. Chez les prématurés, la charge de l'organisme en aluminium est plus élevée que chez les autres nourrissons. On s'efforcera donc de limiter ce genre d'exposition chez tous ces groupes vulnérables.

10.3 *Populations professionnellement exposées*

Le risque est plus important pour les travailleurs exposés pendant de longues périodes à de fines particules d'aluminium. Cependant, on ne dispose pas de données suffisantes pour fixer avec quelque certitude des limites d'exposition qui protègent contre les effets indésirables de l'aluminium.

On connaît des cas de fibrose pulmonaire dus à une exposition à de la poudre d'aluminium à usage pyrotechnique, très souvent enrobée d'huile minérale .En revanche, il n'est pas prouvé que l'exposition à l'aluminium sous d'autres formes puisse également provoquer ce type de fibrose. Dans la plupart des cas de fibrose observés, il y avait eu exposition simultanée à d'autres agents fibrogènes.

On a attribué un certain nombre de cas d'asthme d'irritation à l'inhalation de sulfate, de fluorure d'aluminium ou de tétrafluoraluminate de potassium ou encore à un séjour dans l'environnement complexe des ateliers de production de l'aluminium.

10.4 Effets sur l'environnement

L'aluminium présent dans l'environnement en phase solide est relativement insoluble, en particulier lorsque le pH est voisin de la neutralité, d'où les très faibles concentrations d'aluminium en solution dans la plupart des eaux naturelles.

Dans les milieux acides ou peu tamponnés où l'apport d'acide est important, la concentration de l'aluminium peut atteindre des valeurs nocives pour les organismes aquatiques et les plantes terrestres. Toutefois, la sensibilité à ce métal varie largement selon les espèces, les souches et les stades de développement.

Les effets biologiques délétères de fortes teneurs en aluminium inorganique sous forme monomère peuvent être atténués par la présence d'acides organiques, de fluorures, de silicates et de concentrations élevées de calcium et de magnésium.

Dans les eaux excessivement acides, il y a une réduction sensible de la diversité biologique due à la mobilisation de l'aluminium sous des formes plus toxiques. Cette réduction de la diversité biologique s'observe à tous les niveaux trophiques.

RESUMEN Y CONCLUSIONES

1.   Identidad, propiedades físicas y químicas

El aluminio es un metal blanco plateado, dúctil y maleable. Pertenece al grupo IIIA de la Tabla Periódica, y en los compuestos suele encontrarse como Al^{III}. Forma cerca del 8% de la corteza terrestre y es uno de los metales comunes más reactivos. La exposición al agua, al oxígeno o a otros oxidantes conduce a la formación de una capa superficial de óxido de aluminio que confiere al metal una gran resistencia a la corrosión. El óxido de aluminio es soluble en ácidos minerales y álcalis fuertes, pero insoluble en agua, mientras que el cloruro, el nitrato y el sulfato de aluminio son solubles en agua. Los halogenuros, los hidruros y los alquilos más cortos de aluminio reaccionan violentamente con el agua.

El aluminio posee una elevada conductividad térmica y eléctrica, baja densidad y gran resistencia a la corrosión. A menudo se alea con otros metales. Las aleaciones de aluminio son fuertes, ligeras y fácilmente susceptibles de conformación a máquina.

2.   Métodos analíticos

Se han desarrollado diversos métodos analíticos para determinar la presencia de aluminio en muestras biológicas y ambientales. Los dos métodos más utilizados son la espectrometría de absorción atómica en horno de grafito (GF-AAS) y la espectrometría de emisión atómico-plasmática inductivamente acoplada (ICP-AES). La contaminación de las muestras por el aluminio del aire, de los recipientes o de los reactivos durante el muestreo y preparación constituye la principal fuente de error analítico. En función del tratamiento previo de la muestra y de los procedimientos de concentración y separación, los límites de detección son de 1,9-4 µg/litro en los líquidos biológicos y 0,005-0,5 µg/g de peso seco en los tejidos al usar la GF-AAS, y de 5 µg/m^3 en el aire y 3 µg/litro en el agua cuando se emplea la ICP-AES.

3.   Fuentes de exposición humana y ambiental

El aluminio se libera en el medio ambiente tanto a través de procesos naturales como de fuentes antropogénicas. Está muy concentrado en el polvo de suelos dedicados a actividades tales como la minería y la agricultura, y en las partículas generadas por la combustión del carbón. Los silicatos de aluminio (arcillas), un importante componente de los suelos, contribuyen a los niveles de aluminio hallados en el polvo. Los procesos naturales superan con mucho la contribución antropogénica directa al medio ambiente. El aluminio movilizado por el hombre se forma en su mayoría de forma indirecta como resultado de la emisión de sustancias acidificantes. En general, un descenso del pH ocasiona un aumento de la movilidad y biodisponibilidad de las formas monoméricas de aluminio. La principal materia prima utilizada para producir aluminio es la bauxita, que contiene hasta un 55% de alúmina (óxido de aluminio). La producción mundial de bauxita fue de 106 millones de toneladas en 1992. El metal de aluminio tiene una gran variedad de usos, entre ellos la fabricación de materiales estructurales para los sectores de la construcción, el automóvil y la aviación, y la producción de aleaciones metálicas. Los compuestos y materiales de aluminio tienen también una amplia gama de usos, que incluyen la producción de vidrio, cerámica, caucho, conservantes de la madera, preparaciones farmacéuticas y tejidos impermeabilizantes. Los minerales de aluminio naturales, especialmente la bentonita y la zeolita, se emplean para depurar el agua, para refinar el azúcar, y en las industrias papeleras y de la fermentación.

4. Transporte, distribución y transformación en el medio ambiente

El aluminio es un metal ubicuo en el medio ambiente, donde se encuentra en forma de silicatos, óxidos e hidróxidos, combinado con otros elementos como el sodio y el flúor, y formando complejos con materia orgánica. No se halla como metal libre debido a su reactividad. Sólo tiene un estado de oxidación (+3) en la naturaleza, por lo que su transporte y distribución en el medio ambiente dependen tan sólo de su química de coordinación y de las características físico-químicas del sistema ambiental concreto. A valores de pH superiores a 5,5 los compuestos naturales de aluminio aparecen predominantemente en forma no disuelta como gibbsita ($Al(OH)_3$) o como aluminosilicatos, excepto en presencia de grandes cantidades de material orgánico disuelto, que se une al aluminio y puede dar lugar a un aumento de la concentración del aluminio disuelto en lagos y cursos de agua. La movilidad del aluminio y su ulterior transporte en el medio ambiente dependen de varios factores, entre los que cabe mencionar el tipo de especies químicas, los cursos hidrológicos, las interacciones suelo-agua y la composición del sustrato geológico. La solubilidad del aluminio en equilibrio con la fase sólida $Al(OH)_3$ depende en gran medida del pH y de agentes complejantes tales como fluoruros, silicatos, fosfatos y materia orgánica. La química del aluminio inorgánico en los suelos y los cursos de agua ácidos depende de la solubilidad de los minerales y de los procesos de intercambio y de mezcla de las aguas.

La acidificación del suelo libera aluminio disolviéndolo, y el metal llega así a las corrientes de agua. La movilización del aluminio por precipitación ácida permite que haya más aluminio disponible para captación por las plantas.

5. Niveles ambientales y exposición humana

El aluminio es uno de los principales constituyentes de varios componentes de la atmósfera, en particular del polvo procedente de suelos (tanto de fuentes naturales como de origen humano) y de partículas generadas por la combustión del carbón. En las zonas urbanas los niveles de aluminio en el polvo de la calle van de 3,7 a 11,6 µg/kg. Los niveles de aluminio en el aire varían desde 0,5 ng/m^3 sobre la Antártida hasta más de 1000 ng/m^3 en las zonas industrializadas.

Las concentraciones de aluminio en las aguas superficiales y subterráneas son muy variables, dependiendo de factores geológicos y físico-químicos. El aluminio puede estar en suspensión o disuelto. Puede estar en forma de ligandos orgánicos o inorgánicos o de ion aluminio libre. En las aguas naturales el aluminio existe tanto en forma monomérica como polimérica. Las especies de aluminio dependen del pH y de las concentraciones de carbono orgánico disuelto (DOC) fluoruros, sulfatos, fosfatos y partículas en suspensión. Las concentraciones de aluminio disuelto en las aguas de pH aproximadamente neutro suelen ser bastante bajas, entre 1,0 y 50 µg/litro. En aguas más ácidas se alcanzan valores de hasta 500-1000 µg/litro. En condiciones de acidez extrema provocadas por el avenamiento ácido de minas se han medido concentraciones de aluminio disuelto de hasta 90 mg/litro.

La exposición humana no ocupacional al aluminio en el medio ambiente se produce principalmente a través de la ingestión de agua y alimentos, sobre todo de estos últimos. La ingesta diaria de aluminio con los alimentos y bebidas es en los adultos de entre 2,5 y 13 mg. Esto representa un 90%-95% de la ingesta total. El agua de bebida puede contribuir con unos 0,4 mg diariamente, según los valores de las actuales directrices internacionales, pero más probablemente se sitúa en torno a los 0,2 mg/día. La exposición pulmonar puede contribuir hasta con 0,04 mg/día. En algunas circunstancias, como la exposición ocupacional y el uso de antiácidos, los niveles de exposición pueden ser mucho mayores. Con dos tabletas antiácido de tamaño medio, por ejemplo, se puede consumir más de 500 mg de aluminio. La evaluación de la captación consecutiva a ese tipo de exposiciones plantea algunos problemas debido a dificultades analíticas y de muestreo. Las investigaciones isotópicas realizadas con Al^{26} indican que una de las formas más biodisponibles del aluminio es el citrato, y que cuando el aluminio está en dicha forma podría darse hasta un 1% de absorción. No obstante, los seres humanos absorben al parecer sólo el 3% de la cantidad total de aluminio ingerida diariamente con el agua de bebida, una fuente relativamente secundaria en comparación con los alimentos.

6.   Cinética y metabolismo

6.1   *Ser humano*

El aluminio y sus compuestos parecen ser mal absorbidos por los seres humanos, pero no hay estudios adecuados sobre la velocidad y el grado de absorción. Las concentraciones de aluminio en la sangre y la orina se han empleado como una medida fácilmente obtenible de la captación de aluminio, habiéndose observado niveles elevados en la orina de soldadores de aluminio y de productores de polvo de escamas de aluminio.

El mecanismo de absorción gastrointestinal del aluminio todavía no ha sido totalmente dilucidado. La variabilidad se debe a las propiedades químicas del elemento y a las diversas especies químicas formadas en función del pH, la fuerza iónica, la presencia de elementos competitivos (silicio) y la presencia de agentes complejantes en el interior del tracto digestivo (p.ej., citrato).

Se ha empleado el isótopo radiactivo Al^{26} para estudiar el destino biológico y la absorción gastrointestinal del aluminio en el hombre tras la ingestión de compuestos de aluminio. Se ha detectado una variabilidad significativa entre los individuos. Se han notificado fracciones de captación de 5 × 10^{-3} para el aluminio como citrato, 1,04 × 10^{-4} para el hidróxido de aluminio y 1,36 × 10^{-3} para el hidróxido administrado con citrato. Un estudio sobre la captación del aluminio del agua de bebida reveló una fracción de captación de 2,35 × 10^{-3}, llegándose a la conclusión de que en la población general los individuos que consumen 1,5 litros/día de agua de bebida con un contenido de 100 µg aluminio/litro, absorben un 3% del aluminio total ingerido diariamente a partir de esa fuente, dependiendo de los niveles presentes en los alimentos y de la frecuencia del uso de antiácidos.

La proporción de Al^{3+} plasmático normalmente unido a proteínas en el ser humano puede ser hasta del 70%-90% en los pacientes sometidos a hemodiálisis con niveles moderadamente altos de aluminio en el plasma. Los niveles más elevados de aluminio suelen encontrarse en los pulmones, donde puede hallarse en forma de partículas inhaladas insolubles.

La orina es la vía más importante de excreción del aluminio. Tras la administración por vía oral de una dosis única de aluminio, pasados 13 días se había excretado un 83% por la orina y un 1,8% por las heces. La semivida de las concentraciones urinarias en soldadores expuestos durante más de 10 años fue de 6 meses o superior. Entre trabajadores jubilados expuestos al polvo de escamas de aluminio, las semividas calculadas se situaban entre 0,7 y 8 años.

6.2 Animales

La absorción por vía gastrointestinal es normalmente menor del 1%. Los principales factores que influyen en la absorción son la solubilidad, el pH y las especies químicas. Los compuestos complejantes orgánicos, sobre todo el citrato, aumentan la absorción. La absorción del aluminio puede interferir en los sistemas de transporte del calcio y el hierro. La absorción cutánea y por inhalación no han sido estudiadas con detalle. El aluminio se distribuye en la mayoría de los órganos del cuerpo, y cuando las dosis son altas se acumula principalmente en los huesos. De forma limitada pero aún no determinada con precisión, atraviesa la barrera hematoencefálica, y llega también al feto. El aluminio se elimina eficazmente por la orina. El periodo de semieliminación plasmática es de aproximadamente 1 h en los roedores.

7. Efectos en mamíferos de laboratorio y en sistemas de pruebas *in vitro*

La toxicidad aguda del aluminio metálico y de los compuestos de aluminio es baja; los valores notificados de la DL_{50} oral están comprendidas entre varios cientos y 1000 mg aluminio/kg de peso corporal. Los valores de la CL_{50} por inhalación no han sido establecidos.

En estudios a corto plazo en los que se examinó una gama adecuada de variables de evaluación después de exponer ratas, ratones o perros a diversos compuestos de aluminio (fosfato sódico de aluminio, hidróxido de aluminio, nitrato de aluminio) a través de los alimentos o del agua, sólo se observaron efectos muy discretos (disminuciones del aumento de peso corporal, asociadas generalmente a un descenso del consumo de comida, o efectos histopatológicos leves) a las dosis más altas (70 a 300 mg aluminio/kg de peso corporal al día). Los efectos sistémicos que siguieron a la administración parenteral incluyeron también disfunción renal.

No se han hallado estudios de inhalación adecuados. Después de la administración intratraqueal de óxido de aluminio se observó fibrosis asociada a partículas, parecida a la hallada en otros estudios sobre el sílice y el polvo de carbón.

No se observaron signos manifiestos de fetotoxicidad, ni alteraciones de los parámetros reproductivos generales después del tratamiento de ratas con 13, 26 ó 52 mg aluminio/kg de peso corporal al día (en forma de nitrato de aluminio) mediante alimentación forzada. Sin embargo, se observó un retraso dosis-dependiente del crecimiento en la descendencia, a dosis de 13 mg/kg en el caso de las hembras y de 26 mg/kg en el caso de los machos. El nivel mínimo con efectos adversos observados (LOAEL) en el desarrollo (disminución de la osificación, aumento de la incidencia de defectos congénitos en las vértebras y el esternón y peso fetal reducido) fue de 13 mg/kg (nitrato de aluminio). Estos efectos no se observaron a dosis mucho más altas de hidróxido de aluminio. Se detectó una reducción del crecimiento posnatal al emplear 13 mg/kg (nitrato de aluminio), aunque no se analizó la toxicidad materna. En estudios sobre el desarrollo cerebral se detectó una disminución de la fuerza de aprehensión en la descendencia de hembras a las que se administraron con los alimentos 100 mg aluminio/kg de peso corporal en forma de lactato de aluminio, no observándose signos de toxicidad materna.

No existen indicios de que el aluminio sea carcinógeno. Puede formar complejos con el ADN, así como enlaces entre las proteínas cromosómicas y el ADN, pero no se ha demostrado que sea mutágeno en bacterias o que induzca mutaciones o transformaciones en células de mamífero *in vitro*. Se han observado aberraciones cromosómicas en células de la medula ósea de ratas y ratones expuestos.

Hay indicios fundados de que el aluminio es neurotóxico en animales de experimentación, aunque se da una considerable variabilidad entre especies. En especies susceptibles, la toxicidad que sigue a la administración parenteral se caracteriza por un deterioro neurológico progresivo, conducente a un estado epiléptico que acarrea la muerte (DL_{50} = 6 µg Al/g de peso seco del cerebro). Morfológicamente, la encefalopatía progresiva se asocia a una patología neurofibrilar de las neuronas grandes y medianas, sobre todo en la médula espinal, el tallo encefálico y determinadas zonas del hipocampo. Estos ovillos neurofibrilares son morfológica y bioquímicamente diferentes de los que caracterizan la enfermedad de Alzheimer. En animales de experimentación expuestos a sales solubles de aluminio (p.ej., lactato y cloruro) a través de los alimentos o el agua, a dosis de 50 mg aluminio/kg de peso al día o mayores, se ha observado un deterioro de la conducta sin signos concomitantes de encefalopatía o cambios neurohistopatológicos manifiestos.

La osteomalacia que afecta al hombre se observa también sistemáticamente en las especies de cierto tamaño (p.ej., el perro o el cerdo) expuestas al aluminio; en los roedores se observan manifestaciones parecidas. Estos efectos parecen darse en todas las especies, incluido el hombre, a niveles de aluminio de 100 a 200 µg/g de cenizas óseas.

8.   Efectos en el hombre

No se han descrito efectos patógenos agudos en la población general como consecuencia de la exposición al aluminio.

En Inglaterra una población de aproximadamente 20 000 individuos se vio expuesta durante por lo menos 5 días a niveles elevados de sulfato de aluminio, debido a la contaminación accidental de unas instalaciones de agua de bebida. Se informó de casos de náuseas, vómitos, diarrea, úlceras bucales, úlceras y erupciones cutáneas y dolores artríticos. Se comprobó que los síntomas eran en su mayoría leves y de corta duración. No se pudieron atribuir efectos duraderos sobre la salud a las exposiciones conocidas al aluminio del agua de bebida.

Se ha propuesto la hipótesis de que el aluminio presente en el agua potable es un factor de riesgo por lo que se refiere al desarrollo o la aceleración de la enfermedad de Alzheimer y al deterioro senil de la función cognitiva. Se ha sugerido también que el polvo y los vapores de aluminio fino apisonado son quizá factores de riesgo que propician el deterioro de las funciones cognitivas y la aparición de enfermedades pulmonares en determinados trabajos.

Se han llevado a cabo unos 20 estudios epidemiológicos para comprobar la hipótesis de que el aluminio del agua de bebida es un factor de riesgo de la enfermedad de Alzheimer, y dos estudios han evaluado la asociación entre el aluminio del agua de bebida y el deterioro de las funciones cognitivas. El diseño de estos estudios abarcaba desde el control ecológico hasta el control de los casos. Se consideró que 8 estudios realizados en poblaciones de Noruega, el Canadá, Francia, Suiza e Inglaterra tenían la calidad necesaria para satisfacer los criterios generales establecidos a fin de evaluar la exposición y los resultados y de poder efectuar ajustes por lo menos en algunas variables de confusión. De los seis estudios que analizaron la relación entre el aluminio del agua de bebida y la demencia o la enfermedad de Alzheimer, tres hallaron una relación positiva, pero no así los otros tres. Sin embargo, todos los estudios presentaban algunos fallos de diseño (relacionados por ejemplo con la evaluación de la exposición ecológica, la no consideración de todas las fuentes de exposición al aluminio y de factores de confusión importantes como la educación, la situación socioeconómica y los antecedentes familiares, el uso de medidas indirectas de la evolución de la enfermedad de Alzheimer, o unos métodos sesgados de selección). En general, los riesgos relativos determinados eran inferiores a 2, con grandes intervalos de confianza, a concentraciones totales de aluminio de 100 μg/litro o superiores en el agua de bebida. Sobre la base de los conocimientos disponibles acerca de la patogénesis de la enfermedad de Alzheimer y de todas las pruebas aportadas por estos estudios epidemiológicos, se llegó a la conclusión de que los datos epidemiológicos actuales no respaldan la hipótesis de una relación causal entre la enfermedad de Alzheimer y el aluminio del agua de bebida.

Además de los estudios epidemiológicos realizados para analizar la relación entre la enfermedad de Alzheimer y el aluminio del agua de bebida en otros dos estudios se examinó la relación entre los casos de disfunción cognitiva y de enfermedad de Alzheimer en poblaciones de ancianos y los niveles de aluminio en el agua de bebida. Los resultados fueron una vez más contradictorios. En un estudio realizado en 800 octogenarios varones que consumían agua de bebida con concentraciones de aluminio de hasta 98 μg/litro no se halló relación alguna. El segundo estudio utilizó "cualquier indicio de deterioro mental" como criterio de seguimiento, calculando así un riesgo relativo de 1,72 para concentraciones de aluminio superiores a 85 μg/litro en 250 varones. Tales datos son insuficientes para demostrar que el aluminio sea una causa de deterioro cognitivo en los ancianos.

Los datos sobre el deterioro de la función cognitiva en relación con la exposición al aluminio son contradictorios. La mayoría de los estudios se han hecho en poblaciones reducidas, y la metodología utilizada es cuestionable en lo que respecta a la magnitud del efecto estudiado, la evaluación de la exposición y los factores de confusión. En un estudio comparativo del deterioro cognitivo entre mineros no expuestos y mineros expuestos a un polvo que contenía un 85% de aluminio molido muy fino y un 15% de óxido de aluminio (como profilaxis contra el sílice), los resultados de las pruebas cognitivas y la proporción de personas con dificultades en al menos una de las pruebas fueron peores entre los mineros expuestos. Se detectó una tendencia al aumento del riesgo relacionada con la exposición.

En todos los estudios ocupacionales de los que se tiene noticia, la magnitud de los efectos observados, la presencia de factores de confusión, los problemas relacionados con la evaluación de la exposición y la probabilidad de exposiciones mixtas hacen que, en conjunto, los datos sean insuficientes como para extraer la conclusión de que el aluminio es una causa de deterioro cognitivo en los trabajadores expuestos al aluminio en su trabajo.

En estudios limitados con trabajadores expuestos a vapores de aluminio se ha informado de síndromes neurológicos que incluyen el deterioro de la función cognitiva, disfunciones motoras y neuropatía periférica. Se ha informado de una pequeña población de soldadores de aluminio que, comparados con soldadores de hierro, presentaron un ligero deterioro de la función motora repetitiva. En otros estudios realizado con cuestionarios se detectó un aumento de los síntomas neuropsiquiátricos.

En los pacientes con insuficiencia renal crónica, la exposición iatrogénica a líquidos de diálisis o productos farmacéuticos con aluminio puede producir encefalopatía, osteomalacia resistente a la vitamina D y anemia microcítica. Estos síndromes clínicos pueden prevenirse reduciendo la exposición al aluminio.

En los niños prematuros expuestos a fuentes iatrogénicas de aluminio puede producirse un incremento del contenido de aluminio de los tejidos, particularmente en los huesos, incluso cuando la disfunción renal no es lo suficientemente grave como para provocar un aumento de los niveles de creatinina en sangre. En caso de insuficiencia renal pueden aparecer convulsiones y encefalopatía.

Aunque la exposición humana al aluminio está muy extendida, sólo se ha informado de unos cuantos casos de hipersensibilidad consecutivos a la aplicación cutánea o la administración parenteral de algunos compuestos de aluminio.

Se ha informado de casos de fibrosis pulmonar en algunos trabajadores expuestos a polvo muy fino de aluminio apisonado utilizado en la fabricación de explosivos y material pirotécnico. Casi todos los casos estaban relacionados con la exposición a partículas de aluminio cubiertas de aceite mineral. Dicho procedimiento ya no se utiliza. Otros casos de fibrosis pulmonar se han relacionado con exposiciones a otros agentes minerales como el sílice y el asbesto y no pueden atribuirse exclusivamente al aluminio.

Algunos casos de asma inducida por sustancias irritantes se han asociado a la inhalación de sulfato de aluminio, fluoruro de aluminio o tetrafluoruro potásico de aluminio, así como al ambiente cargado de los cuartos de calderas utilizados en la producción de aluminio.

La información disponible es insuficiente para poder clasificar el riesgo de cáncer asociado a las distintas formas de exposición humana al aluminio y sus compuestos. Los estudios en animales no indican que el aluminio o los compuestos del aluminio sean carcinógenos.

9. Efectos en otros organismos en el laboratorio y en el campo

En las algas acuáticas unicelulares se ha detectado una mayor toxicidad a pH bajo, circunstancia que aumenta la biodisponibilidad del aluminio. Estas algas son más sensibles que otros microorganismos, y de 19 especies lacustres la mayor parte presentaron una inhibición completa del crecimiento a una concentración total de aluminio de 200 µg/litro (pH 5,5). Es posible seleccionar cepas tolerantes al aluminio; se han aislado algas verdes capaces de crecer en presencia de 48 mg/litro a pH 4,6.

En los invertebrados acuáticos la CL_{50} está comprendida entre 0,48 mg/litro (poliquetos) y 59,6 mg/litro (dáfnidos). En los peces, la CL_{50} a las 96 horas va desde 0,095 mg/litro (pez estandarte americano) hasta 235 mg/litro (gambusia común). Sin embargo, estos resultados deben interpretarse con cautela dados los importantes efectos del pH en la disponibilidad del aluminio. El amplio margen de valores de la CL_{50} se debe probablemente a la distinta disponibilidad. La adición de agentes quelantes, como el NTA y el EDTA, reduce la toxicidad aguda del aluminio para los peces.

Los macroinvertebrados responden de diversa forma al aluminio. En el margen normal de pH la toxicidad del aluminio aumenta al disminuir el pH, sin embargo en aguas muy ácidas el aluminio puede reducir los efectos del estrés ácido. Algunos invertebrados son muy resistentes al estrés ácido y pueden llegar a ser muy abundantes en aguas ácidas. Se ha informado de un aumento de la tasa de deriva de los invertebrados en cursos de agua en condiciones de estrés por pH o por pH/aluminio; esa es una respuesta común a diversos agentes estresantes. Invertebrados lacustres sobrevivieron en general a la exposición al aluminio en la naturaleza, pero sufrieron en condiciones oligotróficas debido a la disminución del fosfato inducida por la precipitación con el aluminio.

Se han llevado a cabo pruebas de toxicidad en peces a corto y largo plazo en muy diversas condiciones y, lo que es más importante, a distintos valores de pH. Los datos muestran efectos significativos a niveles de aluminio inorgánico monomérico de tan sólo 25 µg/litro. No obstante, la compleja relación entre la acidez y la biodisponibilidad del aluminio dificulta la interpretación de los datos de toxicidad. A niveles de pH muy bajos (inhabituales en aguas naturales) la concentración de hidrogeniones parece ser el factor tóxico, y la adición de aluminio tiende a reducir la toxicidad. En el margen de pH 4,5 a 6,0 el aluminio en equilibrio ejerce su máximo efecto tóxico. Se ha visto que la toxicidad también aumenta a niveles crecientes de pH en la región de pH alcalino. El mecanismo propuesto para explicar la toxicidad del aluminio en los peces es la incapacidad de los animales a mantener el equilibrio osmorregulador, y los problemas respiratorios asociados a la precipitación del aluminio en el moco de las branquias. El primero de estos efectos se asocia a niveles bajos de pH. Estos datos de laboratorio han sido confirmados por estudios realizados en la naturaleza, especialmente en zonas sometidas a estrés ácido.

Los huevos y las larvas de los anfibios se ven afectados por la acidez y el aluminio, y se da una interacción entre estos dos factores. Se ha informado de fenómenos de disminución de la incubación, retraso de la eclosión, retraso de la metamorfosis, metamorfosis con tamaño reducido y aumento de la mortalidad en diversas especies a concentraciones de aluminio inferiores a 1 mg/litro.

La exposición de las raíces de plantas terrestres al aluminio puede frenar el crecimiento radicular, la captación de nutrientes y el desarrollo de la planta. Se ha demostrado la tolerancia al aluminio tanto en el laboratorio como en la naturaleza.

10. Conclusiones

10.1 Población general

Los estudios realizados en animales acerca de la exposición al aluminio han revelado riesgos para el desarrollo neurológico y las funciones cerebrales. Sin embargo, no se ha demostrado que el aluminio entrañe riesgos para la salud de las personas sanas y no expuestas en el trabajo.

No existen pruebas de que el aluminio tenga un papel causal primordial en la enfermedad de Alzheimer, patología que el metal no induce *in vivo* en ninguna especie, incluido el hombre.

La hipótesis de que la exposición de la población anciana de algunas regiones a niveles elevados de aluminio en el agua de bebida puede exacerbar o acelerar la enfermedad de Alzheimer no está avalada por datos válidos.

Tampoco hay datos válidos que corroboren la hipótesis de que determinadas exposiciones, ya sean ocupacionales o a través del agua de bebida, pueden asociarse a un deterioro inespecífico de la función cognitiva.

No existen datos suficientes relacionados con la salud que justifiquen la revisión de las actuales directrices de la OMS respecto a la exposición al aluminio de individuos sanos no expuestos ocupacionalmente. Así, por ejemplo, no hay una base científica sólida para establecer una norma basada en criterios de salud sobre el aluminio en el agua de bebida.

10.2 Subpoblaciones con un riesgo especial

En pacientes con trastornos de la función renal, cualquiera que sea su edad, la acumulación de aluminio provoca un síndrome clínico caracterizado por encefalopatía, osteomalacia resistente a la vitamina D y anemia microcítica. Las fuentes de aluminio son los líquidos de hemodiálisis y las preparaciones famarcéuticas que contienen aluminio (p.ej., aglutinantes de fosfato). Los productos que contienen citrato pueden aumentar la absorción intestinal. Los pacientes con insuficiencia renal corren por tanto el riesgo de sufrir neurotoxicidad por aluminio.

La exposición iatrogénica al aluminio entraña riesgos para los pacientes con insuficiencia renal crónica. Los lactantes prematuros tienen en su organismo una mayor carga de aluminio que los otros lactantes. Deben tomarse toda clase de precauciones para limitar la exposición de esos grupos.

10.3 Poblaciones expuestas ocupacionalmente

Los trabajadores que han estado expuestos durante largo tiempo a niveles altos de partículas finas de aluminio corren quizá un mayor riesgo de sufrir efectos nocivos para su salud. Sin embargo, no hay datos suficientes para fijar con cierto grado de fiabilidad unos límites de exposición ocupacional en relación con los efectos adversos del aluminio.

La exposición al polvo de aluminio pirotécnico apisonado, recubierto casi siempre de aceites lubricantes minerales, ha provocado fibrosis pulmonar (aluminosis), pero no se ha demostrado que la exposición a otras formas de aluminio produzca fibrosis pulmonar. En la mayor parte de los casos notificados había habido también exposición a otros agentes potencialmente fibrogénicos.

Algunos casos de asma inducida por sustancias irritantes se han asociado a la inhalación de sulfato de aluminio, fluoruro de aluminio o tetrafluoruro potásico de aluminio, así como al ambiente cargado del interior de los cuartos de calderas utilizados en la producción de aluminio.

10.4 Efectos ambientales en el medio ambiente

Las fases sólidas que contienen aluminio en el medio ambiente son relativamente insolubles, en particular a un pH aproximadamente neutro, de ahí las bajas concentraciones de aluminio disuelto que tienen la mayoría de las aguas naturales.

En los entornos ácidos o escasamente tamponados que reciben aportes muy acidificantes, las concentraciones de aluminio pueden aumentar hasta niveles perjudiciales tanto para los organismos acuáticos como para las plantas terrestres. No obstante, existen grandes diferencias en la sensibilidad a este metal según la especie, la cepa y la etapa de la vida.

Los efectos biológicos adversos de las concentraciones elevadas de aluminio monomérico inorgánico son menores en presencia de ácidos orgánicos, fluoruros, silicatos y niveles altos de calcio y magnesio.

En las aguas sometidas a estrés ácido se produce una reducción sustancial de la diversidad de especies, asociada a una movilización de las formas más tóxicas de aluminio. Dicha pérdida de diversidad se observa en todos los niveles tróficos.